Praise for *Kickass Healthy LADA*

"Haskins's advice to advocate for yourself is very valid, the nutritional information she provides is extremely helpful, and advice to TEST, TEST, TEST is critical. She writes so clearly and wittily that one can also recommend this book as a 'good read.'"

— MAYER B. DAVIDSON, MD, Professor of Medicine,
Charles R. Drew University and David Geffen
School of Medicine at UCLA

"Very entertaining and scientifically accurate, *Kickass Healthy LADA* navigates the nuances of diabetes diagnosis through the eyes of a patient. I recommend this book to all newly diagnosed patients with type 1 diabetes or LADA and their family members."

— LORENA ALARCON-CASAS WRIGHT, MD,
FACE, Clinical Associate Professor, University
of Washington School of Medicine

KICKASS
HEALTHY
LADA

HOW TO THRIVE WITH
LATENT AUTOIMMUNE DIABETES IN ADULTS

JACQUELINE HASKINS

FOREWORD BY MAURY HAFERMANN, MD

hachette
BOOKS

NEW YORK

Hachette Go, an imprint of Hachette Books
Hachette Book Group
1290 Avenue of the Americas
New York, NY 10104
HachetteGo.com
Facebook.com/HachetteGo
Instagram.com/HachetteGo

First Edition: April 2023

Hachette Books is a division of Hachette Book Group, Inc.
The Hachette Go and Hachette Books name and logos are trademarks of Hachette Book Group, Inc.

Hachette Go books may be purchased in bulk for business, educational, or promotional use. For more information, please contact your local bookseller or the Hachette Book Group Special Markets Department at Special.Markets@hbgusa.com.

LCCN: 2022032753

ISBNs: 9780306830730 (trade paperback); 9780306830747 (ebook)

Printed in the United States of America

LSC

Printing 1, 2023

To Mom and Dad, to R, K, and S,
to BVD, BK, MO, and TNH . . .
thank you for your footprints in the snow.

CONTENTS

PART III. JOYFUL CARB-CRAFT

PART IV. CRUISING WITH CARB-CRAFT

TABLES

FOREWORD

LADA (LATENT AUTOIMMUNE DIABETES IN ADULTS) IS AN IMPORTANT but under-recognized medical condition superbly illuminated by the wonderfully engaging and eminently readable book you hold in your hands.

Upon being diagnosed with LADA, Jacqueline Haskins—a biologist and creative writer by trade—was struck by just how little information was available on her condition. This was a call to take action. The resulting book reflects her sharp intellect, strong desire to understand her condition, and determination to participate in her wellness on her terms.

Kickass Healthy LADA explains the background and fundamentals of LADA, and comprehensively reviews treatments and new technologies. With clear explanations and practical, concrete examples, Ms. Haskins respectfully allows room for a wide variety of individual preferences. Most refreshingly, she does not shy from the fact that the majority of care is built upon the foundation of healthy choices in diet, activity, and stress management. I particularly enjoyed her description of developing a new, healthier relationship with food in a manner she delightfully terms Carb-craft. The feather in this book's cap is that it is not delivered as a dry medical tome of admonitions and lists, but in lively, humor-filled prose.

Accessible and relevant to readers from a variety of backgrounds, this book is truly a pleasure to read. I found myself in turn commiserating, chuckling, and cheering as she recounts rushed, too-brief doctor visits; the mental load of carrying an "invisible" condition like diabetes; and the need for self-advocacy and perseverance to connect with a like-minded provider.

Written from the heart and with deep honesty, Ms. Haskins's well-organized and well-researched information, reinforced with essential bullet points and chapter summaries, creates a thoroughly useful how-to manual for LADA. Throughout, her ability to look at life with a wry, very human smile shines brightly through.

In *Kickass Healthy LADA*, Ms. Haskins has woven a scientist's sensibility with an artist's appreciation for the color and humor present in even the vicissitudes of life. She successfully takes a medical condition, LADA, that has largely flown under the radar, and gives it the recognition it deserves. I hope this book helps you on your LADA journey.

—*Maury Hafermann, MD*

Dr. Hafermann attended Dartmouth College, graduating summa cum laude, and medical school at the University of Washington, graduating with honors. He chose to enter the specialty of Family Practice based on a strong desire to understand, support, and include the whole person in their pursuit of wellness and health. He enjoys how Family Practice blends not only continuity—getting to know people over time—but also contiguity, the vital and essential aspect of learning about the breadth of a person and their health, and how this informs creating a complete yet personal wellness and treatment plan.

PART I

WHAT TYPE OF DIABETES DO I HAVE?

1 WHAT THE HECK IS LADA?

*Seeing ourselves as whole and healthy is an act
of pure rebellion.*
  —Natasha Marin

AVA LAUGHS, JOKING WITH THE BARISTA AT THE COUNTER OF GOOD Mood Food, our favorite coffee shop, as she orders coffee and a blueberry nectarine scone. I stand behind my friend, my arms crossed, scowling.

My eyes and nose feast on sugar-shiny, gingery pear scones; on still-warm cookies—each a mini Japanese garden filled with chocolate boulders; and on lemon poppy bread whose lemon will make your tongue curl while the tiny seeds explode with flavor. The café brims with scents of cinnamon, whipped cream, and coffee, the hiss of espresso machines, and the chatter of happy customers.

I glower.

"So," Ava asks over her shoulder as she signs the touch screen, "how is the diabetes going?"

I glare at the drinks board. My just-diagnosed diabetes now bans my favorite fragrant, house-made chai. Or so I believe.

"What would you like, Jackie?" Ava prods. The server's hand hovers, waiting.

My shoulders clench. I didn't come to our special Sunday getaway just for some tea bag dangling in tepid water. I want a *treat*.

"Jackie, what would you li—" Turning, Ava sees my face, and her voice falters.

"I mean . . ." She hesitates. "What can you eat?"

Boom. Ava just lasered the question always rolling on repeat, like an annoying song stuck in my head. What can I eat?

It isn't that there are no answers, it's that there are too many—a different answer from the *Mayo Clinic Diabetes Diet* than from *Dr. Bernstein's Diabetes Solution*; a different answer from doctor-authored *The End of Diabetes* than from "scientifically proven" *Aging Well with Diabetes* with its "146 eye-opening secrets." And on and on, shelf after shelf. Add to this: dickering websites, disagreeing nutritionists, and a stew of physicians barely reining in their contempt for the guidelines of the American Diabetes Association. What's *that* about?

Then add one more little problem: ***I've been misdiagnosed.*** I've been told I have diabetes type 2. But that's not true. ***Like one in ten diagnosed type 2***, I actually have (but don't know I have) a very different diabetes, with different causes and treatments than type 2.

I'm a fit, active biologist who worked in the woods for decades; a backpacker, skier, and mountain biker. A month ago, "You have diabetes" landed on my head like a cartoon falling anvil. I turned to my doctor, my library, and the internet for answers, but only came away with more questions.

As the caffeine-hungry in line behind me twitch and jingle their keys, I don't yet know all the ingredients of my paralyzing confusion. I've never even heard the name of the disease I actually have (LADA). But I have been told I must eat *"exactly right from now on"* or I could go blind . . . while having a stroke . . . with a side of heart attack . . . and for dessert, some toes chopped off.

I'm scared. I'm ready to live clean. But who do I trust when so many reputable sources completely disagree? What *can* I eat?

That long-ago morning at the counter of Good Mood Food, I did the grown-up thing.

I wailed, "Nothing!"

And I stormed out of Good Mood Food. I left Ava flat, a swirly art-topped coffee in her hand.

LADA—LATENT AUTOIMMUNE DIABETES IN ADULTS—IS CONFUSING

Imagine if 3.4 million Americans had a life-threatening chronic disease—yet lacked straight-talking resources to understand it, and on top of this were routinely misdiagnosed. Amazingly this is true for LADA, latent autoimmune diabetes in adults, sometimes called diabetes 1.5.

You may know there's more than one type of diabetes; many have heard of type 1 and type 2 (T1 and T2). Turns out there are other forms as well, including LADA, which is actually *more common* than T1.[1] And yet, like me at the counter of Good Mood Food that day, many people who have LADA have never even heard of LADA.

LADA has been well-known among medical researchers for four decades,[2] but it's frequently overlooked by doctors and only beginning to be known to the general public. "LADA is an important form of diabetes, which should be recognized, understood and managed . . . yet, in many ways, it remains an enigma," to quote one of the many medical journal articles deploring this toxic information gap.[3]

LADA's inaccurate alphabet-soup name doesn't help: Forget "latent" because it's not; forget "in adults," because although it's frequently diagnosed in middle age and beyond, a person of any age can have LADA.[4] Focus on "autoimmune." This word is accurate! And important. This word is the reason *so much advice* claiming to be for diabetes in general *doesn't always apply* to those of us with LADA.

"At diagnosis, patients with [LADA] are . . . clinically indistinguishable from patients with type 2 diabetes, though they tend to be younger and leaner. Only with screening for autoantibodies . . . can they be identified with certainty," writes Dr. Hawa of London's Queen Mary University.[5]

LADA was described in the 1980s,[6] before the Berlin Wall came down, before the first *Simpsons* episode aired, and before disposable contact lenses. Yet still today, 10 percent of diabetics told by a doctor, "You are type 2," are in fact LADA.[7] We misdiagnosed millions often receive inadequate or incorrect medical advice, because **LADA has a fundamentally different underlying cause than T2, and T2 treatments may harm us.**[8]

LADAs have to filter through diet and treatment advice very carefully. Some T2 treatments will make us sicker, not better.

TOP 10 THINGS TO KNOW ABOUT LADA

1. **LADA is not your fault.** It's one of more than a hundred autoimmune diseases. *Autoimmune* means the body gets confused and we mistakenly attack ourselves: with LADA, we attack our cells that make insulin.

2. Active, fit people with healthy lifestyles develop LADA. We can **remain or become healthy** with LADA.

3. **Many with LADA are undiagnosed or misdiagnosed**, due to lack of awareness. Ten percent of people told they are type 2 are misdiagnosed LADAs. **Misdiagnosis is dangerous,** as we may be given treatments that make us sicker, or not be offered the treatments we need.

4. **Simple, affordable lab work**—an antibody test—shows whether you have LADA.

5. Diabetes is an **umbrella disease** of several types that are very different, just as skin cancer is different from lung cancer.

6. Many common beliefs about diabetes **do not apply to LADA**. Our culture misunderstands diabetes.

7. LADA (and all diabetes) becomes **dangerous/deadly if untreated**. Uncontrolled diabetes attacks our brain, heart, eyes, kidneys, liver, nerves, and more.

8. On the other hand, **well-controlled** diabetes is the leading cause of . . . **nothing**.

9. **You can enjoy delicious food** while keeping your LADA well controlled.

10. It's easier than you might think to be **happy and healthy with LADA**.

∘ ∘ ∘

That morning in Good Mood Food, I didn't know any of this. Quite a few surprises were headed my way, and thanks to my winning personality, I was about to smash into them like brick walls. I would have to relearn so much I thought I knew about food, learn to advocate for myself, and come face-to-face with my own prejudices. Eventually, thanks to brick-wall therapy, I'd realize that "eating healthy" is about more than carbs and protein: It's a cultural, psychological, and social justice issue.

IS THIS BOOK FOR YOU?

Interweaving my personal story with the latest medical and health information, this book explains what LADA is, when to suspect you have it, treatment options, and the medical catch-22 that makes misdiagnosis so pervasive. Plainspoken, medically researched, and extensively footnoted, it lays out how Carb-craft—fine-tuning the carbohydrates in our food—helps us live our best life. Along with "What can I eat?" I answer other big questions that once obsessed me, from "Why me?" to "Can I cure my LADA?" (Spoiler alert: It depends.)

Many with diabetes are not yet aware—diabetes has been called one of the most underdiagnosed diseases in America. One in three Americans will have diabetes by 2050, the CDC projects.[9]

- This book is for you if you were fairly lean and fit when told you had "diabetes type 2."
- This book is equally for you at any weight. Being lean is one clue we may be LADA, but a LADA can be anywhere on the weight spectrum.
- This book is for you if you have been told that you have reduced insulin production, or that there is an autoimmune component to your diabetes.
- This book is for you if you have tested positive for GAD antibodies,* or another diabetic antibody, or had a low fasting C-peptide.
- This book is for you if you've been told you have LADA or diabetes type 1.5.
- This book is for you if you believed you were type 2 but discovered that your blood sugars go surprisingly high when you eat lentils, black beans, hummus, and similar "healthy" foods that doctors and nutritionists keep recommending.

---

* Antibodies to glutamic acid decarboxylase.

- This book is for you if you've walked out of a type 2 diabetes class thinking: What they just taught is the way I've been eating for the past decade—and it was *while eating this way* that I developed diabetes . . . what's going on?
- This book is for you if your diabetes "just doesn't fit."

While this book is dedicated to LADA diabetics, it will also be useful to type 1s, type 2s, those with other forms of diabetes or prediabetics, and anyone who wants to learn more about food and their body. This book will assist doctors, loved ones, and advocates: anyone who desires greater understanding of a diabetic's struggle and the best way to support us.

This book is for the stunned-bunny newbie or for the long-diagnosed who hasn't found support and information. It's for those struggling to gain weight, those at their weight goal, and those wishing to lose weight. It's for the diabetic who wants to stop gritting her way through holiday meals, dreading dinner dates, and barely surviving the banquet table at wedding receptions—who is ready to start dancing.

This book is for you if you want to be in charge of your own life—if you want to feel good, be healthy, and eat delicious food.

BIG PICTURE 1.
ROAD MAP: WHERE WE'RE HEADED

To live well with LADA, we need to understand what it is, and what it's up to in our body. Part 1 of this book explains what's going on inside of us, why, and how to work with that. In part 2, we gather the tools for good health. Part 3 looks at food—a key tool—and how to enjoy favorite cultural and heritage foods while protecting health. Part 4 ponders the long term— how to stay healthy for the rest of our life—and closes with thoughts on access and equity.

Part 1: The big picture of diabetes, and how LADA fits within it.
Part 2: The biology of getting healthy: tools for health.
Part 3: Carb-craft in two dozen rules.
Part 4: The psychology of staying healthy: saying no to "the yo-yo," and yes to *long-term* health.

As we go, we'll discover:

1. LADA means *doing for ourselves* what our body's automatic systems once did. We've lost the autopilot button, but not our ability to drive and thrive.
2. There is *no magic pill* ("just eat foods that start with Q!") to make this go away. We'll win by playing all the cards in our hand; using all our tools in combination.
3. One definition of diabetes is "difficulty processing/digesting carbohydrates." That's why you'll hear a lot about carbs (carbohydrates) in this book, and why our healthy eating tool is called Carb-craft.
4. Carb-craft will mesh with your heritage, religion, and ethics and with the foods you love. *Carb-craft is compatible* with halal, kosher, vegan, meat-loving, paleo, keto, Mediterranean, anti-inflammatory, and other healthful ways to eat.

5. Stress, fever, steroids, and other surprises can affect blood sugars *as much as food*.
6. LADAs are often misdiagnosed as T2 even though we have the *opposite* underlying cause; this misdiagnosis jeopardizes our health.
7. LADAs must *advocate* for ourselves.
8. LADAs often wait too long to *begin insulin*.
9. Nurture your garden (microbiome), understand inflammation, and *pamper your beta cells* (insulin-producing cells).
10. With LADA we can be healthy, avoid food obsession, feel good, and eat delicious food.

2 DIABETES? INCONCEIVABLE!

How My Bias and My Body Set Me Up for a Fall

LADA is often misdiagnosed and treated as type 2 diabetes.
This results in . . . harm to patients.
—Professor Katherine O'Neal[1]

"DIABETES? HOW DID YOU KNOW? WHAT WERE YOUR SYMPTOMS?" friends asked.

"I . . . um . . . didn't have any symptoms," I mumbled, confused.

"Okaa-ay . . ." My friend would roll her eyes. "Then how did you get diagnosed?"

Oh, that. That's an embarrassing story.

ONE NEW YEAR'S DAY I CALLED A FRIEND JUST TO SAY HELLO.

"I'm great, thanks," Jayson said. "Except I just had a heart attack."

Since he's a nurse, Jayson realized what his vague, barely noticeable symptoms pointed to. So my hiking, biking, Grand Canyon–paddling friend got himself right to the hospital. He survived because he went in time.

That scared the @#!$ out of me.

After we hung up, I looked out from the ridge where my house perches and across our town dotted on a valley between ridges draped in larch and Douglas fir, homeland of the P'Squosa. I live in Washington State's Cascade Mountains. This winter, it kept raining the minute after it snowed, so my house was knee-deep in soft-serve slush with freezer-burn patches of ice. For me, weather is more than conversational because the dirt road to my house doesn't get plowed; in winter I get home every evening by snowmobile, a once-red disco-era snowmobile with a scrounged beige hood, duct-taped windshield, and slowly fatiguing right front ski.

Staring out at the ridge, I thought about Jayson, a little, but I'm ashamed to say I mostly thought about myself. I saw my life suddenly at a distance. Jayson's news shone a spotlight on things I'd shrugged off— low energy, brain fog, and a middle-of-the-night racing heart. Meh, it's been too dark, too rainy, and I miss my son, off to college, that's all. But another part of my brain whispered that I hadn't had my choles- terol checked in twenty years, and my hands had pins-and-needles some nights. "Silent heart attack" began to dance before my eyes like a soft- serve sugar plum fairy.

Monday morning I hurried through the doors of my local clinic. Your heart sounds good, a doctor reassured me, but let's follow up with a tread- mill test, EKG, blood panel . . .

At the last minute I mentioned, "You know, a couple of relatives have diabetes." So the doctor tacked on one more test, a test he wouldn't have done otherwise.

And that was how I got diagnosed—and misdiagnosed—the first time.

FIVE DAYS LATER, I STOOD IN A GAS STATION, STARING AT A LETTER I'D just picked up from my in-town mailbox. The three-sentence form letter said: "You have type 2 diabetes."

Wait, whaaaat? No heart attack? In a tizzy, I phoned a medically astute friend I'll call Rose.

"Did they do an A1c?" Rose asked.

"A what?" The gas pump was singing at me—yikes. I walked over to the dumpster so I could hear. My car was packed with tent, sleeping bag, and suitcase I'd shuttled down by sled and snowmobile. Diabetes! Should I panic . . . or should I continue on with my plan to drive across the moun- tains to my Whidbey Island writing class I'd been looking forward to for so long?

"Ask for an A1c," Rose patiently repeated.

I called my clinic, made the appointment, and requested they mail all my test results. Then, reassured by Rose that I wasn't going to topple over that afternoon, I headed out of town.

Diabetes? Doesn't that happen to people who eat wrong? It can't be true: I'm fit, active, shop at health food stores, eat 90 percent vegetarian. There must be some mistake, said a part of my brain that was not merely arrogant, but profoundly mistaken, setting me up for the first brick wall I would shortly be smashing into.

When I got home from Whidbey Island, the test results waited in my mailbox, pages of columns, numbers, and puzzling names. I googled each mysterious word and number, scribbling questions. I didn't see A1c in my stack but I googled that, too.

I walked into my doctor's appointment clutching my scribbled pages, grateful I wasn't having heart attacks. On the other hand: Diabetes? Ridiculous. I'd request an A1c and clear up this little mistake.

THANKS FOR DISCOVERING INSULIN, SIR EDWARD

We have known about diabetes for four thousand years. The ancient Greeks described diabetes, as did physicians of ancient India, Egypt, and China.[2] One form of diabetes was called *wasting disease* because people wasted away, breaking down their own muscles, literally eating their own bodies, as starvation victims do. Curiously, people suffering from wasting disease excrete a lot of sugar, so the condition was named diabetes ("siphoning") mellitus ("honey"), meaning: "sugar is pouring out in your pee." A mystery: What makes people starve to death while swimming in, and dumping out, sugar?

For centuries diabetes was mysterious, painful, and ultimately fatal because people starved to death while swimming in blood sugar—unless this toxically high blood sugar first killed them in some other way (heart attack, stroke, liver failure, kidney failure, eeny, meeny, miney, mo).

Then in 1910, a researcher with the absolutely fabulous name Sir Edward Albert Sharpey-Schafer isolated a natural chemical produced by our pancreas and said, "Let's call this insulin." Scientists soon figured out that insulin is like a key that unlocks the doors of our cells so that sugar can be pulled out of our bloodstream and into those hungry cells.

Insulin is what allows sugar—our body's main fuel—to move from our bloodstream into all our hardworking cells, like our muscles and brain.

Insulin is a specialty key *only for sugar*. We only need it when we eat things our body breaks down into sugar. Which, it turns out, includes almost all of our food. All carbohydrates (except fiber) and much of the protein we eat can turn into sugar in our body.

DR. ALASKA

We'll call him Dr. Alaska: John Lennon glasses, trim salt-and-pepper hair, a kind man with a cheery smile. My valued doc for over a decade; I really appreciated how he always heard and respected my input. It's no wonder there's a waiting list to be Dr. Alaska's patient.

"How are you today?" Dr. Alaska shook my hand, his brown eyes warm, smile lines crinkling.

"Thanks." I managed a half smile back. "Confused." Clutching my scribbled pages, I started in on my questions: What does this test mean? What does that test mean?

He patiently answered each question while I scribbled more notes. He asked: Had I been thirsty a lot? Peeing a lot?

I shook my head. Nope.

"Okay." Dr. Alaska leaned forward. "We should start you right away on metformin."

"Um, actually, I was hoping we could do an A1c test."

"We already did."

How did I miss that? I thrust the fistful of pages at him. "Which one is that?"

He flipped through the papers, then back through the papers, then frowned. "Hang on."

He left the room and was back in a few minutes with a new piece of paper. My A1c test. Apparently the nurse forgot to mail one test.

Dr. Alaska handed me the paper. I stared at it. I had been reading online about A1cs, so I knew this number was clearly over the line, well above the prediabetes zone.

Holy @#!$! I have diabetes.

3 WHY ARE THERE MANY TYPES OF DIABETES?

Locks Versus Keys

Diabetes rejoices in silly names . . . MODY is no doubt the*
silliest, but . . . latent autoimmune diabetes in adults (LADA)
comes close.
>—Dr. Edwin Gale, Southmead Hospital, Department
>of Diabetes and Metabolism[1]

Alternative terms that have been used to describe [LADA]
include type 1.5 diabetes, latent T1D, slowly progressive
Insulin Dependent Diabetes Mellitus (SPIDDM), or youth
onset diabetes of maturity.
>—Dr. Chiara Guglielmi, Campus Bio Medico,
>Department of Endocrinology and Diabetes[2]

AS I SAT WEDGED BETWEEN DR. ALASKA'S MAGAZINE RACK AND blood pressure machine, in a chair that smelled of lemon apple sanitizer, the part of my brain singing "La, la, la, not me," was silenced. A new flock of fears began to flap around in my head. *What exactly is diabetes? Is this for life?*

Dr. Alaska reached for his prescription pad. "We'll start you on metformin and a statin, and see how—"

"Wait. Can't people get better just with diet and exercise?"

---

* Maturity onset diabetes of the young.

"Well . . ." His frown deepened. "In some cases. Unlikely for you."

"Why?"

"Usually the people that works for are pretty overweight when they start." He snapped the computer shut.

Whaaat?

"I don't . . ." I shook my head, dazed. " . . . I don't think . . ."

"Listen, diabetes is deadly. You don't want to delay. The earlier you get going on a good program, the better your success rate."

Dr. Alaska stood in the doorway, prescription pad in one hand, pen in the other, the minute hand on a big round clock ticking emphatically over his shoulder. I didn't summon the courage to launch into another hundred and one questions, but among all the thoughts banging around in my head, I discovered one piece of clarity: If it was *possible* to heal myself through diet and exercise, I wanted to try that first.

His pen began to hurry across the paper. "I'm writing you a prescription for—"

"No," I said. "No, let me go home and . . . think."

Dr. Alaska stopped mid-jot, disapproval etching his face. "I strongly recommend you start these medications right away. They're effective and safe. Delay can be deadly."

But in the end I left with just a prescription for a blood glucose meter. Plus Dr. Alaska's warning that this was against his professional judgment, and his strong urging to talk to the hospital nutritionist.

"The nutritionist session is *free*," he emphasized.

Free, great, but I didn't want to waste it. The next time I walked into this building, I was going to have done a lot more reading. I'd know what the heck a statin was, and all the pros and cons of metformin.

As for nutrition? Please. I knew my elbow from a doughnut.

The words of a woman with so much more to learn than she could even imagine.

THERE ARE ONLY THREE THINGS TO EAT

There are only three things to eat: protein, carbohydrate, and fat. *Any bit of your food that's not fat or protein is a carbohydrate.*

A carbohydrate is built from sugars like a Lego castle is built from Lego bricks. Some like to picture a carbohydrate as a train, a string of boxcars (sugars).

There are simple carbohydrates (short trains) and complex carbohydrates (long or branched or complicated trains where the cars are double- or triple-locked together). It doesn't take long to uncouple a short train. Done! All the sugars flood into your bloodstream quickly. But it takes a while to uncouple the complicated trains. Their sugars move out into the bloodstream more slowly, with less of a sharp peak.

If sugar is like saying "tree," glucose is like saying "tupelo." Tupelo is a type of tree, and glucose is a type of sugar. So the term *blood sugar* is correct. Not all sugar is glucose, so the term *blood glucose* (BG) is more precise.

YES *AND* NO

Diabetes is complicated. The answer to almost every important question I've ever had about diabetes has been: yes *and* no.

Wait, what?

Is blood sugar (blood glucose) bad? Yes *and* no. The human machine runs on BG like your car runs on gas. Sugar is our main fuel. If your BG drops too low, you die. If your BG stays too high too long, this creates damage that will ultimately kill you as well. **BG peaks *or* valleys**, either one, if they go beyond what your machinery is designed to handle, **will harm you**. And insulin, as we saw in chapter 2, is the crucial gatekeeper, the only thing that allows sugar to move out of our blood and into our hungry cells.

When it comes to blood sugar, staying healthy is all about avoiding blood sugar peaks and valleys. In my fit teenage son, BG barely jiggles—his internal checks and balances smooth the curve regardless of what he eats. But for me, now, BG is constantly rising and falling, a wave, always on the move.

Here are three definitions of diabetes, all true, all connected:

1. Diabetes is an insulin problem.
2. Diabetes is a problem processing/digesting carbohydrates.
3. Diabetes is a problem regulating blood glucose.

The first thought that popped into my head was: *I won't eat anything that turns into blood sugar.* But that doesn't work. We need BG. We will die without BG. Also, virtually anything we eat can ultimately be turned into BG by our resourceful body.

Which is not to say that everything we eat is the same. The devil is in the details. What, when, why, how, and how much you eat—as well as whether you go for a bike ride, run a fever, worry for a lost pet, and so much more—affect whether your BG will stay stable, spike, or crash. No sound bites.

DIABETES: ONE DISEASE OR MANY?

Diabetes is an umbrella condition, composed of many types. What all types of diabetes have in common is: The way our body processes food is getting messed up.

The exact way it gets messed up varies. Some who have diabetes try to build muscle but stay "skinny as a coat hanger" (as a T1 described himself). Others of us eat one bite of lettuce and watch it turn into three pounds of fat. (Okay, not quite, but it can feel that way.)

Why? What's going on inside?

Our cells need to eat constantly; they're always at work, always burning fuel. Yet we can't eat all the time—we have to hunt, gather, fill out tax forms, and help our species continue through . . . ahem . . . fun stuff. You know.

While our cells eat all the time, we eat meals. This works because our body can store food and then move it to exactly where it's needed at exactly the right time. Like breathing, we never have to think about this essential process of food shuffling—until something goes wrong.

Diabetes is one of those ironic diseases. We eat, but our cells struggle to eat. The food that goes into our mouths doesn't get where it should, when it should. Our diabetic body is like a weird El Dorado where the streets are paved with gold (sugar), but only because the people there can't hold on to gold, can't carry it to the store or the bank. The people are starving, and the streets are clogged with shimmering beauty so deep it becomes toxic. Some of us are barely eating yet bloating; others are starving yet peeing sugar.

We can think of diabetes as an insulin problem. Or as a problem eating carbohydrates and sugars. Toe-may-toe, toe-mah-toe.

AS FAR BACK AS THE FIFTH CENTURY, PEOPLE HAD AN INKLING THAT two opposite-looking kinds of people became ill and peed sugar. Some spoke of diabetes of the young versus the old. The mechanism for the difference was unearthed in 1936 by—are you ready for another fabulous name?—Sir Harold Percival Himsworth.

Big picture, there are two ways to have an insulin problem. One, you can run out of insulin. Or two, you can have oodles of insulin that has *lost its effectiveness*. Back in Sir Harold's day this was a revolutionary insight.

These two types came to be called:

1. Type 1s, the ones who run out.
2. Type 2s, who have abundant or even excessive insulin that struggles to do its job.

Why do people run out of insulin? (Type 1, T1)

Friendly fire, sadly. We mistake our own body for the enemy and attack our own crucially important cells: our precious beta cells, the cells that make insulin. Running-out-of-insulin diabetes is an *auto-immune* disease. As we go to press the Autoimmune Association (formerly AARDA) lists over a hundred autoimmune diseases, including multiple sclerosis, lupus, celiac, and several forms of arthritis. Why would a body attack itself? And how can we wave the white flag and get ourselves to cease and desist? These remain medical mysteries.

T1s are losing insulin, losing the crucial key to open the locks that let blood sugar out of blood and into hungry cells.

Why does insulin sometimes lose power? (Type 2, T2)

Our bodies can become resistant to insulin. Picture living with a teenager whose music, already not to your taste, keeps getting louder and louder. First you try earplugs, then acoustic tiles, and finally you begin thumbing brochures with pictures of palm trees. When insulin is too high too long, cells can become insulin-resistant. At a physical level, the locks on the cell wall where the insulin "key" needs to fit break, get gummed up, or disappear.

T2s are losing or breaking the crucial locks that let blood sugar out of blood and into hungry cells.

Keys, locks, or both?

While T1s and T2s start out with opposite causes of the same problem (keys versus locks), they can become more similar as their disease progresses. T1s can develop insulin resistance (lock issues). And poorly controlled T2s may burn out their pancreas, and reach a point where they no longer make enough insulin (keys) and need to inject insulin.

LADA

Then in the 1980s, type 1.5 was discovered. Scientists are still bickering about what to name us. Most call our disease LADA, latent autoimmune diabetes in adults. LADA is like T1 played at very low RPMs, or T1 mellow. It's autoimmune (friendly fire), but it's a meadow path—rather than a cliff—down to the river of no-insulin, perhaps offering opportunities for prolonging the descent.

Just like a T1, a LADA is losing her keys. (Some LADAs also have insulin resistance, but as in T1, losing our keys is what drives our disease.) **With LADA, *we expect to run out of insulin*** at some point. But if we act early and use all our tools, we can pamper our insulin-making cells and we might increase the amount of time we'll still be able to make insulin: adding more months, years, perhaps (for some) decades after diagnosis to our "insulin honeymoon."[3]

MODY

Maturity onset diabetes of the young: another silly name for another important form of diabetes. MODY is not autoimmune; it is caused by a genetic variation that reduces insulin production. For MODY, genetic testing shows which of the fourteen (at last count) genetic variants is at work, and which treatment is recommended.[4]

THE BIG FOUR

T1, T2, LADA, and MODY are the big four. And as scientists dig deeper into genetics and antibodies, diabetes can be split into ever-finer subtypes. There's more and more and more, all hopping through the frothy waves and scrambling to the shore (as Lewis Carroll's walrus told his carpenter). T1 and MODY are more commonly diagnosed in youth, and T2 and LADA more commonly in adults, but *every type of diabetes can occur at any age*.

LOCKS VERSUS KEYS

In the lock-and-key analogy: A T1 lost his keys, while a T2 broke her locks. Both are sitting on the front steps waiting for the locksmith. But when that professional arrives, they're going to need very different kinds of help.

We LADAs keep dropping our keys, too, but we're slower about it, and many of us are also getting gummed-up locks (in LADA, our lock situation is variable).

MODYs get handed a genetic key ring with not quite enough keys on it.

This book will focus on T1, T2, and LADA, the three most common types of diabetes.

MISDIAGNOSIS HEIGHTENS RISK

"Unfortunately, patients with LADA are often misdiagnosed as having type 2 diabetes," writes Dr. Ernesto Maddaloni of Sapienza University. "This translates into a significantly increased risk of complications."[5]

If a LADA is misdiagnosed as T2, and is doing things to reduce insulin *resistance*, but his problem is he's *running out* of insulin (losing his keys), he may be wasting time while the clock runs out, losing opportunities to protect and nurture his insulin-making beta cells.[6] Even worse, he may be doing **active harm** to his beta cells, because some type 2 treatments that don't harm a robust pancreas can hit a struggling pancreas hard, and **burn out beta cells more quickly,** pushing a LADA off the cliff faster (see chapter 12 and note 7).[7]

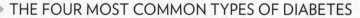

THE FOUR MOST COMMON TYPES OF DIABETES

T1. Autoimmune. Friendly fire destroyed your insulin-making beta cells. Now (or soon) every day and every time you eat, you will need to inject insulin.

T2. Your pancreas and its beta cells are fabulous, darling. You have oodles of insulin. Unfortunately, you've become resistant to insulin. Your body is like a coffee addict who needs ten cups a day to wake up. So your pancreas pours out more and more insulin, but even this large amount of insulin struggles to do its job.

MODY. Low production of insulin caused by genetics. There are many types, some milder, some more impactful; genetic testing shows the best treatment.

LADA. We're autoimmune, like T1, but we may be mistaken for T2, especially if we're middle-aged or older and not yet in insulin crisis. We're the friendlier friendly fire. The good news: We may be able to loiter in our "honeymoon" (the period where we still make insulin) and have a long last slow dance with our insulin before we join the T1 crowd.

If we're running out of insulin but don't know it, we're losing precious time and perhaps causing active harm; some T2 treatments will burn out a LADA's insulin-making cells more quickly.

o o o

We make insulin in just one place: the special cells called beta cells within our small but mighty pancreas. What your pancreas does for you, no other organ can.

If you have some working beta cells left, be good to them! How? That's what this whole book will be about.

4 FROM BURNOUT TO HOPE

Why Burnout Is So Common, and the Promise of New Research

> LADA . . . *represents a considerable proportion (about*
> *5–10%) of all diabetic patients . . . phenotypical*
> *characteristics of these patients do not allow the correct*
> *identification without screening of GAD antibodies . . .*
> *Early identification of LADA patients will . . . [allow]*
> *prevention of the beta-cell destructive process.*
> —Dr. Guntram Schernthaner, Rudolfstiftung Hospital,
> Vienna[1]

AS THE SNOW MELTED AND SPRING BREAK NEARED, MY FOLLOW-UPS with Dr. Alaska just . . . hadn't felt right. Back in the good old days, Dr. Alaska always seemed to really hear me, really see me as an individual. Now, in a way that was hard to put into words, in his office I felt like a generic interchangeable diabetic. It felt like he had a script for T2 that I was being slow to follow: "non-compliant."

While the day would come when I'd think to myself, *If I were a doctor, I'd probably have a script for T2 also*, at that moment what I felt was: *not heard*.

I felt something was off—but I didn't know enough yet to know what or why.

I'd always trusted my doctor as blindly as I trusted my car mechanic; thanks to good luck and privilege, both had worked out for me. Educate myself? Advocate for myself? Huh?

DID YOU KNOW THERE'S SUCH A THING AS . . . ?

"Has anyone talked to you about LADA diabetes?" asked Rose.

"Talked to me about *what*?"

Like so many of us, it was not from my doctor that I first heard about LADA. Nor from the excellent hospital nutritionist. Nor the blogs I clicked through online, the books in my local library, or the University of Washington bookstore's five long shelves of books on diabetes. For weeks I'd been poring through all kinds of references on diabetes, but it was only the extraordinary good luck of having a knowledgeable friend that put me on the road to health. Which seems crazy considering LADA came onstage with Hall & Oates and Guns N' Roses, shoulder pads and Cosby sweaters, Joan Jett and Mudhoney.

Once I knew the word *LADA*, I started finding it all over the place! Not with much information attached, but enough to be intriguing. Misdiagnosed LADAs might be slender, I read; might be younger and have better lipid profiles; and might find it much harder to control their blood sugars than a T2.[2]

Could this be me? When I tried to talk about LADA with Dr. Alaska, I left confused and frustrated.

"You know, it is absolutely your right to request a second opinion," Rose said as I dithered on the phone with her. "There's nothing weird or wrong about that."

Wasn't there, though? Dr. Alaska had been my trusted doc for a decade—I couldn't be *rude*. Plus . . . insurance . . . would I have to pay for a second opinion myself?

ON THE SPECTRUM

Diabetes is a spectrum: *How* resistant to insulin are you or *how* fragile are your beta cells; *how quickly* are your beta cells dying; *how many* had you already lost when you were diagnosed?

All of us with diabetes have much in common, and we are each unique. I like to picture diabetes like the view on a favorite hike: Silver Pass. At the summit you can turn in a circle, 360 degrees, and see mountains in every direction, range after range. To the west, the mountains glow blue; moving east the blue tints with purple; and even farther east the mountains are a pinkish tan. If you're a "lumper," you see three types of mountains: blue, purple, tan. If you're a "splitter," you see an intricate and infinite variation. That's why some people will tell you there are four types of diabetes, and some will tell you there are twenty. Neither lumpers nor splitters are wrong. There is no wrong. There are only mountains, grasshopper.

If you want to get somewhere, you need to know which mountain you're standing on. You're not judging or dissing the other mountains. In fact, you're learning from them. You just need to know where you are.

NOT ONLY IS DIABETES A SPECTRUM—LADA IS A SPECTRUM ALL BY itself. LADA is a much more mixed bag than T1 or T2. "Despite high prevalence of LADA . . . the treatment of LADA patients is far less elucidated than is the case for T1D and T2D. Finding a treatment strategy for LADA . . . that can reduce the decline of beta cell function, ensure adequate metabolic control and thereby reduce the risk of diabetic complications is . . . an important clinical challenge," endocrinologist Ingrid Hals wrote in 2019.[3]

> ⟩ T1s start out just autoimmune.
> ⟩ T2s start out just with insulin resistance.
> ⟩ Most LADAs, on the day we are diagnosed, have a bit of both things going on.

o o o

All LADAs have the T1 problem (running out of insulin), but we vary a lot in how much *resistance* to insulin we have. And each LADA's degree of insulin resistance typically changes over time.

Some LADAs, when we're first diagnosed, are very T1-ish, with little insulin resistance. Many others are solidly T1-ish and also have a big scoop of insulin resistance on top. A few of us are more to the T2 side of life, both in our genetics and in how our disease behaves, and have just a touch of autoimmunity gilding the lily.

This doesn't mean no one knows what you should do; it means that to learn *your* best treatment plan, you need to dig deeper than the label LADA, and learn which mountain you're standing on.

WHEN WILL MY HONEYMOON END?

I finally worked up the courage to ask, and Dr. Alaska was quite happy to refer me to an endocrinologist (a doctor who specializes in diabetes). Oh. Turns out when I advocate for myself, people act like that's normal. Huh.

The endocrinologist's earliest appointment was three months away. While I waited, I kept reading and researching.

My reading confirmed that yep: I should expect to completely run out of insulin, and reach a point of needing to take insulin every day, and every time I eat. My next urgent question, of course, was: **When will I run out?**

The answer I got was: Who knows?*

People call it our honeymoon—the time when our pancreas is still making some insulin but not enough to fully manage the job, so our body begins to struggle every time we eat. This impacts our body, it's picked up in tests like the A1c, and we get diagnosed.

Typically by the time a LADA is diagnosed, she has permanently lost three-fourths of her insulin-making ability.

Ouch.

How long does a LADA honeymoon last? We're so varied that there's a huge range: Our honeymoon might last six months, six years, twelve years, or more. And the comments I read online from T1s and others who had lost all insulin production were so wistful: "If only I'd known to value and protect my honeymoon."

Yikes—it had already been months since my diagnosis, and now I had months to wait to see the specialist—would my precious honeymoon expire while I waited?

I called Dr. Alaska's office. Could they schedule me for the test for LADA?

"No."

The answer was conveyed by a nurse to my voicemail. "We'll let the endocrinologist decide whether to do the test."

---

* Fasting or stimulated C peptide, and levels of antibodies like GADA, can give a hint, but it's very imprecise (chapter 13).

A wall, sometimes, is a moment of decision.

I made another appointment, walked in, sat down, and threw a fit. It wasn't pretty. But I was completely clear: I wanted to walk into that endocrinologist appointment with all relevant test *results* in hand. Enough waiting!

Dr. Alaska eventually conceded, maybe just because it was clear I wouldn't leave until he did. I walked from his office to the lab one floor down. A simple blood draw—standard, easy, covered by insurance—to check GAD antibodies and C-peptide.

Weird. When I advocate for myself, the things that I'm needing happen . . . and I'm not kicked off insurance, and I don't get frowny faces in my chart . . . everyone acts like it's normal.

A FEW DAYS LATER, WHEN THE BLOOD WORK CAME BACK, I WAS DIagnosed: LADA.

TESTING FOR LADA

> - GAD antibodies (glutamic acid decarboxylase autoantibodies; sometimes written GADA or GAD-A) are found in 90 percent of LADA patients. They are the "footprints" left by the autoimmune attack, the evidence that our diabetes has an autoimmune cause.
> - Not every LADA has GADA (sounds like the start of a limerick!) but most do. A LADA might instead (or also) have islet cell antibodies (ICA) such as islet antigen 2 (IA-2A), zinc transporter antibodies (ZnT8), or insulin antibodies (IA).
> - A LADA may have only one antibody, or more than one.
> - T1s often have multiple antibodies; T2s do not have any of these antibodies.
> - C-peptide, a protein involved in the creation of insulin, indicates how much insulin you recently made. It is often measured at the same time you are tested for antibodies. (More on the C-peptide test in chapter 13.)

o o o

A SECOND OPINION WILL FIX EVERYTHING . . . RIGHT?

Having snowmobiled through mushy January to hear Dr. Alaska tell me I had **T2**, I drove past May's blossoming cherry orchards to the clinic of "Dr. Hawaii."

"Yep, you're LADA," Dr. Hawaii told me. "And LADA is really just **T1**."

A cheery, efficient, no-nonsense person with arching eyebrows and dainty earrings, Dr. Hawaii didn't want to perplex me with self-care strategies. I should eat any old thing, she said, fall off the insulin cliff, then hook up for life with an insulin machine.

"They're wearable!" she enthused.

I stared back like a deer in the headlights, aghast, holding back tears. This was the happy ending I'd waited months to hear? To be cheerily told I'd soon be wearing a machine the rest of my life?

I'd walked into her office with a spring in my step, so thankful the waiting was over, hoping for that magic pill, maybe *Only eat foods that start with a vowel*. Instead, I'd smacked hard into another brick wall. Ouch.

To be honest, in the months since my diagnosis, I'd been flailing. I'd been spinning bald tires on ice as I raced to . . . I wasn't sure where . . . pursued by the fear that any and every bite of food added another nail to my coffin, my impending heart attack, my foot chopped off.

I'd brought home a giant stack of books. Each one swore it was the truth, the whole truth—and proceeded to contradict the other books in the stack.

I'd swallowed cod liver oil, chanted ohmmm, fasted, fretted, and weighed myself more in the past five months than in the previous five years. One knowledgeable friend had suggested, in utter seriousness, that I should roll in snowbanks and eat worms to reset my immune system.

Testing my blood sugars till every finger ached, I could tell that— absolutely!—*food and exercise had a huge impact* on my blood sugars, and on how I felt. But I was just guessing, trying this, trying that, always wondering: *What can I eat?*

I had been sure *the specialist* would answer this nagging question for me and make all well in my world again.

Guess I shot my second opinion on the wrong doctor.

Insurance would never cover *another* visit to a *different* endocrinologist . . . would they? And . . . was I sick enough to be worth it? Was I making a big deal out of nothing?

Once again Rose reassured and encouraged me. Absolutely, she said. Get a second second opinion.

JULY FOUND ME DRIVING HALFWAY ACROSS THE STATE TO SEE "DR. Chicago" at Virginia Mason Medical Center, a top-notch research hospital. Maybe I'd get into some cutting-edge study!

You have **neither T1 nor T2,** said Dr. Chicago, a low-key man with a deep brow and trim beard. After scolding me for "testing too often" (he disapproved of testing BG more than once a day—a discredited attitude some unfortunately still hold), Dr. Chicago handed me a long list of T2 medications and circled a few we could try "when you're sicker."

Dismissive is the word that comes to mind.

Like an opposites version of Dr. Hawaii, he leaned T2 where she leaned T1. What they shared was a vibe of: *Come back when you're sick.*

But what if a person living with diabetes *wants to be healthy*?

My hopes splintered again, I stumbled out of another doctor's office.

"Come on, peoples," I muttered as I wound out of the hospital parking maze onto a traffic-jammed highway, "isn't *prevention* still a thing?"

BURNOUT

I was as confused as ever, still scared, and suffocated by a fog of weary dread that I'd never figure this out—that diabetes was a death sentence with no reprieve, no parole.

Nonsense, piped up my intuition. How I live, what I eat: These *must* matter!

Or if not, I wanted to hear that from an expert so I could run straight to my favorite ice cream shop and order a Lalapalooza.

Why were my mediocre partial successes at controlling my glucose levels, attained at an eating-disorder-like cost (although to be fair, I hadn't tried worms yet), making me invisible? How does a person *prove* they need help?

Stupid tears crept down my cheeks.

A DIAGNOSIS OF DIABETES CAN DOUBLE OR TRIPLE OUR LIKELIHOOD of depression. Many of us become clinically depressed when diagnosed.[4]

Shock. Loss. All the stages of grief, including anger and denial. On top of confusion, isolation, and lack of support. I found myself in a toxic stew, much too common in all types of diabetes. Burnout is an enormous problem, as you'll see within minutes of surfing any online diabetes forum. Burnout may strike immediately or repeatedly, even years after diagnosis--please reach out for help.[5] Is the pleasure of eating, one of the most basic human delights, robbed from us forever?

I imagined I'd never again fit in with friends: *Hey, let's all go out for pizza, let's all go out for ice cream—aww, come on, don't be a Debbie Downer!* Our friends may feel we are judging them when we simply, quietly, take action to care for ourselves. Meanwhile we're feeling left behind, watching the rest of the world frolic past without us.

On my bad days: frustration and tears. Other days I was too exhausted for that. Some days I read everything I could find about LADA. Other weeks I binge-watched rom-coms.

At parties and potlucks I gritted my teeth, carefully keeping my back to the buffet table, and too often afterward slunk into the grocery, skulking out with forbidden carbs, glancing around the parking lot as if the dark chocolate hiding in my bag was a very dark crime.

I rarely admitted that my diagnosis left me feeling bereft, adrift, a failure, a loser, trapped, and hopeless. Since it is "bad" to be depressed, and worse to be self-pitying, and since my disease was less awful than so many other horrible things, with no lack of people excited to point that out to me, I kept these "unacceptable" feelings to myself.

IF AT FIRST YOU DON'T SUCCEED . . .

In December, eleven months after my initial diagnosis, I drove across the mountain pass once more, slept on the floor of a friend's daughter's apartment, fought rush-hour gridlock, got lost (thanks for nothing, Siri), parked randomly and illegally, and dashed out-of-breath into the office of Fabulous Doctor Five.[*]

---

[*] Yes, I'd met with a Dr. Four as well! Moving on . . .

"Yes, what Dr. Chicago said, that you are *neither* type, is technically true," said Dr. Five, "but in terms of treatments and outcomes, it can be helpful to think of LADA as having aspects of **both** types 1 and 2."

Then Fabulous Doctor Five, as if there were all the time in the world, answered every question I had. And her answers made sense. And offered hope, clarity, and direction.

No, she said, right now we can't revive beta cells that have died, so yes, *let's focus on protecting the beta cells you still have*. Yes, there probably is an insulin cliff in your future. No, there's no test to say *when* you'll hit the cliff. Yes, absolutely, there are *things to do right now to help delay the cliff and to improve immediate and long-term quality of life*.

"*Pamper the beta cells*," said Fabulous Doctor Five.

Dr. Five approached the inevitable uncertainty of medicine from the opposite direction as Drs. Hawaii and Chicago. Her approach: If there are indications something may well help the beta cells, and no risk—then why not?

I walked out of her office feeling light, like someone who's just taken off a backpack after a ten-mile climb. The Seattle rain, so soft on my cheeks, was the most beautiful rain in the world. And I didn't even have a parking ticket.

BEST OF ALL: BOMBSHELL BETA NEWS

Our beta cells, the source of all our insulin, are extraordinary. When we call on them, they can crank up insulin production fiftyfold; they can pump out a million insulin molecules per minute. Our beta cells are both powerful and fragile, more vulnerable than other cells in our pancreas.

In LADA, our cherished honeymoon (the time when we still produce some insulin) will end, and we can't know exactly when. Scientists once thought that our honeymoon ends the day our confused immune system hunts down and kills our last beta cell. But . . . is this really true?

Researchers, bless them, question the obvious, and have discovered an amazing source of hope. In both T1s and T2s (so presumably also in LADA), a few wily beta cells hide from our immune system by *dedifferentiating*. A dedifferentiated beta cell can't produce insulin, but it's still alive. Scientists now hope to revive these "sleeping beauty" beta cells. No success stories yet, but revival looks *more promising during the honeymoon* than in later stages, and more promising for those of us who were older when our symptoms began.[6]

"The presence of dormant ('hibernating') beta cells that evade immune attack . . . might lie at the heart of . . . both T1DM and T2DM," writes Dr. Bart Roep of the Beckman Research Institute. His research group favors "beta cell therapy to improve beta cell stamina and vitality and to protect these cells . . . to achieve durable remission."[7]

Some of our beta cells may be hiding from attack, especially if we're still in our honeymoon, and perhaps even years after. These sleeping beauty beta cells can't produce any insulin while asleep, but—they're not dead yet. Showing our beta cells some love might have big payoffs, both right now and to keep the door open for future possibilities.

PERSIST, EDUCATE, ADVOCATE

There are too many stories of LADAs remaining misdiagnosed for a decade or longer. If not for my wise friends, and if not for persisting and insisting on answers, today I would be bitter, burned out, and very sick.

Thankfully, the tide is starting to turn. An international panel of experts recently recommended that anyone diagnosed as T2 be tested for LADA.[8] So far this recommendation hasn't been widely adopted; we can advocate to help these scientists be heard.

Diabetic burnout is predictable. But not inevitable. Some burnout comes from bad information. We may be struggling with an inappropriate approach intended for a completely different type of diabetes.

Keep looking—your Fabulous Doctor Five is out there. You won't sink the ship of medicine by searching for her. Instead you'll be helping, because a diabetic who isn't getting good support tends to be a sick diabetic. And when we're sick diabetics, we're expensive. To ourselves and to society. That's right, this whole book is about saving money! Along with your eyesight and your brain.

Best of all: Because some of our beta cells may be alive but hiding, pampering our beta cells can have huge payoffs. Pampering our beta cells can moderate BG swings, lengthen the honeymoon, and make daily life easier . . . and might keep more sleeping beauties around for exciting future possibilities!

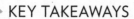 KEY TAKEAWAYS

1. Healthy people become diabetic, and we can become or remain healthy with diabetes.

2. Diabetes is a spectrum. All diabetics have a great deal in common; yet we are each unique.

3. In the different types of diabetes, different causes lead to a similar result: Blood sugar, which was once on a fairly even keel, now swings through peaks and valleys.

4. After diabetes is discovered (typically, based on A1c), LADA is diagnosed by testing for antibodies. The typical first test is a simple blood draw to measure GAD antibodies and C-peptide.

5. Most LADAs have lost (or dedifferentiated) three-quarters or more of their beta cells when diagnosed and can no longer produce as much insulin as they once did. As we go to press, beta cells cannot be replaced, regrown, or "woken up"—but this is an area of active research.

6. Finding the right doctor matters. Be prepared to advocate for yourself.

7. My LADA diagnosis felt like an enormous loss. Anger, denial, depression, and burnout are common when a person learns she has diabetes.

8. While I would have slapped someone who said so in the early days of my diagnosis—the day would come when I'd realize that, like many difficult things, LADA brought surprising hidden gifts.

o o o

Jackie, you have type 2—no, type 1—no, neither—no, both. Let me just say: It was a confusing first year. If I had stopped with my first doctor, I would have believed (been told) I was T2. If I had stopped with my first specialist I would have believed (been told) I was T1.

Instead, thanks to a bit of ~~stubbornness~~ perseverance, and a huge amount of support and encouragement, I learned *so much* (starting with the word *LADA*) that I felt ***should be much more widely known***! I felt this so strongly, I sat down and wrote a book.

5 SYMPTOMS? WHAT SYMPTOMS?

Why Diabetes Is One of Our Most Underdiagnosed Diseases

Signs that you may have LADA, instead of type 2,
include being thin, having a personal or family history of
autoimmune disease, [and] blood sugar levels that keep rising
despite a healthy lifestyle.
　　—Sari Harrar, author and journalist[1]

The only way to identify [LADA] is by antibody testing.
　　—Professor Katherine O'Neal[2]

I'D KNOWN "BETH" FOR TWO DECADES. EVERY SUMMER OUR KIDS played together along cobbly Kitsap beaches. Yet it wasn't until I was outed as diabetic myself that I learned she has diabetes.

Today, out the window behind Beth, a weathered cedar boathouse built by a great-grandfather leans over the water, its roof glowing with emerald moss and dotted year-round with chili pepper Christmas lights. Beth's tiny house, more window than wall toward Miller Bay, enfolds you in that wild world of water always in motion, always dotted with goldeneyes, harlequins, or the quick scribble of an otter.

"Sometimes I almost wish I *did* have symptoms," Beth says.

Symptoms other than her blood glucose, she must mean. She just told me that most days her fasting glucose is over two hundred, sometimes over three hundred.

It's just the two of us at breakfast. As she stares down at her plate, a small sigh escapes. Instead of her usual lively face, I see the vulnerable, in-private face of someone who has slammed into a brick wall and given up trying to get past it.

I take her hand. I nod. I completely get it.

When I was diagnosed by random luck, friends asked me, "How did you know, what were your symptoms?"

I'd shake my head, bewildered. "I didn't *have* any symptoms," I'd insist.

I never added: Well, it's true I've felt tired . . . no, not tired: weary, list-less . . . I don't feel the energy, the joy, the bright alertness, the playfulness of my twenties . . . of course that's just normal aging . . . plus life circumstance, living alone now after thirty years . . . but that's on me. I just need to take a class, join a gym, do yoga, meditate, weave baskets, volunteer with children, write a book, lead a revolution, invent a better solar battery, train in parkour and plyometrics, and then I'll feel better. Sure, I'm gonna start on all that. Next week.

What kind of idiot would I be to complain about "not feeling twenty" to a friend or a doctor?

I take another bite of this glossy-magazine-gorgeous breakfast Beth pre-pared: an egg baked in the bowl of an avocado half, sprinkled with sharp cheddar and pan-fried ham. Delicious, fun, "zero"-carb.

When Beth was diagnosed, she fully committed to her doctor's rec-ommended diet for about six months, and her health markers improved. "The doctor said if I kept it up, I could stop all my meds. It felt so great to know that I *could* do it. But then . . . I gave myself a break . . . and I just . . . never started again."

Again, I nod. Heart attack, stroke, dialysis, lions, tigers, and bears—the scary list smashes onto our life and then . . . life goes on. And on. Beth feels "fine." Fine enough, at her day job, her desk job—not the dream job she pursued in her twenties but . . . she has a family now. Maybe she doesn't have the energy of her twenties but—pish—who does?

Her diabetes, well of course it's real but . . . it just doesn't *seem* real. Her doctor's advice comes across as muted, halfhearted: Just do the best you can.

Not that Beth hasn't made *any* changes: She avoids sweets, pours a lot of mental struggle into not yielding to their tantalizing whispers. (Aunties live all around Beth's tiny home and are always bringing by something to share: spicy warm gingerbread made from garden-grown ginger, fudge stirred with a wooden spoon in a copper pan, or sea-shell-shaped sugar cookies bright with pastel sprinkles.)

Other than avoiding sweets, Beth is mostly back to eating the way her family has always enjoyed: fish, crab, and clams fresh from the bay; veggies from Grandma's fabulous garden; homemade bread from the new bread machine. Beth's nod to diabetes is to throw in an occasional Whole30 or keto meal like the one on our plates. She adds fat bombs. And skips the homemade pie from backyard berries.

How often does Beth think about diabetes, about food? Pretty much . . . always. It is right under the surface, all day, every day. The worry is like poison ivy beneath the skin, itching, itching.

"I almost wish I *did* have symptoms," she says again, quietly. "Real, in-your-face symptoms. It would be easier, then."

Outside the window, a drifting osprey suddenly plummets, bursting the water in a fountain of spray. When it lifts off, its talons drip, empty.

OR: YEAH, I HAD SYMPTOMS—I ALMOST DIED!

The first African American to win the Academy Award for Best Actress, Halle Berry was also a Miss USA contestant, and regularly on lists like *People*'s "Most Beautiful." (Yes, that's code for: She was slender as heck. *And* beautiful.) When she was in her twenties, during filming for her first big break, Berry began to feel fatigued. She passed out on the set, went into a coma, and could not be woken for seven days. This was how she learned she had diabetes.

Author Anne Rice, whose books have sold nearly one hundred million copies, awoke at age fifty-seven to a painful headache and trouble breathing. Shortly afterward she fell into a coma and nearly died. This was how she learned she had diabetes.

"If you think you have any chance that you might have diabetes, for God's sake, go get the blood sugar test," Rice told ABC News. "It's a simple test."

My friend "Charlie" had been to the doctor twice already, complaining of the flu. Just . . . I don't know, Doc . . . tired. Listless. No energy. The doctor kept sending him home—how many people get the flu in winter? Get some rest. When a diabetic friend heard Charlie's story . . . she wondered. She brought her BG meter to his house and—yikes! Charlie was in an ambulance to the hospital.

Telling me the story years later, Charlie's wife shivers. "He almost died," she whispers.

THIS "OPPOSITE" STORY IS REALLY THE SAME STORY. DIABETIC symptoms, like the infamous iceberg, are 90 percent underwater. Low-energy, listless, fog-brained . . . with America chronically exhausted, who notices that?

Way too commonly, diabetes is diagnosed not by the smoke but by a five-alarm blaze. *One in four diabetics, and over half of prediabetics, don't know they have it.*

Why does diabetes sneak up on us like this? What's going on inside?

LET'S GET HORMONAL

Insulin is a hormone. Hormones are chemical messengers.

But we've got nerves for sending messages, you may be thinking. What's the point of a whole second message system—what's the point of hormones?

Our nerves are like the phone or telegraph system of the body. Some messages demand the high-speed line direct to President Brain. Messages like: *Jump! Tiger! Ouch fire hot!*

Our body also has a very different messaging app, more like a fleet of bicycle couriers. Our bicycle couriers, aka hormones, are good for bulky, complicated, or enduring messages. They're for pizza and flowers, not four-word telegrams; for messages that don't need micro-second delivery, and need to linger.

A hormone is produced by one organ to send a signal to other organs. Your brain, gut, thyroid, pancreas, liver, and others are always chattering together on this chemical Instagram. Hardy, hopeful hormones carry messages that are more about perseverance than about instantaneous zap delivery. Hormones ignite powerful emotions and persistent cravings.

Our bicycle couriers carry messages like: *My tummy's rumbling and that's making me want to trek down to the marsh, stand ankle-deep in cold water, dig cattail roots out of the goopy mud, gather firewood, build a fire, roast those roots for a long time, then peel those roots, then pound those roots . . .*

Sadly, T1s have an immune system that keeps screaming *You're fired!* at our insulin bicycle messengers, shooting out their tires, and burning down their homes—the fabulous beta cells. There's hardly an insulin bicycle messenger to be seen on T1 streets anymore.

T2s have plenty of insulin bicycle messengers. Their streets are swarming with them. But their cells have built a gated community with armed guards and barred windows (insulin resistance), and refuse to open the door.

As for LADA: We lucky ducks get both problems at once—the barricades and the shot-out tires! While this sounds like a raw deal, the upcoming chapter will reveal why having both problems holds a hidden blessing.

INSULIN RESISTANCE—WHY?

We can all understand running out of something (our T1-ishness). But what's up with insulin resistance? Why would our wise body do that?

Too much of a good thing can be deadly. People have killed themselves by drinking too much *water*. Most medicines, at higher doses, are poisons. Many of us have taken two aspirin at some point in our lives, but I hope none of you ever contemplate swallowing the entire bottle. Even our body's basic coin-of-the-realm, blood sugar, can become damaging and then deadly at too-high amounts.

High BG can damage our cells, silt up our bloodstream, and wallop our organs. Causing oxidative stress, increasing free radicals, destroying antioxidants, and triggering dangerous chronic inflammation, high BG threatens virtually every important system in our body. Insulin resistance can develop as a protection. Our cells self-quarantine, lock their doors, put up defensive barriers.

INVISIBLE SYMPTOMS?

Insulin is a hormone, and a hormone problem can be weirdly hard to notice. It's not like hitting your thumb with a hammer; it's very compelling yet somehow non-obvious.

The best analogy I can give is being premenstrual. (Gentlemen, please roll with this. Gents are just as hormonal as women, of course, but because your hormones don't cycle, you may be less tuned in to hormonal effects.)

After we've lived in our body awhile, we notice changes happening in the days before our menses. For some women these are subtle, and for some they're loud and proud. Even the women with sledgehammer symptoms are sometimes surprised by their period. Or by a friend asking: "Is it possible you're . . . ?"

"Oh, right, of course. Duh."

Yes, these symptoms are absolutely real. *Subtle* would be the wrong word. But still they can be somehow missable, blending into the background of life.

Now that I know my body well, I know why I fell asleep at the surfing pizza party, to the enduring ridicule of my friends. When I over-carb, I may nod off or get spacy—cotton-brained, like I feel with the flu—my pee smells funny, and I sometimes get a funny-tasting dry mouth.

I didn't notice these when I had them *all the time*. (Imagine if you had your period *all the time*.) I notice my high-BG symptoms now, because most of the time I control my BG. So now these symptoms stand out.

We can think we don't have symptoms because for so long we've been on a treadmill that other people never experience. It's hard to have any idea how much better we *could* feel. How much better we *will* feel after we learn to Carb-craft, and get off this treadmill.

What is normal? Normal is what we don't notice. It's crazy, but sometimes we have to get well to notice we've been sick.

I THINK BACK TO BREAKFAST WITH BETH AND HOW MUCH I DON'T know about her situation. I don't know if we're in similar or very different places on the spectrum. Maybe Beth is classic T2 and, if she became significantly more physically active every day, might slash her health risks, feel great, and keep her BG in an excellent range while eating the normal-healthful way she's always enjoyed . . . including a small slice of that homemade pie.

If Beth is like me, there's a sad irony in her bullet-sweating diligence in avoiding one square of dark chocolate, and the next morning eating several slices of homemade bread along with her keto egg-and-avocado. Because each slice of bread contains many more carbs—therefore much more sugar—than that mouth-melting chocolate.

Beth is a smart, strong, competent person. But does she have the information and support she needs?

1. Diabetes is one of the most underdiagnosed diseases in America.
2. Its symptoms are so missable that many of us think we don't have any. Too often we're only diagnosed by a medical crisis.

o o o

For me, having normal-ish BG again is like being twenty years younger. I can't believe how much better I feel now. It would be nuts to say I feel lucky to have LADA. But . . . I really like my life now. Better than in the draggy, listless months before I was diagnosed. Huh. What's that all about?

Accepting *Esquire* magazine's "Sexiest Woman Alive" award, Halle Berry said: "I don't know exactly what it means, but being 42 and having just had a baby, I think I'll take it."[3]

Berry was asked: Did diabetes make it hard for her to achieve her dreams?

"[Diabetes] gave me strength and toughness," she told the *Daily Mail*. "Diabetes turned out to be a gift."[4]

6 CAN I CURE MY DIABETES?

*5 million people die from diabetes every year, most often
because of cardiovascular events.*
  —Dr. Charlotte Ling, Lund University
  Diabetes Centre[1]

*The risk of both micro- and macro vascular complications is at
least as high in LADA as in type 2 diabetes patients, in spite
of [LADA patients'] generally healthier metabolic profile.*
  —Dr. Sofia Carlsson, Karolinska Institutet[2]

DAPPER GRANDPA JACK, FOR WHOM I AM NAMED, WAS A RAGTIME
fancier, fingers rippling up the piano as he crooned Sinatra in a smoke-
husky voice. In my memory, he and ferret-fierce Grandma Dorothy live
in a firefly-enchanted garden of tire swings, persimmon trees, and magnolia blossoms bigger than my head dangling down like self-peeling piña-
tas. Inside the house, everywhere, is smoke: from Grandma's constantly
smoldering cigarette and Grandpa's cherrywood pipe. Smoke hangs like
fog in the kitchen where my grandma makes preserves; it chokes the air
inside cars, and drifts above the dining room's lace cloth and polished
silver. The curtains, the couch, the pillows, the towels, and both of my
grandparents reek of smoke.

Grandpa once told me a story from their courtship days: Dorothy dives
into the Missouri River, grabs the lead rope of the canoe, and as her friends
in the canoe laugh and splash her, not-quite-five-foot Dorothy swims, rope
in one hand, towing them half a mile across the Missouri to the far shore.

I HAD BEEN AT COLLEGE JUST A MONTH WHEN I OPENED THE LETTER: Doctors had removed one and a half of Grandpa's lungs. "There's nothing they can do. They've sent him home to die."

But Grandpa astounded the doctors, and all of us. He lived another decade. Jubilantly. On half a lung. That surgery was his wake-up call, a bucket of ice water straight to his face: After his surgery, he never smoked again. He lived to receive a treasured award, revel in camping adventures, and travel all across the West with his children and grandchildren.

But Grandpa's surgery wasn't an ice-bucket moment to his wife. She kept right on smoking . . . until she had a smoking-related stroke and lingered, drooling, confined, and begging to be allowed to die, for an eternity of months. We were powerless to intervene as the facility tied Dorothy's hands to the bed rails so she wouldn't keep pulling out her feeding tube.

Watching Grandpa's joy and Grandma's agony has made me a believer in buckets of ice water. When I was diagnosed with diabetes, it was my wake-up call; and if I could give you each one gift, it would be to throw a bucket of ice water into your face. The rest of this book will focus on hope and solutions, but this chapter will take an icily cold look at the risks of diabetes.

OUR RISKS

LADAs get it from both sides: both autoimmune attack and insulin resistance. So we have to worry about:

- Toxically high blood sugar; or dangerously low blood sugar.
- Too-high insulin; or too-low insulin.
- Chronic systemic inflammation.
- Ketoacidosis (very high blood sugar *combined with* very high ketones).

The risks of low blood sugar, like the risks of running out of oxygen, are scary but simple: Drop too low and you die.

Ketoacidosis is also a medical emergency, requiring immediate hospitalization. In ketoacidosis, a combination of high blood sugar and high ketones makes your blood dangerously acidic. **Ketoacidosis is different from ketosis.**

Later in this book we'll look at keto diets: a range of high-fat diets that emphasize replacing carbs with healthful fats and obtaining the majority of our food energy from fat. Keto diets involve ketosis but *not* ketoacidosis. In the Carb-craft section we'll discuss why **reputable keto diets are perfectly safe**.

> › **Ketosis:** A healthful condition where the body burns moderate amounts of ketones (derived from fat) for fuel instead of sugar.
>
> › **Ketoacidosis:** A life-threatening condition: Much higher levels of ketones, combined with very high levels of sugar, cause the blood to become acidic.
>
> › **Keto or ketogenic diet:** Replaces carbs with healthful fats. Reputable keto diets are perfectly safe.

o o o

In part 2, "Tools for Good Health with LADA," we'll talk about self-care to prevent BG lows and ketoacidosis, and we'll take a good look at inflammation: why it happens, why it matters, and tools to fight it. For now let's look at the problem that gets most of us diagnosed, too-high BG, along with a less commonly discussed problem: overachiever insulin.

HIGH INSULIN

"Not only too low, but also too high systemic insulin levels are detrimental," writes Dr. Hubert Kolb of the University of Duesseldorf's Faculty of Medicine. "The phenomenon of insulin toxicity . . . [happens because] there are additional cellular responses to elevated insulin levels which are not toned down during insulin resistance."[3]

Hang on, I said, when I first heard this: We LADAs are *running out* of insulin—so how can our insulin be too high?

"Persistently elevated" insulin might be a better way to explain this problem. When insulin levels never drop, this can disrupt important maintenance activities, especially lipid processing and protein synthesis; can interfere with the action of our kidneys; and can cause buildup of gunk on the walls of our blood vessels (atherosclerosis). The longer such damage goes on, the harder it is to reverse.[4]

In LADA, our insulin production begins to struggle to meet demand; our response falls behind the curve. Like a three-year-old chasing too many chickens, a LADA's diminished insulin can take a lot longer to deal with the normal daily surges of sugar. In other words, because our insulin couldn't get quite high enough quite fast enough, it stays elevated, still chasing those last few chickens, for a long time. So our insulin switch doesn't get thrown to "off" often enough or long enough.

Chronically elevated insulin interferes with our body's maintenance. It's like a parade that keeps going down Main Street 24/7, preventing the maintenance crew from getting in there to fix the potholes. Our body needs to take breaks from insulin. If it doesn't, we'll soon find medical frowny-faces on our cholesterol tests and lipid profiles.

Many forms of diabetes can lead to *dyslipidemia*: a fancy term meaning our cholesterol and triglycerides get out of whack. Lack of downtime from insulin can interfere with removal of triglycerides from our blood, and inhibit our liver from making healthier forms of cholesterol.[5]

CHRONIC INFLAMMATION

A vast body of scientific research shows that inflammation is "the man behind the curtain" for many diseases.

When you catch a cold or flu, *short-term* inflammation is a fabulous friend. And if a splinter infects your finger, short-term inflammation brings extra blood and healing cells to the area. But *chronic (long-term, persistent)* inflammation is a whole different beast. It wears away at your body, and after years can have devastating effects. We can think of inflammation like fire. We like it when it's contained and appropriate, in the same way we willingly build a campfire to cook our dinner, and after the last marshmallow is roasted, we pour water on the coals and put the fire out.

With chronic inflammation, our body *fails to put the fire out*, and fire begins to creep everywhere, destructively. Chronic inflammation can make everything from our gums to our bowels leak; then bacteria from both ends start partying together in our bloodstream. Chronic inflammation dysregulates our immune system, making us more vulnerable to all kinds of diseases, from coronavirus to cancer. Chronic inflammation *triggers autoimmune diseases*, such as LADA. This may be the reason people with LADA are more likely to have additional autoimmune diseases, such as Crohn's or thyroid disease.

Chronic inflammation is a huge risk factor for heart disease, dementia, kidney and liver disease, and more. As Harvard Medical School puts it: **"The four horsemen of the medical apocalypse—coronary artery disease, diabetes, cancer, and Alzheimer's—may be riding the same steed: inflammation"**[6] (my emphasis).

We'll look at inflammation in more detail in part 2, where we'll discuss tools for tamping down the flames.

HIGH BG

As we saw in chapter 5, insulin resistance is a protective response: a barrier our body puts up to try to protect us from the oxidative stress, free radicals, and chronic inflammation triggered by high BG.

When barricaded cells refuse to take BG from our blood, where will it build up? Yep, our blood. Our blood vessels and our nerves are particularly vulnerable to high BG. That's why diabetes is especially hard on our circulatory system, nerves, brain, heart, kidneys, and eyes.

This is the reason diabetes raises our risk of Alzheimer's and other dementias. It's why in the US most diabetics will die of a heart attack or stroke; it's why diabetes is the number one cause of blindness in adults over thirty, the number one cause of kidney failure, and (outside of accidents) the number one reason for foot/leg amputations.[7]

Did that feel like a bucket of ice water in your face? I did that for Grandpa Jack.

Circulatory System

Too-high insulin, too-high BG, and chronic inflammation together cause plaque buildup on the walls of our blood vessels (atherosclerosis). This increases our risk of blood clots, blocked blood vessels, heart attacks, other heart damage, and strokes.

"Atherosclerotic cardiovascular disease (ASCVD) is the commonest cause of death in the United States and western world," writes Dr. Jialal.

"It claims around 2300 lives in the United States every day . . . [in diabetes] it is the leading cause of mortality, and diabetic patients are 2–4 times more likely to die from ASCVD as compared to non-diabetic patients."[8]

Ouch. Then a second way toxically high BG attacks our circulatory system is by causing a proliferation of weak-walled blood vessels. Where there should be a few orderly circulatory "streets" reaching each "house" (cell), there's now a tangled mess of looping blind alleys whose frail walls are at high risk of breaking. When blood vessels break in the eye, this can create a permanent spot of vision loss, which typically grows over time, reducing vision and sometimes ending in blindness.

Our circulatory system feeds and cares for all our cells and organs. And our circulatory system is a key communication system, delivering hormonal messages from one organ to the others. When diabetes attacks our blood vessels, this puts *all our organs and functions* at risk—one reason diabetes's effects are so widespread and so serious.

Heart

Our heart beats 100,000 times a day; 2.5 billion times in seventy years. It's a powerful muscle, and needs more energy than any other organ. Our heart continuously pulls fuel from our blood. Fatty acids are its preferred fuel (up to 90 percent of total energy), and it burns sugar to make up the balance. Our heart is great at taking in fuel; not so great at blocking fuel out. So if our blood gets overloaded with cholesterol or sugar, these stream straight into our heart, and can cause damage. In early phases, this damage is reversible.[9]

LADAs may look fit and active on the outside, but we may have been, unawares, taking damage to our circulatory system and heart.

"Although patients with LADA are leaner and have healthier lipid and blood pressure profiles," writes Dr. Raffaella Buzzetti, "evidence shows that there is **no difference in cardiovascular outcomes** between these patients and those with type 2"[10] (my emphasis).

Nerves

Just to make it a slam dunk, high BG also targets our nerves. Nerve damage develops over time, if we repeatedly allow our BG to go high. Sixty to 70 percent of diabetics develop nerve damage (neuropathy).[11]

Diabetic nerve damage ranges from numbness, to tingling or burning, to disabling pain. Nerve death can lead to loss of function, impacting for example digestion, erectile function, the urinary tract, the heart, even weird things like how much we sweat. Fifty percent of men with diabetes develop impotency due to reduction of nerve function; and women with diabetes are more likely to suffer from vaginal dryness.[12]

Feet

Since one of the longest nerve connections is between toes and brain, communication typically breaks down here first. A common symptom of diabetes is that we lose touch with what's happening in and on our feet. *Hey, this blister is getting infected, hey, ouch, this hurts*, the feet try to yell; but thanks to diabetes you're running a roaring lawn mower while wearing noise-canceling headphones and singing at the top of your lungs. Next thing you know, someone wants to chop off your toes.

Brain

This one's kind of a biggie, right?

It's no mystery why something that attacks nerves and blood vessels would be hard on the brain. Poorly controlled diabetes raises your risk for Alzheimer's disease, vascular dementia, and other dementias. Diabetes increases your risk for mild cognitive impairment (MCI), often a precursor of dementia, and also increases the probability that MCI will progress to dementia.[13]

Have you ever thought . . . *Wow, I was really spacy this afternoon . . . that same sort of spacy as running a fever . . . like my brain just wasn't running at full speed . . . for the first time ever, I couldn't remember my cousin's daughter's boyfriend's name . . . oh well, guess I'm just getting old?* I was having more and more of those moments, never imagining their connection to my blood glucose.

Each spike in BG can give you brain fog. Repeated spikes or sustained high levels of BG can do serious, sometimes irreversible, damage to your brain. In one study, participants who modified their diet in a way that lowered glucose peaks reduced their risk of Alzheimer's by 53 percent. Other studies confirm that Alzheimer's risk can be lowered by avoiding excess calories, by regular exercise, or by maintaining a healthy weight from middle age onward[14]—all things that correlate with controlling BG.

Besides slowly and steadily fogging your brain, eroding neural connections and pushing you toward dementia, high BG can also attack your brain suddenly with a stroke. Blood vessels supply your brain with oxygen; high BG makes these vessels more likely to be blocked or to rupture. That's a stroke. Within three or four minutes without oxygen, the affected part of your brain begins to die. Diabetes raises our risk of stroke by 50 percent.[15]

Kidneys

Elevated BGs make the kidneys work double and triple shifts to pull that "sweet pee" (diabetes mellitus) out and flush it away. Many diabetics can, by the smell of our pee, tell we've allowed our BG to go high. (If that was TMI, beware of asparagus.)

Like a radiator, your kidneys are mainly circulatory systems. Tangles of weak-walled blood vessels don't mix well with working your kidneys overtime. A third of diabetics develop kidney damage (nephropathy) over time.[16]

Liver

Our liver wears two hats. First, it's our Secret Service, leaping on toxic hand grenades (such as five straight shots of tequila), absorbing and defusing them. Second, pencil behind its ear, our liver is our personal Federal Reserve, aiming to keep BG levels in the healthy range, so our cells always have plenty to eat, but are protected from toxically high BG.

In a kid's cartoon our liver would be a friendly treasury-factory-wastedump-postoffice-ninja. Monitoring messages (hormones) from all over our body, the liver keeps the economy flowing, and stores and disassembles toxins. It sequesters excess BG, and releases BG when hormonal messages (like a low level of insulin) inform the liver that the BG economy needs a little boost.

High BG, high insulin, and inflammation increase triglycerides and other fat molecules in our blood. When the liver jumps on these hand grenades and stores them, fat accumulates in our liver. This can progress to disease (NAFLD, nonalcoholic fatty liver disease) and ultimately liver failure. About 70 percent of T2s, and an unknown number of LADAs, have NAFLD. In some this will progress to cirrhosis.[17]

Cancer

Diabetes increases our risk of cancers, including kidney cancer, stomach cancer, liver cancer, oral cancer, breast cancer, leukemia, and more. A recent review of forty-seven scientific studies from across the globe, combining data from almost twenty million people, estimated that diabetes raises our risk of cancer 19 to 27 percent.[18]

NON-NEGOTIABLE

Ouch. That's a lot. Now I'm a blind, brainless, cancer-riddled zombie with no toes, simultaneously dying of liver failure, kidney failure, and a heart attack? Diabetes may lack the panache of "cool" diseases, but it can still pack a punch.

I'm not trying to squash all the hope out of your soul. I'm laying out why **self-care matters** so deeply.

ALL THIS BRINGS US BACK TO . . . THE A1C

It's not so much the one slice of homemade birthday cake yesterday, but the *long-term picture of our BG* across months and years—that's what's behind these scary health effects. That's why doctors focus on our A1c.

Glycosylated hemoglobin A1c (A1c for short) looks at our red blood cells, and how much sugar is stuck to them.* This can be translated into our average BG over the past three months, since a red blood cell typically lives for three months.

We can be diagnosed with diabetes based either on our peak BG or on our A1c.

---

* Throughout this book, I use mg/dL for BG, the standard units in the US. To convert to mmol/L, standard in much of the rest of the world, divide by 18.

DO I HAVE DIABETES?

Peak BG diagnosis: If our BG ever goes above two hundred, we have diabetes.

A1c-based diagnosis: We're put into one of three groups, based on our A1c:

> - A1c of 5.6 or below: *non-diabetic.* A non-diabetic's BG may be rock-steady, or may wander between 80 and 120, with average and fasting BG typically 100 or less. (Fasting BG is our BG taken first thing upon waking for the day, before breakfast.)
> - A1c 5.7–6.4: *prediabetic* (stage one diabetic). BG two hours after a meal may exceed 140 or even 190.
> - A1c 6.5 and above: *diabetic.* BGs may vary extremely.

o　o　o

A1C GOAL

If we've been diagnosed with diabetes, what is our A1c goal?

Wouldn't it be lovely if all authorities agreed on that point?! Some say keep it below 7, some say below 6.5, some say below 6, some say below 5.5, and some say, "It depends."

Diabetes goals are often relaxed for the elderly, or others near their end of life, for two reasons: First, because diabetes complications build over time, and second because for these folks, medication interactions and other treatment complications can be more severe.

7 or below is the goal recommended by the ADA (American Diabetes Association) for all diabetics. Supporters of this goal point to studies like ACCORD, where attempting to lower BG through "aggressive" prescription of multiple medications led to a higher rate of death in older patients with cardiac disease.[19]

6.5 or below usually, but it depends, say the AACE (American Association of Clinical Endocrinologists), ACE (American College of Endocrinology), and many doctors. They recommend that the majority of diabetics aim for this goal, while the goal can be laxer (let A1c be higher) in specific cases: for children, for people with limited life expectancy, or for those with multiple chronic conditions. And they advocate even stricter (lower A1c) goals in particular situations, especially pregnancy.

Below 6 (the 5 percent club). The 5 percent club is an informal group of diabetics who support one another in achieving and maintaining A1cs under 6 percent. A quarter of diabetics meet this goal today.[20]

Even lower? Some studies show increased risk to blood vessels, nerves, and eyes when A1c goes above 5.5.[21]

Different targets are right for different people, different places along the diabetic spectrum. For a person in their last years of life who may be juggling multiple medical issues, piling on meds may not be the right choice, since diabetic health risks depend on the picture of our BG *across months and years*. But as a "young antique," I'm all about achieving my best health: Thanks for the inspiration, Grandpa Jack.

JOINING THE 5 PERCENT CLUB

There are innumerable stories of diabetics bringing their A1c down from 13 to 5-point-something in a matter of months.[22] For any type of diabetes, joining the 5 percent club can be a great goal, helping protect us from that shopping list of horrors. A quarter of diagnosed diabetics are in this club today.

On the other hand, as my yoga teacher reminds stiff-as-a-wilted-carrot me: "Start from where you are." Pick an A1c goal that feels right to you. *Any size reduction in A1c can help your health*: One encouraging study found that each 1 percent reduction in A1c lowered health risks by 21 percent.[23]

WHY SOME DOCS CALL A1C "IMPORTANT BUT INCOMPLETE"

The A1c tells us our average BG, which is a great start. But two people with the same average could have completely different situations, one healthy, one unhealthy.[24] One could have BGs rolling along in a healthy zone, and the other could have BGs careening from dangerously high to dangerously low: These two different scenarios could have the same *average* value.

The A1c, writes Dr. Irl Hirsch of the University of Washington's School of Medicine, "has major limitations and even in the best of circumstances provides only a simplified snapshot of glycemic control. The

[A1c] is **important but incomplete**"[25] (my emphasis). It does not capture *glycemic variability*: the height, depth, and frequency of our sugar *peaks and valleys*.

That's why many focus on *time in range*: on how much of the time our BG stays within a safe range. If we wear a CGM (continuous glucose monitor), we can observe exactly how much of the time BG stays in a healthy range and what specific events drive it high or low. (More on CGMs and other cool diabetic gear in part 2.) There is also a test called GlycoMark that shows how often in the last two weeks BG went above 180.

For people whose red blood cells have a common shape variant—for example, a malaria-protective less round shape more common in people of African descent—the A1c maybe need to be calibrated differently.[26]

The A1c is just an index we all tend to use, but we could just as easily talk about our average BG over the past three months. Like inches versus centimeters, average BG and A1c are different measuring sticks for the same thing. Table 1 shows how A1c translates to average BG and vice versa.

TABLE 1. A1C and Average BG

A1c	4.9 and below									
average BG	94 and below									
A1c	5.0	5.1	5.2	5.3	5.4	5.5	5.6	5.7	5.8	5.9
average BG	97	100	103	105	108	111	114	117	120	123
A1c	6.0	6.1	6.2	6.3	6.4	6.5	6.6	6.7	6.8	6.9
average BG	125	128	131	134	137	140	143	146	148	151
A1c	7.0	7.1	7.2	7.3	7.4	7.5	7.6	7.7	7.8	7.9
average BG	154	157	160	163	166	169	171	174	177	180
A1c	8.0	8.1	8.2	8.3	8.4	8.5	8.6	8.7	8.8	8.9
average BG	183	186	189	192	194	197	200	203	206	209
A1c	9.0	9.1	9.2	9.3	9.4	9.5	9.6	9.7	9.8	9.9
average BG	212	214	217	220	223	226	229	232	235	237
A1c	10.0	10.1	10.2	10.3	10.4	10.5	10.6	10.7	10.8	10.9
average BG	240	243	246	249	252	255	258	260	263	266
A1c	11.0 and above									
average BG	269 and above									

Another way to convert between A1c and average BG is with an online calculator such as the one on the ADA's website (diabetes.org).

THE ACCELERATOR HYPOTHESIS: A MENTAL GAME CHANGER

The accelerator hypothesis—that *insulin resistance accelerates all forms of diabetes, but its relative importance depends on the degree of auto-immunity*[27]—was a mental game changer for me.

For LADA, the accelerator hypothesis would mean: Our insulin resistance determines where on our journey of losing insulin we will hit trouble. If we have more insulin resistance, we'll hit trouble earlier, before our beta cells have taken as much damage. Thus for LADA, insulin resistance becomes an early warning system. As Dr. Ramachandra Naik explains: "Insulin resistance will determine **at what point in the autoimmune process** LADA will become manifest"[28] (my emphasis).

This really turned my thinking around. I'd been feeling sorry for myself for having both the T1 and the T2 problem. But this points out a surprising silver lining: Warned by insulin resistance about the cliff in our future, we can take earlier, more effective action to delay or prevent that cliff; we can start pampering our beta cells earlier, while they're healthier and there are more of them. And since some MIA beta cells are not truly dead, just sleeping (*dedifferentiated*; see chapter 4), the earlier we take action to pamper our beta cells, the better.

"Beta cell dedifferentiation is reversible before the disease progresses to a certain degree. It has been shown that **modulating blood glucose to normal levels can lead to the reversal of beta cell dedifferentiation**" (my emphasis), writes endocrinologist Qiong Wei.[29] With an early and strong start, pulling our BG back into the healthy zone could revive beta cells and perhaps even increase our insulin production.

We've long known that insulin resistance can be rolled back through lifestyle changes—enjoying healthy foods and activity—the subject of the next section of the book. Now it appears that LADAs may be able to impact the T1-ish side of our equation as well!—especially if we start early and hit it hard.

DO LADAS HAVE THE BEST OF BOTH WORLDS, OR THE WORST?

On the glass-half-empty side: Compared with T1 and T2 we have rampant misdiagnosis, less research, and lingering medical confusion about best treatments.

On the glass-half-full: Compared with T1 we have a kinder genetic load (next chapter), later onset, and slower progression. Many of us have resistance on top of autoimmunity, which we could view as adding insult to injury—or as an *early warning system*.

Having fragile beta cells *as well as* insulin resistance means we get alerted to our insulin resistance earlier, before our internal "streets" have become as clogged.

Having resistance on top of the autoimmune attack means our blood sugars get funked up *earlier*, while we still have more and livelier beta cells.

The earlier we get (correctly!) diagnosed, the sooner we can begin pampering our beta cells.

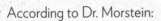

According to Dr. Morstein:

"In conventional care, diabetes is a relentlessly progressive disease invariably causing complications that worsen over the years and then lead to an early death. However, that is not how it has to be!

"If they have not progressed too far, all these degenerations of the body can be reversed. I've seen neuropathy heal and limb numbness return to full feeling; kidneys improve; eyes stabilize, and even improvements in retinopathy; and fatty liver inflammation resolve . . .

"It must be reemphasized that complications should never occur in the first place. Only people with *uncontrolled* diabetes develop these problems . . .

"No diabetic patient willing to follow a comprehensive integrative treatment protocol ever has to develop complications."[30]

o o o

I used to fear diabetes was an inevitable losing battle, ending in either: (a) a slow, hungry death, covered with sores and amputations, or (b) sudden heart attack or stroke. What a relief to hear from medical experts that this is not true. Diabetes is a condition like hearing loss, which people live with either happily or grumpily, depending on our attitude. If LADA is caught early, and addressed head-on with a positive attitude, we can thrive. In the early days of my diagnosis, I couldn't wrap my mind around the term *healthy diabetic*. And now I am healthy with diabetes, and have many friends who are healthy with diabetes. (Some had already been my friends—I'd been completely unaware of their diabetes.)

As one friend says: "*Well-controlled* diabetes is the leading cause of . . . nothing."

LADA IS FOR LIFE

If we've been diagnosed with LADA, it's likely we will always have greater sensitivity to carbohydrates than many other people. LADA will remain part of our journey, even if we eliminate or reverse all symptoms and meds. Although LADA is for life, many risks can be avoided, symptoms eliminated, and damage reversed. What we can accomplish depends on where we are on the spectrum (which mountain we're standing on), how hard we work at it, and whether we have the information and support we need.

HEALTHY WITH LADA

1. We can lower our A1c into the zone of a prediabetic, or even a non-diabetic.
2. We can combat insulin resistance through healthy lifestyle changes. Many can reduce or eliminate medications for insulin resistance.
3. Pampering our beta cells may extend their life, and perhaps even wake a few sleeping beauties.

o o o

REALISTIC LADA GOALS

- *We can **lower** A1C into a healthy range.*
- *We can **lower** risks of cancer, dementia, liver failure, and other complications.*
- *We can **lower** cholesterol and improve lipid panels.*
- *We can **eliminate** many scary symptoms* including depression, loss of feeling in the feet, rampant tooth decay, gum disease, and spiraling damage to major organs.
- *We can **eliminate** nagging daily tribulations* like exhaustion, listlessness, brain fog, a frequent urge to pee, thirst, and dry mouth.
- *We can **reverse** many types of damage,* repairing damaged nerves, proliferating weak veins, and more.
- *We can **reverse** the insulin resistance* of cells throughout our body, repairing and mitigating at a cellular level.
- *We can **shelter** our beta cells,* and perhaps even rebuild beta cells and insulin production, even if we can't halt the immune attack.

o o o

KEY TAKEAWAYS

1. Uncontrolled diabetes is deadly and scary. Too-high insulin, too-high BG, and chronic inflammation together can damage virtually every part of our body.
2. The A1c is a great start but doesn't give the complete picture. We need to know more than our average BG; we need to know our BG highs and lows, both of which can be dangerous.
3. I used to pout about having diabetes from both directions: insulin resistance on top of disappearing insulin. Now I realize: Having it from both directions gives me an early warning system, and twice as many tools for health.
4. Diabetes is for life, but good/bad health is optional. We can have the same health markers as a non-diabetic if: we are diagnosed early; have the support, information, and access we need; and play all the cards in our hand.

o o o

7 IS THIS MY FAULT?

Why Me? What The @#!$ Happened?

Diabetes is a multifactorial disease, caused by a complex
interplay between environmental and genetic risk factors.
—Dr. Mette Andersen, University of Copenhagen[1]

THE DOCTOR IN THE TED TALK LOOKS LIKE HE'D FEEL AT HOME
pumping iron with the guys, or sipping high tea with the queen, or in an
underwear ad. Or, apparently, in a surgery theater, lopping out a chunk of
your colon. And he seems to be on the verge of tears, his voice thick with
emotion.

"Why did I hold her in such bitter contempt?" he asks us, or himself.
"Why did I feel justified in judging her?"

Because, he confesses, the woman he encountered at 2:00 a.m. in the
ER was heavy—obese. He was the surgical resident asked to decide if the
rotting diabetic ulcer on her foot required an amputation. It did.

Seven years later, surprised to find himself wrestling with insulin resistance, Dr. Attia's thinking shifted.

"I wish I could speak with that woman again." Dr. Attia takes a deep
breath, eyes downcast. "I'd like to tell her how sorry I am. I'd say—you
know, as a doctor, I delivered the best clinical care I could. But as a human
being I let you down. You didn't need my judgment and my contempt.
You needed my empathy and compassion . . . If you're watching this now,
I hope you can forgive me."[2]

IT'S TEN MINUTES AFTER MY DIAGNOSIS. TEN MINUTES SINCE I GOT word of my A1c in Dr. Alaska's office. Now I'm wobbling down the sidewalk toward the pharmacy, stunned, clutching a prescription for a glucose meter.

In my small town ringed by mountains, the pharmacy is tucked into a row of Front Street shops where you can buy everything from hiking boots and sunglasses to handcrafted Earl Grey ganache chocolates. But I only half-see the shops and the people walking by. In a cartoon, tweetie-birds and stars would be wheeling around my head and there would be little *x*'s in my eyes.

I—almost literally—bump into an acquaintance.

"How are you today?" she says.

I hesitate. I weigh *Fine, you?* against the truth. Slowly, dazedly, I begin to honestly tell her.

I haven't gotten out more than a few sentences before she snaps: "Well, at least you don't have cancer."

Her words land like the "two" of a one-two punch. My mouth stops making sounds. What can I say? She's not wrong.

I AM A LUCKY, PRIVILEGED PERSON WHO HAS LIVED A LONG LUCKY life. "All" I face is never again enjoying food (or so I believe). I'm not facing chemo, radiation, wig-shopping, brain surgery. I know she's not wrong. I am completely silenced.

Cancer? My God, I'm so sorry. Tell me what's going on.

Diabetes? Dang, dum-dum, maybe you should have thought about that before you pounded down so many doughnuts.

WE'RE RIGHT UP THERE WITH VIAGRA PEDDLERS AND ANCIENT BRITish kings—it's completely socially acceptable to mock diabetics.

I sit down to relax with late-night comedy. Behind the comedian, a screen shows a picture of a chef recently in the news . . . he appears obese. "His superpower is having *all* the diabetes," the comedian jeers.

I flip on a sitcom: Our (overweight) hero is being interrogated by a busybody matchmaker.

"Girlfriend?"

"Um, no."

"Herpes?"

"No."

"Diabetes?"

"Not yet."

Diabetes don't get no respect, as Rodney Dangerfield would remind us if he wasn't under a tombstone that says: THERE GOES THE NEIGHBORHOOD.

But only diabetics are hurt by jokes like these. And we probably just need a good kick in the pants. Since our disease is own fault. Thanks, comedian Michelle, you're helping me turn my life around. I bet you're really good at fat-shaming, too—if the comedy gig doesn't work out, you can always be a diet coach.

One way to ridicule something is to misrepresent or misunderstand it, whether through irony or ignorance. Ignorance sure helps. After you score the fun laugh, we're all left standing in the residue of ignorance: false, hurtful ideas, left unchallenged, propagating.

"WHY ARE YOU SO HESITANT TO TELL PEOPLE YOU HAVE DIABETES?" Ava berates me as we walk a mountain trail. Butter-yellow avalanche lilies punch through the thinning snow to catch the late-slanting sunshine. Ava recently dealt with a serious misdiagnosis—medicated for anxiety when in fact she had a mineral deficiency—and the way she discovered the true cause was through crowdsourcing, talking about her situation with anyone and everyone.

Excuse me? I manage *not* to snap back. *When was the last time you saw a nationally televised comedian ridicule magnesium deficiency?*

I manage not to say that because, like the acquaintance on the pharmacy sidewalk, Ava is right.

I should make noise, speak up, advocate for myself. I should own who I am. Hmm, what might it mean that so many people keep telling me this?

GENETICS LOADS THE GUN AND ENVIRONMENT PULLS THE TRIGGER

But *why*? Why did this happen to *me*? I know, the Dalai Lama wouldn't ask. Still, who can help wondering?

"Genetics loads the gun, environment pulls the trigger," explains the cheerful, glowingly pregnant physician assistant leading my diabetes class.

The answer to nature versus nurture is usually: You're both right. Genetics prints out a dot-to-dot, and environment decides how to connect it. The way the two add together is unique for each of us.

Environment includes so many things. It includes things you can't help, like where you were born; what your mother ate, drank, smoked, or vaped while you were in the womb; and infections you got as a baby. And it includes things you choose: fried chicken, carne asada, or tandoori; boogie-board, body-surf, or couch-surf.

GENETICS LOADS THE GUN

All forms of diabetes are strongly genetic. If two people eat, exercise, and behave exactly the same way, but have different genes, one will develop diabetes, and one will not.

While all types of diabetes are genetic, lifestyle choices play a bigger role in the onset of T2 than of T1 and LADA.

Many of the triggers for T1 happen before age two.[3]

But T2 triggers are predominantly lifelong lifestyle choices. Three-quarters of T2 cases could be prevented through physical activity, healthful food, and healthy body weight.[4]

LADA, per usual, falls between T1 and T2. All LADAs have autoimmunity, but we vary in amount of insulin resistance. LADAs can be sorted into genetic subtypes that align with how our LADA looks and acts.[5]

A decade ago, researchers questioned whether LADA was truly its own disease or "just" a mixture of T1 and T2. Now that researchers have described genes unique to LADA, we're acknowledged as having our very own disease.[6] Awesome. "The genetic signature of LADA is independent and [LADA] should not be considered a hybrid form of T1DM and T2DM," writes Dr. Petr Heneberg.[7]

Many T1 genes are in the HLA (human leukocyte antigen) region, which helps *regulate the immune system*. (Oh. Immune system. Autoimmune disease. I get it.) LADAs share many T1 HLA genes, but typically in a lighter load.[8]

LADA's genetic overlap with T2 is smaller and more variable.[9]

Family history studies align with genetic data. Having a family history of T1 raises our risk of LADA sixfold; and having a family history of T2 raises our risk of LADA twofold.[10]

GENETIC OVERVIEW

T1 is caused by relatively few genes that occur in relatively few people. For those with a known risk of T1 (for example, family history), genetic testing is valuable for early identification.

T2 has more than two hundred genetic loci,[11] each with a real but small effect. T2 doesn't have a simple genetic fingerprint, and genetics alone is only 20 percent of T2 risk,[12] so genetic testing is not very helpful for T2 diagnosis.[13]

LADA overlaps a great deal genetically with T1, a bit with T2, and has some genes all its own. As with T1, both genetic testing and antibody testing can help LADA be diagnosed earlier; and *earlier is better*.

- LADAs share with T1: many genes in the HLA region; PTPN22, INS, and SH2B3.[14]
- LADAs share with T2: TCF7L2.[15]
- LADA-specific: PFKFB3, and subtype-specific signatures in the HLA region.[16]

o o o

EPIGENETICS: OUR ANCESTORS' *ENVIRONMENT* AFFECTS OUR HEALTH

Epigenetics is the study, not of which genes I received, but of how the expression of those genes—the way they turn on and off—has been changed by things my parents or grandparents lived through.

If our predecessors starved *or* overate, this raises our risk of diabetes (all types). If our parents or grandparents, men or women, experienced famine, malnourishment, or obesity, our risk of diabetes rises. The womb environment affects us as well: If a mother is malnourished, overweight, or diabetic while a child is in the womb, the child's risk of diabetes increases.[17]

The epigenetics of diabetes is a relatively new field, which many hope may someday lead to new treatments for diabetes.[18]

... AND ENVIRONMENT PULLS THE TRIGGER

Risk factors being studied for *all types* of diabetes include:[19]

- Toxins in our air, soil, water, and food, including PCPs,* phthalates, organochlorine pesticides, and other POPs.†
- Ultra-processed foods and sweetened beverages.
- Chronic inflammation.
- Body weight / amount of abdominal fat.
- Lack of exercise.
- Health of the mother during pregnancy.
- Early childhood infections.
- The microbiome: tiny helpers, such as bacteria, naturally within the digestive system.
- Leaky gut.
- Deficiency of vitamin D and other nutrients.
- Hormone imbalances.
- Allergens.
- Hepatitis C.
- Lack of sleep / sleep apnea.
- Stress, anxiety, and depression.

A T1's environmental risk usually happens very early. T1 antibodies may peak before age two, says Dr. Marian Rewers, and 70 percent of children with antibodies before age two progress to diabetes over the next ten years.[20] T1 risk has been linked to diet, childhood illnesses, weight gain,

---

* By PCP I mean the pesticide pentachlorophenol, *not* the recreational drug phencyclidine, often called angel dust.

† POPs are persistent organic pollutants: common pesticides and herbicides used on farms or inside and outside our homes. These include PFCs (perfluorinated compounds), phenols, PDBEs (polybrominated diphenyl ethers), polycyclic aromatic hydrocarbons, perchlorate, and other compounds research has linked to diabetes risk.

psychological stress, and the womb environment. For most T1s, these risks happened when they were too young to take preventive action.[21]

Not so for T2. In T2, as in T1, genetics hands out loaded dice. But for T2 a much bigger part of the odds, about 80 percent, come down to lifestyle. The biggest risk factor for T2 is being overweight (increases risk sevenfold). The risk of T2 can be reduced by reducing ultra-processed carbohydrates (Wonder Bread), processed meat (hot dogs, lunch meat), and sugar-sweetened beverages (soda); by increasing whole grains and vegetables; and by not smoking. Physical activity is a very powerful factor in preventing or rolling back T2.[22]

And LADAs—you guessed it—are in between. LADAs are so variable that knowing what's true for the "average" LADA may not tell us much about our own situation.[23] Still, *every LADA has tools* to pamper our beta cells, slow our disease, improve our energy level and mood, and prolong our honeymoon. We'll dive into these tools in the next chapter.

CONNECTED RISKS

Many people with one autoimmune disease are more prone to other autoimmune diseases. Having LADA (or T1) means you are more at risk for Graves' disease, Hashimoto's thyroiditis, Addison's disease, and other autoimmune diseases.[24] These are beyond the scope of this book; this is something to discuss with your doctor.

IS IGNORANCE BLISS?

"Half of Americans Have Diabetes or a High Risk for It—and Many of Them Are Unaware," says a 2017 *LA Times* headline.[25] Until I joined this fun secret club myself, its reality was invisible to me. I interacted with diabetics every day, never knowing they had diabetes, especially if they didn't fit my stereotypes about body shape.

And now people do to me what I once (mentally) did to others. "You don't *look* diabetic," way too many people have said to me. (Referring to my hair color, obviously.) In *Your Diabetes Questions Answered*, author Jenny Ruhl wryly notes that some of her relatives refuse to believe she has diabetes—because she's happy and healthy, and stays active and fit.[26]

Diabetes strikes people who eat wrong, I once ignorantly thought . . . along with: *Diabetes means you never get to eat sweets again.* (Thank goodness that one's wrong!) I once thought: *Because diabetics weren't good boys and girls, Life took away their dessert.* My ignorance was comforting and comfortable. Like platform shoes, it made me feel just a little bit elevated. I wanted to believe diabetics had made poor choices because I wanted to feel safe. I wanted to believe someone who has gained weight is weak-willed because I wanted to feel safe. My ignorance did not make me safe. It made me an asshole in platform shoes. Headed for a fall. I poke fun, here and there, at things friends and strangers have said to me—but none have been more ignorant than myself.

Ouch. Karma can kinda sting.

I CRIED BECAUSE I HAD NO SHOES UNTIL I MET . . .

Driving near Coupeville last week, I flipped on the radio and heard the voice of a teenager, who at age fourteen went through a terrible illness and lost all ability to eat food. Any food or drink taken orally could kill her now. All her nourishment, for the rest of her life, would have to come through a feeding tube. For the rest of her life, not one bite of a crisp fall apple. Not one swallow of cool lemonade on a hot day. She will never enjoy an intimate dinner with a prom date. Never plan her wedding cake. On Thanksgiving, her family no longer shares a big traditional meal: They go to the movies together.

"How has this changed your life?" asked the interviewer.

What a stupid question! Stupid interviewer! I thought.

But it was the right question. Because I would never have imagined the girl's reply.

She really considered the question, in a brief silence, rare on the radio. I signaled, and turned off the highway onto a tree-lined street.

"Well . . . before," said the girl on the radio, "my life was all about soccer. I loved soccer so much. It was all I did. Now . . ."

Around my car, cottonwood fluff flurried, and wild roses and fragrant iris wafted perfume over a long saltwater view. The Port Townsend ferry sounded a plaintive alto call.

"I created a chat space and a blog so teens like me all over the world could support each other, could talk about our experiences . . . Sometimes moms and dads of non-verbal kids write to me to tell me how much it means to them to hear what this experience is like. Every day, people thank me for sharing my story and for letting them share theirs . . ."

I drove past hopeful strawberry beds, aspiring peas beginning to twine up a trellis, and new basil, small but sturdy. The ferry moved slowly out from shore.

" . . . I wasn't doing anything like that before, back when I was just playing soccer all the time. Now I'm really helping people. Now my life, and what I do, really matters."

YOUR FAULT OR YOUR FATE?

America's trend toward abundant, cheap, subsidized, brightly colored, highly advertised, non-nutritious crapola foods is not unconnected from diabetes. Genetics deals out radically different susceptibilities to diabetes and to weight gain; and when we also consider the links of weight gain to poverty, food insecurity, lack of food sovereignty, sexual abuse, emotional abuse, and many other "environments" not of a person's choosing, we see that having a weight that interferes with our health may be on a spectrum toward addiction issues and systemic inequities.

Rates of diabetes vary in different parts of the world, between different ethnicities, and by socioeconomic status. Most of these differences appear linked to poverty, privilege, and status: especially exposure to pollution, and access to healthy food and water.[27] These connections raise diabetes to a social justice issue, as we'll address in the final section of this book.

Nothing can change society's stereotypes except countering the tired jokes with authentic stories. Like the stories of diabetic Olympic gold medalist Gary Hall Jr.; of Supreme Court Justice Sonia Sotomayor; or of Will Cross, the first diabetic to summit Everest, who now gives inspirational speeches (between his extreme climbing adventures), asking audiences: "What's your Everest?"

ONCE UPON A TIME, I USED TO THINK DIABETES WAS LIKE A FIVE-dollar haircut the day after Oktoberfest—something sad-sack people brought on themselves. Ignorant and condescending, I washed along in the mainstream attitude toward diabetes. Doctor Attia, I feel you. Comedian Michelle, I can't point my finger at you—I've done worse.

I couldn't journey into true health until I shifted away from defensiveness, resentment, and self-blame. And I couldn't do that overnight. Like many of us, I fell into the depression that often comes with this diagnosis.

I hope you give yourself time and permission to grieve. And then, when you're ready to be healthy, commit to the difficult process of letting your anger go. There can be a gift of humility and deep connection with others brought about by this life-changing disease, if you choose to let that happen.

No, it's not your fault. It's your fate. It's your peculiar and particular baggage to carry down the road of life. The people around you who don't have diabetes are unlikely to fully understand—and many aren't going to try very hard. If carrying this burden gives insight into the burdens of others, burdens you may have been a little glib about in the past, wonderful.

Beyond that . . . I had to just stop worrying about what others thought. No, they don't get it. You know what? They're going to get something else.

KEY TAKEAWAYS

1. LADA is not your fault. In all types of diabetes, genetics loads the gun and environment pulls the trigger.
2. As recently as a decade ago, some questioned whether LADA was "just" a mix of T1 and T2. Now genetic studies confirm we are our very own disease.
3. LADA has a big overlap with T1 genes, a smaller overlap with T2, and a few genes all our own.
4. A shopping list of environmental risks, some of which we can control, gives us hints for staying our healthiest. All LADAs have tools to improve health—as the next set of chapters will lay out.

o o o

PART I | SUMMARY

1. Half of Americans have diabetes or a high risk of it—and many are unaware. Diabetes is one of the most underdiagnosed diseases in America. Its symptoms, while of enormous consequence, often feel invisible.
2. Three related definitions of diabetes: We struggle with insulin; we struggle to process carbohydrates; we struggle to control our blood sugar.
3. Diabetes feels daunting: it can double our risk of clinical depression.
4. LADAs are often misdiagnosed as T2. Yet we have the opposite underlying cause. Some T2 medications harm us. We must advocate for ourselves.
5. Simple blood work (for antibodies) shows whether we're LADA.
6. LADAs are the largest group of autoimmune diabetics, and the most diverse.
7. Genetics loads the gun and environment pulls the trigger. Typically we have eaten and behaved just like millions of non-diabetics—they began with different genetics.
8. The 5 percent club is a great goal with any type of diabetes. No matter how high your A1c today, *you can* join this club. While this is *my* favorite goal, choose the goal that's right for you.
9. For LADA, insulin resistance might be an early warning system, determining where on our autoimmune journey we hit trouble. It's hard to say if having resistance *on top of* autoimmunity is good or bad . . . but it may help us take action while we have more and healthier beta cells.
10. It's likely that some of your MIA beta cells are not dead, just hiding—dedifferentiated. Keep pampering your beta cells, both the working and the hiding.

Now that it was broken, I began to appreciate that I'd once had a flawless autopilot system keeping my BG safe. With autopilot no longer an option, I'd now have to "drive" my blood sugar consciously, all day, every day.

I'd learned that all LADAs expect an insulin cliff in our future, and some of us may have the power to delay that cliff. If the cliff comes quickly, well, that's how my genetic dice rolled: no shame, no blame. But while my dice are still rolling, with a little luck, and a lot of pampering, I'll try to keep my precious honeymoon going for extra months, years, or perhaps even decades . . . right now, no one really knows the limits.

I was discovering that LADA is not a sound-bite disease; there's no simple fix, no magic pill. But it turns out there's a whole toolshed full of valuable tools. I was over my dumb-bunny shock now, and excited for hands-on how-tos: *Exactly how* do I pamper my beta cells? And how do I reduce my insulin resistance?

Part 2 lays out the tools that can get us through the door of the 5 percent club, explains our diabetic superpower, and delves into these *exactly how* questions. We're about to plunge into (pinch your nose!) the garden in our gut and the biochemistry of our food—the underpinnings of Carb-craft.

In LADA, as in a card game—to win we want to play all the cards in our hand.

PART II

TOOLS FOR GOOD HEALTH WITH LADA

8 OUR DIABETIC SUPERPOWER

Becoming the Expert on Ourselves

We all need to create our own maps and guidebooks.[1]
  —Camille Dungy

*The simple act of paying attention can take you
a long way.*
  —Keanu Reeves

A HANDSOME DIABETES BOOK CAME HOME WITH ME ONE NIGHT. IF
you've browsed diabetes books, you know the type. On the cover, the
doctor-author in his crisp white lab coat and neatly tucked blue-and-red
tie: his head tilted, his smile sincere, sympathetic, and Sears-catalog-level-
of-hotness. You've read similar cover blurbs: "one of the most responsible
and authoritative voices in American medicine today" and "three times
more effective than other diet plans."

But when I tried what he offered, then tested my blood sugar, ouch!

My mistake, I'd think. Wondering what I did wrong, I'd test again
and—strike two!

With a charming smile, this book kept coaxing me in the wrong direction. Still I kept loving it—its promises were so simple and so exactly what
I wanted to hear. I clung to it. I let it gaslight me, again and again. Finally,
though, I started spending time with other books, with different-colored
ties and very different advice. And then I began to hate that first book.

An official postcard from the library knocked on my door, scolding:
Return that book. I set the postcard on my kitchen counter. Dust drifted
across it. Bits of dried rosemary arranged themselves into flowers sprouting

between stray dog cookies. When I glanced at that counter, I frowned. Which would weigh heavier on my conscience? Returning this dastardly, manipulative book, which then might deceive and betray someone else? Or "stealing" from the library . . . that's a crime against humanity, right?

Silly Jackie. I don't know why it took so long before the lightbulb clicked on (and the book returned safely to his Dewey decimal home). Possibly this is a fine book *for a T2*. I wouldn't know. It was a terrible book for me . . . but I'm LADA.

Dozens of books, websites, and classes claim to be about diabetes, plain and simple. But too often they're actually for T2 and never confess it. ***Diet advice for T2 is often inadequate or unhelpful for LADA*** and other autoimmune diabetes.

MY LADA DIAGNOSIS DROPPED ME INTO WHAT FELT LIKE A TSUNAMI of misinformation. So many books were as bad as that first one, but with a differently striped tie—different advice, same spirit-breaking disappointment. Three things muddy these waters. The first is how often "experts" believe type 2 advice will help a LADA, when in fact it's like bringing a grapefruit spoon to a knife fight. If, like most LADAs, you've lost three-quarters or more of your beta cells by the time you're diagnosed, switching to whole wheat bread won't stop your BG spikes. Standard food rules for T2s (limit pasta to a quarter of your plate; eat lots of beans and oatmeal; snack on fruit) send my BG right through the roof.

Second, research on LADA has lagged behind T1 and T2 research. "There is a shortage of randomized clinical trials in LADA and the optimal treatment regimen is still unknown," Dr. Sofia Carlsson of Karolinska Institutet wrote in 2019.[2]

The third problem? We live in a time of diet culture wars.

Because I'm a nerd, I'd come home from the library with armloads of books about "healthy food" or "being healthy with diabetes" (as if there were only one type). Pick a topic, any topic, say the question of fat: While knowledgeable experts agree that adding healthy fats can help us manage blood sugars, you can find a noisy handful calling this "pathological." Similarly, while true experts agree that eating low-carb helps diabetes, you can find medical authors with national followings writing, "Say no to low-carb diets."

As a beginner this made me crazy. How could I know who to trust?

 For a LADA, food advice for T2 is like bringing a grapefruit
spoon to a knife fight.

o o o

OATMEAL? BEANS AND GREENS?

Every diabetes cookbook I flipped through showcased berry-studded oatmeal. Yet every online LADA forum I visited heaped scorn on oatmeal, oat
groats, or any variation. "I don't think any hot-grain breakfast is good for
any diabetic," one wrote, summing up the feelings of the group.

Dr. Barnard's book on diabetes puts "old-fashioned oatmeal" at the
top of his list of recommended foods.[3] But Dr. Morstein's book echoes the
LADAs: "Foods that do not necessarily contain refined sugar but are very
high in carbohydrates (a bowl of oatmeal, for example) will break down
into glucose that will overwhelm your system, too."[4]

One book, highly recommended by my local clinic's dietitian, prom-
ised I could "cure" my diabetes by eating beans and greens. But my blood
meter kept telling me a different story.

Every single time I ate beans, say a half serving of a favorite brand
of vegetarian chili, my blood glucose went way too high. This happened
repeatedly: with black beans, garbanzos, hummus, pinto beans, refried
beans, lentils . . . dang, if *lentils* aren't healthy for me . . . *what can I eat?*
What's going on?

In the next session of diabetes class, the instructor told us how wonderful beans are for diabetes, and passed out a handout of recommended
foods, featuring beans at the very top.

I raised my hand and described my experience—that beans sent my
BG soaring.

The T2s sitting around me looked blank. But one student—a misdiagnosed LADA, I already suspected from other remarks—leaned forward,
eyes bright, nodding vigorously.

"Why?" I asked.

"I don't know." The instructor's forehead crinkled. "That's strange.
Beans are a great food for a diabetic. Maybe you should test again."

BECOME THE EXPERT ON YOURSELF

One reason experts can disagree is that diet research can get distorted by hidden patterns. People who eat more tempeh might also buy more jogger-strollers and bus passes. People who eat more beef may buy more king-cab pickups and garden gnomes. People who have ashtrays in their homes might be more likely to develop lung cancer than people without ashtrays—but that doesn't mean banning ashtrays will lower cancer rates. With a human diet study, it's very difficult to separate cause-and-effect from accidental association.

And while many scientists and nutritionists truly want to understand food science and support human health, not every single human is equally pure at heart. Purse strings are sometimes in the hands of opinion makers with an economic interest in stirring the pot, perhaps to create confusion, hype a personal agenda, or sell a product. In *Your Diabetes Questions Answered*,[5] Jenny Ruhl dishes dirt, uncovering some of the shenanigans behind "Dr. ____'s Diet."

When comedian Michelle mocked, "His superpower is having *all* the diabetes," those words planted like a seed in my mind, and blossomed in the middle of the night. She's right. My diabetes does give me a superpower.

Thanks to our superpower, when food experts contradict each another, we don't have to try to guess who's right. We can test for ourselves how their plan impacts our blood sugar. *We only have to learn what's right for one body: our own.*

BG IS A ROLLING WAVE

If we draw a graph of our BG across time during a day, we'll typically see it rise and fall. We may see a bump up after a meal, or a dip with exercise.

The difference between a diabetic and a non-diabetic is not whether our BG has waves; many people's do. The difference is that with diabetes our waves now go very high and sometimes very low. Very high and very low BGs have big health risks (chapter 6), so we set a goal to keep BG mostly within a safe range ("time in range").

The *size* of a BG wave reveals if a meal or other impact swamped our system and our insulin couldn't keep up. By size of the wave, I'm referring to the area under the curve.

The *spikiness* of the wave—whether it is a sharp peak or a long smooth swell—indicates fast or slow. A sharp spike shows we ate a fast carb like fresh cherries from the farmers market or sweet London Fog tea. A longer, flatter wave indicates a slower carb like whole wheat pizza or kung pao quinoa.

We've talked about carb speed using the analogy of trains: Fast carbs (simple carbs) are like short trains our body can take apart quickly, while complex carbs are like long, triple-linked trains which our bodies need more time to decouple (digest).

Cherries versus pizza might give you the same size wave (same area under the curve). Size is determined by the *number* of cherries, or the number of slices. Shape is determined by food *type*. Together, the combination of size and shape determines whether and for how long BG rises above the safe zone, into dangerous territory.

FAST (SIMPLE) CARBS (SUGAR, HONEY, COOKIES, FRUIT JUICE) RAISE our BG quickly, spiking high and fast. Slower complex carbs make the BG wave roll up slowly, then stay up at that broader peak longer (oat groats, brown rice, whole wheat bread).

Which are better, fast carbs or slow? The answer's not as simple as you'd think.

Imagine all your BGs for a day plotted out on a graph: a line rolling up and down. Imagine choosing a BG that you don't want your BG to go above, and drawing a line straight across the graph at this height: Call this your danger line. Now imagine coloring in red every part of your BG picture that's under your rolling BG line and above your danger line. In other words, coloring red all your excursions above your target BG.

Two aspects of high BG matter: the height of our highest peaks, and the total real estate we colored red. Think of a car overheating. A *quick high* temperature spike causes one type of damage. Other types of damage depend on *how much time* the car spent in the red.

A fast carb may spike you higher than a slow carb would. A slow carb may *keep* your BG elevated for a long time, giving you more time overall in the red.

WINDOWS INTO HEALTH: GLUCOMETER AND CGM

Today's technology lets us peer inside ourselves, and see what's happening in our blood, any time we choose. This is recent, revolutionary, slightly miraculous—and one reason that today so many with LADA are healthy.

A **glucometer** (blood sugar tester) is half the size of a cell phone, can talk to you in six languages, costs as little as twenty bucks (the real cost is the test strips at a buck a pop), and is available to anyone over the counter; for those diagnosed with diabetes who have insurance, a glucometer, and at least one strip per day, should always be covered. A LADA should be allowed more strips, at least four per day; if your doctor isn't aware of this, press the issue.

We have many fewer nerve endings *on the sides of our fingers* than on the pads: when I prick my finger to get a blood sample, I poke the side of the tip of my finger, and try to vary the exact spot, and to vary the finger.

o o o

CGM stands for continuous glucose monitor. The CGM is like taking your little handheld glucometer and attaching it to your body, so it can automatically take a reading every five minutes. With a CGM, you don't need to poke your finger and squeeze out blood—hooray! A CGM shows the full picture of your BG, giving *context*: Instead of one lone number, you see the full picture, all day long; you know whether BG is rising or falling and how fast, and can forecast where your BG is heading and whether to adjust.

There are different brands, and like most people I'm convinced that *my* brand is the best. The best CGMs store a month or more of data and offer easy download of summaries and reports to your phone, computer, or doctor's office. They have customizable alarms to warn of highs and lows and can also notify distant caregivers. Studies show that using a CGM typically lowers our A1c, no matter what type of diabetes we have.[6] A CGM is expensive, and most cannot afford one unless it's covered by insurance; this may require a doctor who can be a good advocate.

Expect your CGM reading to lag about twenty minutes behind your finger poke, because it monitors the BG level in tissue beneath the skin, and BG in this tissue lags behind the BG level in your blood. I missed this memo when I first got my CGM, and worried mine was inaccurate, especially when my blood sugar was rising or falling rapidly. Once I understood the time lag, the numbers made sense and tracked beautifully.

I love my CGM.

For me, not-testing BG is like driving with my eyes closed. And a handful of finger pokes a day feels like, while driving, opening my eyes a few times a day—certainly better than driving blind! My glucometer kept me on the road to health for many months. But it can't compare to the view I have now: With my CGM, I get to see the entire road.

This was not how I felt when I first heard about CGMs. My initial reaction was a combination of *ick* and *ouch*. I was weirded out by the thought of "wearing a machine." Today that sounds as silly as being weirded out by carrying a cell phone in my pocket. I forget my CGM is there—I pat myself down to remember which side it's on today.

Mine is the size of four quarters: so slim, it's hidden by my clothes. I've worn it spluttering through white water clutching an upside-down raft, and in other adventurous settings, and it's come through just fine.

THIS ISN'T ABOUT STRAIGHT A'S AND BUNNY STICKERS

Whether we're using a CGM or glucometer, watching how foods, activities, stress, and so on impact our BG is the way we become the expert on ourselves.

We test-test-test to answer our questions. Questions like: Oatmeal? Beans and greens? Each meal is an experiment, and sometimes we're going to get surprising results: *Oh, I can't eat a whole apple at lunch now, I didn't know that. Oh, cottage cheese is a very fast carb, who knew?* While we're discovering what works and what doesn't, sometimes we land it and sometimes we don't. As my ski-instructor friends say: "If you're not falling, you're not learning."

A single BG reading is never a reason to say *Yay, I'm cured*—and it's never a reason to throw ourselves under the bus, either. The *pattern of many BGs over time* builds the road map to get us where we want to go.

HEALTHY–ER, HEALTHFUL–FOOD

I need to eat really healthy now, I thought. Then three strawberries sent my BG high. Hummus dipped on carrots sent my BG high. A small bowl of vegetable soup sent my BG high. I hadn't yet absorbed that *for me, now, healthy is different than when I had a normal amount of insulin.*

I'd grown up supposing we could draw a line, write HEALTHY on one side and UNHEALTHY on the other, and push any food item to one side or the other. Surprise! I discovered that **there isn't one universal "healthy" when it comes to food.**

But we can each find meals and foods that—for us—protect and promote our health.

MY IMMIGRANT GRANDMA INGFRIED LEARNED ENGLISH THE MOST fun way: put a twelve-year-old in with kindergartners and let them laugh at her while she tries to puzzle her way through app-leh pee-eh. So it's no surprise that adjectives could deeply irk imperious Ingfried. "Healthful food," she'd insist. "Not healthy, healthful."

This from someone who ate pickled herring. Still, fair point. If I were eating a herring, or any fish, I'd be happy for it to be alive and healthy before I ate it, but not during.

Big picture, we absolutely can sort out healthful from unhealthful food. Recent research shows that one of the best predictors of health is simply: the percentage of your meals that are home-cooked. Start there, and then add Michael Pollan's rule of thumb: If you "shop the edge" of the grocery and bring home items that look like themselves—whole vegetables, fruit, nuts, and the like, items our great-grandmothers would recognize, as opposed to shelf-stable things in colorful boxes—**you are 90 percent of the way to healthful**.*

In that last 10 percent, our individual differences really begin to matter. I'm not allergic to eggs, so when my neighbor offers me eggs from the happy hens who wander her garden by day and roost under her porch at night, I think: healthful food! But for my allergic friend, eggs are not healthful, even though the rest of his family eats and enjoys eggs.

There is no universally healthful diet for every human on Earth. Within the last 10 percent, I do my best to tune out the bickering, incorporate the good ideas, and focus on *what works for me.*

"A variety of dietary approaches is acceptable for [diabetes] and prediabetes," writes Dr. Andrea Bolla of the IRCCS Diabetes Research Institute, adding "a higher focus should be placed on the **quality and sources**" of our foods[7] (my emphasis).

DIABETES IS AN ELEPHANT

The tale of the elephant described by blind men originated around 1000 BCE—in the Indian subcontinent, unsurprisingly—and is found in Buddhist, Hindu, Jainist, Sufi, and Baha'i lore. Each blind man touches the elephant and then tells the others what an elephant is like. One says snake, one says wall, the next tree, then fan, then rope—depending on whether the man has touched the elephant's trunk, torso, leg, ear, or tail. Each man, knowing his own experience to be true, wonders why the other men are lying.[†]

Diabetes is an elephant. Some have ahold of the elephant's tail, others have ahold of the trunk, and a steaming pile more have ahold of something else elephant-related. Many are good people saying true things (sometimes about a trunk, while using the word *elephant*).

When I grasped the elephant dilemma, I understood why I'd heard so many conflicting "facts" about diabetes, and such contradictory advice:

---

* Pollan's *Food Rules* is a great compact guide, while his *Omnivore's Dilemma* gets deeper into whats and whys.

† A companion tale declares that when seven blind elephants want to know what a man is like, the first elephant touches a man and says: "Men are flat." All the other elephants agree.

Many who say, "This is good for diabetes," really mean *for T2*, but rarely bother to say so—or worse, are arrogantly assuming that what works for T2 must work for all.

I was beginning to see that while I did have things in common with T2 and could learn from it, I also had important differences. I began to mentally add *in some cases* to all the advice I heard, even advice declared as thunderously as if it were carved on a stone tablet.

SHOULD WE TRUST THE AMERICAN DIABETES ASSOCIATION (ADA)?

And how can that even be a question, right?

Many, many researchers, doctors, diabetes educators, books, TED Talks, and online forums insist that the number of carbs per day recommended on the ADA website is way too high. Dr. Morstein, a measured, careful researcher and documenter, writes: "The ADA's recommendation is terrible and even dangerous."[8]

The number of carbs the ADA recommends *per meal* is *higher* than the amount my little blood meter repeatedly and consistently tells me I can eat *per day* and keep my BG in a healthy range.

Of course 80 percent of diabetics are T2, so the ADA's advice may be adequate for 80 percent of their public, and they may feel that's good enough. Also, organizations tend to be cautious, and to wait until new information has fully suffused through the mainstream. Many say that while the ADA is making progress, its recommendations are a decade or more out of date.[9] If we have LADA today, those are decades that you and I can't afford to wait.

No problem because: We have a superpower. We can look inside out blood, any moment of the day, and see what's up.

KEY TAKEAWAYS

1. There is no single universal healthful food plan.
2. For a LADA, most T2 diet advice doesn't go far enough, or is just plain wrong.

3. With LADA, we don't have to take diet preachers on faith.
   We can test food claims for ourselves.
4. We only have to learn what's right for one body: our own.

○ ○ ○

For me, the hardest part of LADA wasn't finding advice—it was learning which huge steaming pile within the advice to ignore. Which I could never have done without my superpower.

What really causes trouble "is not what we don't know—it's what we know for sure that just ain't so." As Mark Twain famously either did or did not say—no one knows!

BIG PICTURE

BIG PICTURE 2.
WHO CAN AFFORD DIABETES?

No one can afford diabetes . . .

. . . and the less we can afford it, the more likely we are to have it.

In the US, average medical costs with diabetes are thousands of dollars a year: double the costs for a person without diabetes. Also, in the US, diabetes tracks income: The less wealth in our bracket, the more diabetes, and the worse our health with diabetes. Poverty makes diabetes more likely and more deadly, and diabetes makes poverty even more challenging and full of risk. This is especially true for T2, and also true for T1 and LADA.[1]

People without health insurance, people without housing, people with food insecurity, people who don't have a primary provider (regular doctor), and others who struggle monetarily have higher rates of diabetes, have worse health with diabetes and worse outcomes, and are more likely to die. *Every year in the US, children die from cost-related lack of insulin.*[2]

We'll talk more about all this, in a solutions-oriented way, in chapter 24. For now, as I get ready to sling a bunch of advice at you about foods, vitamins, medical equipment, and more, I want to take a moment to acknowledge that some of us will struggle much more than others to afford these things.

9 ROAD MAP, NOT REPORT CARD

Letting Blood Sugars Be a Friendly Guide

Test, test, test!
   —Jenny Ruhl[1]

THE FIRST DAY I WALKED INTO MY DIABETES CLASS, I BLINKED IN surprise: There sat one of my son's elementary teachers, a warm, fun, energetic woman. I always loved dropping my son off at her classroom: desks often shoved against the walls so the kids could play alphabet hopscotch or stretch out on the floor drawing cooperative crayon murals on long rolls of paper. Diabetic? I would never have guessed.

This day, in a roomful of diabetics and doctors, the teacher raised a hesitant hand. "My daughter keeps telling me about protein and, uh, probiotics," she said. "So I was going to make a Reuben sandwich for dinner. But I'm not sure . . . should I use one piece of bread or two?"

The class leader turned to the dietitian.

The dietitian's eyes got wide. "Well, I . . . I don't know," she said. "That sounds like a lovely sandwich, though."

The elementary teacher lowered her hand. The next week, when class began, she wasn't there. She never came back.

If I had a different superpower, time travel, I'd go back in time and say to her: "My dear K___, the dietitian can't answer your question because she doesn't have your superpower. But there *is* an answer to that question. You are the one with the power to answer it. Try that Reuben sandwich with one piece of bread. Try it with two pieces of bread. Try it with a half piece of bread. Try it without bread, as a salad or lettuce wrap. Experiment. Test-test-test."

Naturally the diabetes instructors couldn't answer K___'s question. That question was like Dorothy asking the Wizard of Oz how tightly she should cinch her ruby slippers: which hole on the strap to stick the little metal thingy through. A question that specific, Dorothy can answer better than anyone. Experts can offer the big picture, but only you—and your superpower—can determine what size piece of bread to eat Tuesday night.

FASTING BG: OVEREMPHASIZED, AND TOO OFTEN A "REPORT CARD"

Fasting BG is our BG taken upon waking for the day, before breakfast. There's nothing magical about it; it's just slightly more constant from day to day than a BG taken at any other time of day. Doctors focus on it because they are looking for an index—a report card.

In diabetes class, a retired rancher raises his hand to confess that he and his wife had a bowl of ice cream the previous night. "And this morning, my fasting BG was the same as ever!" he says, arms crossed, exasperated.

As I look around the room, heads are nodding; you can feel the frustration in the room. Why give up ice cream if it doesn't change our health? No one explains to these students that fasting BG is a bit like the average monthly temperature outside: an index that gives a big-picture overview but doesn't show each and every peak and valley.

With LADA, fasting BG is not enough information. We need to know about the peaks and valleys of our BG.

If I improve my exercise and eating for several weeks, my fasting BG may go a little lower (healthier) . . . or it may not . . . and it tells nothing about how my BG bounces around during the rest of the day.

My fasting BG is highly influenced by my personal pattern of morning hormones, as well as by what I ate yesterday, how I slept, what time I woke up today, what I ate last week and the week before, the worries weighing on my mind, how much insulin my cells still make, how much I exercised recently, whether I have a morning caffeine habit . . . all kinds of things.

A once-a-day BG measurement gives us a report card. And that's **helpful to our doctor**: a grade that says whether we're doing okay or whether the doctor should intervene. What **we as patients** want is completely different. We want timely specific guidance as we move through each day.

o o o

I might be wondering: What should I eat for lunch today? Perhaps I used to just open a can of soup, zap it in the office microwave, and get back to work—but now that I have LADA, what will this can of "healthy organic" soup do to my blood sugar? Or in the grocery store: Are these "insoluble fiber" tortillas going to affect my BG differently than regular tortillas? Should I buy them?

Thankfully many doctors understand that *frequent BG testing helps the recently diagnosed or anyone trying to link their eating patterns to their BG patterns.* When we are on a learning curve, frequent testing (or a CGM) helps us keep BG in a safe zone.

My first doctor believed that my insurance would only pay for one glucometer test strip a day. My second doctor understood that because LADA is autoimmune, insurance would pay for several strips a day. Dismissive Dr. Chicago scolded me for "testing too often" (more than once a day). Luckily I knew enough by then to ignore this ridiculous statement. When I added insulin to my self-care, Fabulous Dr. Five worked with my insurance company to qualify me for a CGM (continuous glucose monitor), which for me was life changing.

If your doctor is old-school, be prepared to advocate for yourself.

WHEN SHOULD WE TEST BG?

Whenever we have a question.

If we're wondering—*One piece of bread or two?*—we can test and find out. If we're wondering about pizza, we can test before and after eating pizza, on several days. If we're wondering how to adjust insulin and food on a fifteen-mile-run day, we test before, during, and after the run.

While I was relearning how to eat—how to eat as a LADA—I often checked my BG before and after a meal, during exercise, upon waking, or at bedtime. Times we may want to check include:

- Before each meal and two hours after.
- Before driving.
- Before and after exercise.
- Before going to sleep.
- Upon waking.
- Periodically, in the middle of the night.

Of course we can't do all of those every day—that would be too many finger pokes! Good thing we have ten fingers. Frequent testing can make BG control easier—but don't do it so often you make yourself nuts. Pick your most urgent question, and start there.

EXACTLY WHEN AFTER A MEAL SHOULD WE TEST?

The most common answer is: two hours after the beginning of a meal. This may or may not catch your highest peak, but it's a standard interval, which helps your doctor make sense of it.

The timing of the BG peak after a meal is affected by how fast the carbs are and by how much fat is in the meal. **Fat can slow and spread out the curve.** Tomato soup made with a splash of cream will have a slower, lower, longer peak than water-based tomato soup. A glass of juice or a piece of fruit will peak earlier than cheesy whole-grain pizza (which is both slower-carb and higher-fat).

For some meals (fruit smoothie), BG may be higher at one hour after the meal than at two. However, when all the carbs are starch (oatmeal, brown rice), the peak may be highest at two hours. And occasionally I've had a meal peak even later than two hours after the meal. When I made my burrito from a "carb-balance insoluble-fiber" tortilla, I found my BG peaked at three hours after the meal—and just as high, interestingly, as it peaked at two hours with a normal flour tortilla. High-fat desserts like ice cream also give me a very delayed peak.

Bottom line: Testing two hours after the beginning of a meal is a good starting point. Later, you may choose to fine-tune timing to answer *your particular question.*

WRITE IT DOWN

The best way to discover the patterns is to track your results in a journal.

"It's a fact: people who keep written records have better glucose control than those who don't," writes diabetes educator Gary Scheiner.[2]

A good BG journal notes meals, exercise, stress, and other things you think are relevant. I put different types of BG in different columns, so I can quickly scan for patterns (one column for fasting BG, one for post-meal BG, one for BG during exercise, et cetera). Your food journal might be an index card in your wallet, a mini journal in your glucometer pouch, or an app or list on your phone. (Is there another new free diabetes app every day, or what?) You can keep your journal simple, or tailor it toward specific questions.

In recent journals, I write down the date, time, my BG reading, and a comment: quick and easy. But in my early months I spent a lot more time on my food journal. Back then I had so many questions and so much to learn. My food journal was *how* I learned.

TIME IN RANGE

In chapter 8, we talked about making a picture or graph of our BG, and drawing a straight line across it: our danger line. Our goal would be to prevent (or minimize) our BG going above this line. But where should we draw that line? Where's the cutoff between healthy BG and too-high BG?

That's a genuinely complicated question, a bit like asking: How much sunshine gives you a sunburn? How much whiskey makes you drunk? How much K-Pop makes you dress like NCT Dream?

The answer—"It depends"—is not a cop-out, but a recognition that different LADAs are in different places on the spectrum, standing on different mountains. Just as with target A1c (chapter 6), different people will make different choices for valid reasons.

A person correctly diagnosed early who is feeling healthy and ambitious may set a strong goal such as keeping BG mostly under 140 or 120. A person who took significant damage before they found the information and support to achieve good health might set an iterative goal: at first, working to stay mostly under 200; and when feeling practiced and successful there, aiming for mostly under 180; and so on.

Here are things to consider when choosing *your* time in range (TIR) goal:

180. When your blood sugar spends significant time above 180, you are damaging your body. This number represents a renal threshold, changing the behavior of your kidneys. If you're over 180 a lot, your doctor will likely suggest an intervention.

150 or 160. Above 150 many experience mind fog, dullness, sleepiness, thirst, or frequent need to pee.

140. Staying under 140 is our ticket into the 5 percent club. Some research suggests that damage to the veins, nerves, and eyes begins above 140.[3] Today I keep my BG rolling along 95 percent of the time between 70 and 140.

120. In non-diabetics, BG typically rolls along between 80 and 120. Some advocates insist this should be the goal for everyone with diabetes.[4] This was the goal I set when I was first diagnosed, and I did achieve it, through diet and exercise alone. But it's worth noting that to do so I was obsessing about food so much I made myself and those around me slightly bananas. More important, back then I had more and stronger beta cells. It's the rare *autoimmune* diabetic who can stay in this zone consistently and forever, but while you can—congratulations!

Time in Range Includes Staying Above Dangerous Lows

We need to be careful not to focus so much on bringing down BG peaks that we increase dangerous BG lows. Now that I supplement insulin, I've sometimes congratulated myself on perfectly guessing how much insulin to inject, based on a stellar upper limit to my after-meal wave . . . only to find myself crashing into a scary hole three or four hours after the meal. When we're using insulin, there's an art to getting BG to settle, I've found, which includes not chasing it too hard. It's more like catching a butterfly than like clubbing a velociraptor to death.

Glycemic Awareness?

We may feel BG changes strongly, or we may not feel any different at 250 than at 100. Early in my diagnosis, back when my BG rose and fell more slowly, I felt high BGs very strongly: BGs over 150 used to give me brain fog or make me doze off in the middle of a lively party. Today my BG zips around like a firefly, and it's impossible for me to guess my numbers without testing.

Evolving Goals

Many LADAs are fit, healthy people. When first diagnosed, we may set a strong goal, work hard to meet it, and feel deservedly proud. Then time, like a little mouse, keeps nibbling away at our pancreas. Our beta cells weaken, then wink out.

It's sadly common for a LADA to blame herself for beginning to "fail" at her BG goal. If she's still misdiagnosed as T2, her doctor may unintentionally pile on extra guilt, asking why she's not able to maintain past successes. Months or years along, a LADA may be making Herculean efforts to achieve the unattainable.

WHY DOES 2 + 2 SOME DAYS = 6?

"Why," diabetic Gary Scheiner wondered in the early days of his diagnosis, "can the same type of bagel from the same shop make my glucose go very high one day but not the next?"[5] Such puzzles led Gary to become a CDE (certified diabetic educator) and to write the excellent book for insulin users *Think Like a Pancreas*.

Forecasting how a food or event will impact our BG isn't rocket science, but it's not third-grade flash cards either. When I began, I naively expected I could check once or twice what my common foods did to my BG, and from then on, simply add them up. I thought: *It's just arithmetic, right?*

I expected: BG-before-meal + bagel + orange juice = BG-after-meal.

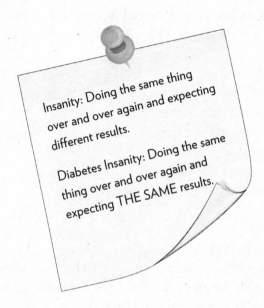

Insanity: Doing the same thing over and over again and expecting different results.

Diabetes Insanity: Doing the same thing over and over again and expecting THE SAME results.

But no. Meal spacing, stress, sleep, vitamin C, lag effects, shadow effects—a lot of things besides that one bagel are always pushing on the sugar waves now rolling through our blood.

Vitamin C. Our glucometer can misread vitamin C as blood sugar. When we eat a food that's high in vitamin C, the meter may display a number higher than our true BG.

Dawn effect. We wake up perky—or at least with enough energy to feel our way to the coffee grinder—because of circadian rhythm. Each morning wake-up hormones zing through our blood: cortisol and growth hormone increase and *insulin decreases,* giving us more blood sugar and more pep.

Somogyi effect. The Somogyi effect can occur in the middle of the night (or during another long pause from eating) if BG drops very low, prompting our liver to dump a big slug of BG into our blood. When we wake up, this big slug will still be cruising around. The Somogyi effect can be confused with the dawn effect; to know if it's Somogyi, you'd test BG after the liver dump but before you normally wake up—for example, 3:00 a.m.

Grab bag. Many things can raise our BG as much or more than a meal, including fever, prednisone/steroids, stress, sleep deprivation, and more.

Our BG can vary with:

> + Sleep quality/quantity.
> + Dawn hormones.
> + Vitamin C.
> + Prednisone and other steroids.
> + Fever / catching a cold / similar illness.
> + Exercise.
> + Stress.
> + Meal spacing.
> + The health of our liver, gut, and body-fat-as-an-organ (all closely intertwined, as we'll explore in upcoming chapters).
> + Lag effects from preceding days.

o o o

There are many reasons your favorite bagel may have a different effect on your BG on Friday than on Tuesday. This doesn't mean give up. It means: **Repetition is the key**. When you've tested your favorite bagel *several times*, you'll have a better understanding of what it typically does to your BG.

Your favorite bagel is not a yes/no question. It's a how-much, how-often, and with-which-other-foods question. Maybe for you it works well to eat a half bagel as long as you skip any fruit or fruit juice. Maybe your body handles a half bagel better at lunch than at breakfast.

Eating well when we're low-insulin is about trade-offs, not prohibitions.

OUR WACKY LIVER

Our liver is so smart. There's just one problem: Sometimes it's too smart for its own good.

As we saw in chapter 6, our liver is amazing: a Federal Reserve ninja warrior. Our liver bankrolls us, tossing stockpiled sugar into our blood when we're sprinting away from a saber-toothed tiger, or when a toxic friend telephones. Thanks, liver. And thanks, pancreas, for pumping out insulin to meet that big sugar surge. Er . . . pancreas? Hello? Hello?

Later we eat a tyrannosaur with fries, and sugar from this meal starts pouring into our blood. Our pancreas wants to release a slug of insulin to match the slug of sugar from the meal. These big slugs of sugar, and matching big slugs of insulin, are called *bolus* BG and *bolus* insulin.

During the downtimes between boluses—between tiger, telephone, and *T. rex*—our liver has us on a constant glucose drip, because it's critical that we never run out of BG: If we did, we'd die. This glucose drip is called *baseline (or basal)* BG. Our pancreas wants to match the liver and constantly drip *baseline insulin* into our blood so our cells can take up the baseline BG.

I was surprised to learn that baseline BG and baseline insulin *make up about half* of our daily BG and insulin.

THIS ALL USED TO WORK PERFECTLY. ON AUTOPILOT.

Now with LADA, most of our insulin-making cells are dead. We're insanely understaffed. The pancreas works like gangbusters to keep up but . . . picture a three-year-old chasing too many chickens.

When an insulin-normal person gets a stressful phone call, they get a spike in BG; as they calm down afterward, abundant effective insulin sweeps the BG from their blood and gets them back to normal. When we LADAs get a stressful phone call, even after we've calmed down afterward, our inadequate insulin is still running after those BG molecules like that three-year-old chasing chickens. Our BG and our insulin can stay high for a long time, much longer than they should, after stress or other surges, and this can damage our body (chapter 6).

I APPRECIATE THAT MY LIVER IS A BRILLIANT FEDERAL RESERVE NINJA warrior. And yet. Perhaps every hero has an Achilles' heel. Our liver has a blind spot. It outsmarts itself.

The liver is packed with stored sugar, mostly in the form of glycogen. It's hard for the liver to monitor sugar in the blood when it's got a lot of sugar around getting packaged or unpackaged. So, genius idea: To know how much sugar is in the blood, the liver measures how much insulin is in the blood! These will always match perfectly, right?

Er . . . unless we have diabetes.

When the liver doesn't see much insulin, it gives us more basal sugar. Now that I'm LADA, and have *chronically low* insulin . . . that's a problem. My liver will keep thinking I need *more* BG, and even further overload my already overloaded pancreas.

Even scarier: Have you ever wondered why, once we inject insulin, our liver may just lounge on its stockpile of sugar and not come to our rescue while we are literally dying from lack of sugar? Because the liver *reads insulin* to see if you need sugar. If you injected a bit more insulin than you needed, and so have plenty of insulin cruising in your system, the liver concludes that you are fine. Sometimes that's a really, really big problem.

Diabetes means: We have to consciously get involved. No more autopilot.

> Our first tool for health is to recognize that our BG autopilot is gone, and begin to drive our BG manually, with our eyes open. This simply means paying attention: what's our BG getting up to, when, and why.

o o o

SAME BASIC APPROACH ONCE WE START USING INSULIN

The majority of LADAs will ultimately need to supplement insulin, should we live long enough. With insulin, we'll use this same BG-mapping approach to gauge our success making *insulin-dosing decisions*. We'll track the picture of our BG, aim for good time in range, and watch for and make note of things that sharply peak or plummet BG. And if you thought it was tricky enough to track the simultaneous effects of dawn effect, sleep quality, exercise, fevers, foods, and more—yep, now add on top of that your changeable insulin doses.

For me, it was a gift to have gotten at ease with this process before beginning insulin. But that's not a luxury we all have—more on this in the insulin chapter.

We can set a cycle spinning either toward, or away from, health. ***Avoiding high BGs pampers our beta cells, and pampered beta cells make it easier to avoid high BG.*** Pampered beta cells means more ability to generate insulin when we need it; a more helpful, less confused liver; a longer honeymoon; and more latitude to eat a wider range of foods and still stay in our safe BG zone.

o o o

FEELING HESITANT TO SLIP ON THOSE RUBY SLIPPERS

People are funny. We'll spout the old "Don't give us a fish, teach us to fish" chestnut, then add: "And could you just cut to the chase? Give me a list of things to eat." Many would rather be given a rule, no matter how silly—Eat only yellow foods! Never eat foods beginning with Q!—than be handed the ability to find the answer themselves.

IN MY DIABETES CLASS, EACH SESSION BEGINS WITH A ROUND-ROBIN: We go around the room announcing our morning fasting BG. (Fun!) We're all obedient, except one woman. I glance down the row to where she sits, already checked out, staring at the floor. Every class, this woman says the same thing: She hasn't tested her BG, and she never plans to. Each time, the psychologist, the nutritionist, and the rest of the instructors try to gently encourage her: Knowledge is power. Every class, she shakes her head and glares at the floor, lips clamped tight. She won't do it, and she won't say why.

My heart goes out to her. I have struggled with emotional eating; feeling judged or like I've failed can push me into self-harm. Even while self-harming, I know what I'm doing doesn't "make sense" . . . we may self-harm when overwhelmed by emotional pain.

For too many of us, the BG meter hurts not only our finger, but also our heart. I still wince when I see a BG number I don't like. My BG numbers can seem to scold me when I am trying so very hard.

Driving blind, never looking at your instrument panel, never testing your blood—that's bad. But squeezing your eyes shut and stomping the gas pedal to the floor, knowing your car is pointed at a cliff, is worse. And this is what emotional eating, triggered by feeling shame or "failure" over a BG reading, might prompt some of us to do.

It's sadly common to be taught to view our BG numbers as a shaming report card when what we want is a road map. Perhaps that strong, quiet woman in class was resolutely saying no to being shamed.

When I start to feel scolded by my BG measurements, I remind myself of something a dear friend says: "No failure, only feedback." (Thanks, Susan.) I focus on big-picture patterns, not one disappointing reading. I'm gathering the information I need to build my road map.

Whether our BG meter feels like a dreaded report card filled with *Fail, fail, fail!* or like Siri's calm alto, "At the next intersection, turn right," is entirely up to each of us.

KEY TAKEAWAYS

1. A report card doesn't help us navigate our day. Test your BG to answer questions and create a road map.
2. Be ready for a grab bag of things—dawn, fever, stress, prednisone, and more—to affect BG.
3. Don't be surprised when 2 + 2 = 6; test each food several times; look at the big picture.
4. Total carbs make the size, while carb speed makes the shape, of an after-meal BG wave. Slower carbs and more fat delay, flatten, and lengthen the wave.
5. When taking a blood sample for a glucometer, prick the side of the tip of your finger.

You're in Charge

6. LADA is a very DIY disease. Doctors can support us with the big picture, but we have to fill in the details and become the expert on ourselves.
7. When you're learning, take notes. Create a system that fits *your* life and answers *your* biggest questions.

8. A CGM shows the whole picture of your BG. If you have the opportunity to use a CGM, choose one that collects data automatically, 24/7. An up-to-date doctor should support every LADA getting a CGM, but some of us will need to advocate for ourselves.
9. Our awesome liver has a vulnerability with diabetes. With LADA our liver may daily overload us with unneeded BG, then not rescue us when we're in sugar crisis. In upcoming chapters we'll discuss tools (such as metformin) to calm our liver when it goes overboard, and tools (medic alerts, glucagon kit) to rescue ourselves when the liver is out to lunch.
10. Eating well when you're low-insulin is about trade-offs, not prohibitions.

Expect Change

11. For most with LADA, the autoimmune attack will continue. As time passes, foods and meals that used to stay safely "in range" will begin to spike BG higher.
12. We expect to run fully out of insulin someday. Still, we know that each time we moderate our BG, we're pampering our beta cells, and delaying our insulin cliff that much longer.

o o o

10 WHY DO WE HAVE FAT?

Do We Need It? How to Love Your Fat and Keep It Healthy

*With its secretion of over 100 different [hormones], [fat] is the
largest endocrine organ and links metabolism and immunity.*
—Dr. Farah Omran of Warwick Medical School[1]

IT'S UNFORTUNATE THAT WE USE ONE WORD, FAT, FOR SO MANY DIF-
ferent things. Fat is:

- A type of molecule in our food and in our bodies, built of fatty acids.
- One of the three basic food types (protein, carbohydrate, fat).
- An organ in our body, just like our skin, heart, and brain.
- A hurtful insult.

The many meanings of the word *fat* create confusion and undeserved
stigma. Take a moment to thank your wonderful fat: your pantry, body
armor, thermal quilt, and more—*you could not survive without fat.* Fat
stores energy, strengthens bones, allows puberty and reproduction, helps
wounds heal, and literally allows us to think, coating the neurons in our
brain. Fat-the-organ controls our appetite, influences our emotions, and is
a key part of our immune system.

We literally can't survive without fat because:

> The membrane around each cell in our body contains
> cholesterol.

> › Fat enables puberty, allows healthy sperm, allows secondary sex characteristics (facial hair, muscle development), allows women to become pregnant, and facilitates labor.
> › In the womb, we develop fat at fourteen weeks. Breast milk is packed with fat.
> › Eating too little fat can increase our risk of dementia. Eating sufficient fat can boost our brain size.
> › Our brain is about 60 percent fat. Myelin, the sheathing our brain cells require so that we can think, is made of fat.
> › Fat promotes healing, and is a crucial part of our immune system.

o o o

FAT THE ORGAN

I was surprised to learn that fat is an organ: It has key roles and functions, produces many hormones, and is constantly chatting with our brain and other organs via hormone-Instagram. Fat-the-organ has a powerful effect on our psyche. It impacts our energy level, metabolism, and mood.

It's not a newsflash that individuals vary. But as I learned more about fat, my biggest surprise was how very, very much we vary. I was surprised to learn that I could eat a muffin, and you could eat an identical muffin, and we'd each get different amounts of calories from it, and then do different things with those calories. Even if that muffin is the only thing we each eat for breakfast, some of us will store more of its calories as fat, while others will burn more of them. Depending on our genetics, sex, age, hormones and microbiome (more on the microbiome in chapter 11), we each process food differently, with some bodies turning more of a given food into fat than other bodies.

"Counting calories is very crude and often misleading," writes London journalist Peter Wilson. "Two items of food with identical calorific values may be digested in very different ways. Each body processes calories differently. Even for a single individual, the time of day that you eat matters . . . research shows that when different people consume the same meal, the impact on each person's blood sugar and fat formation will vary according to their genes, lifestyles and unique mix of gut bacteria."[2]

The latest research shows that **body fat is not a simple matter of calories in versus calories out.**[3] Mood, stress, activity level, and sleep affect fat-the-organ almost as much as what goes into our mouths.

Fat-the-organ is a key component of our immune system, and if fat-the-organ grows too large, our immune system can become imbalanced. Body fat is wonderful unless it gains too much dominance and overpowers other health systems.

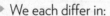

We each differ in:

> Our genetic propensity to store fat.
> Where in our body we store fat.
> How our stored fat affects other body functions.

Each of these depends on our genetics, sex, age, hormone levels, metabolism, and more.

o o o

Too often, our society "grades" people on body shape. Doctors may de-legitimize important health concerns simply based on a person's weight compared with some standard table. That's not my intention here.

Our fat is as active as our liver or pancreas; it's a key organ, actively influencing the brain, liver, insulin, blood sugar, and more. We need to get to know our fat, learn how it supports us and how we can support it, to be our healthiest with LADA.

In this chapter we will use the terms *underweight*, *overweight*, and *obese* to mean falling within weight ranges as classified by modern Western medicine. These are descriptive terms, not judgments. Their use allows us to report on research findings.

o o o

HOW ARE BODY FAT AND DIABETES LINKED?

Being "overweight" does not mean a person has diabetes, and having diabetes does not mean a person is overweight. Six million lean Americans are insulin-resistant, and thirty million obese Americans are *not* insulin-resistant. Thirty percent of obese people are metabolically healthy, while 20 to 30 percent of the non-obese suffer from cardiovascular and heart disease.[4]

The health effects of body fat vary with our genetics, and with whether our fat is "well behaved." Well-behaved fat grows in size by making new cells. Poorly behaved fat grows by supersizing existing fat cells; this can trigger whole-body chronic inflammation.[5]

In some situations, fat increases our longevity. Within the group that modern Western medicine typically labels overweight is a subgroup who have *lower* risk of some modern diseases. Western medicine calls this an *obesity paradox*.

For some, but not all, a fat organ grown too large can no longer support healthy functioning. People who are significantly over their healthy weight are *seven times more likely* to develop insulin-resistant diabetes. Gaining *as little as ten pounds* can cause insulin resistance to double. Excess body weight appears to be a particularly strong risk factor for LADA.[6]

In one recent study, 82 percent of T2s and 31 percent of LADAs had a high BMI (body mass index).[7] T1s may be *underweight* at the time they are diagnosed, because their body may have been struggling to utilize their food, struggling to transport BG from blood to hungry cells. Yet over time T1s may find that hormonal changes or aging may set in motion insulin-resistance issues, weight concerns, or both.

INSULIN RESISTANCE CAN PROGRESS TO METABOLIC SYNDROME (A CLUSter of symptoms associated with frequent/prolonged high blood sugars), and then to T2 diabetes. Any of us can get caught and pushed by this current.

Each time our BG *or* our insulin go high, we tip our body's processes toward making more fat. *It's a cycle*: Insulin resistance increases the proportion of our food that turns into fat, and having extra fat increases our likelihood of insulin resistance. Having more body fat can prompt our liver to dump more sugar into our blood, which sends our BG higher, which prompts more fat creation.[8] Around and around it goes, with every step down the path making it harder to step off. How do we step out of this loop and onto the path to health?

FAT: THE GIFT OF GENERATIONS

Since we need fat to survive, our bodies are built to crave fat. Genetically each person is different, and some crave and create fat much more than others. If you've ever thought, *I swear it's just harder for me to lose weight than it is for her!*—you are absolutely right.

Genetically, some bodies are fat hoarders and some are fat burners. Evolutionarily, either could have its advantages. Some of us (fat hoarders) survived famine after famine and came back strong. Some of us (fat burners) outran famine, and discovered new worlds.

One classic story of genetics and famine resistance compares the Akimel O'odham ("River People," formerly known as the Pima), who traditionally lived along the Gila River in Arizona, to the Maycoba, who lived farther south in Mexico. These two peoples, closely related "cousin tribes," are very similar genetically. Both have a genotype sometimes described as "thrifty" because it excels at storing calories and at surviving famine.

When the O'odham were forced off their land onto a distant reservation that lacked their traditional resources, they had to adopt "Western" foods and a more sedentary lifestyle. This did not happen to the Maycoba, who retained their traditional lifestyle and foods.

Today the Maycoba are healthy: Their rates of weight gain and diabetes resemble the national average. But the genetically similar O'odham are overweight at three times the national average. O'odham men have ten times more obesity than Maycoba men, and O'odham women three times more obesity than Maycoba women. The rate of diabetes among the O'odham is radically higher than the national average, and five times higher than among the Maycoba.[9]

This study tells us that genetics are huge. And that lifestyle—physical activity and processed foods—is equally powerful.

YOUR FAT IS DIVERSE: LOCATION AND COLOR

Just as different parts of your brain have different functions, the same is true for fat-the-organ. Fat in different places on our body, and fat of different colors, do different things and have different health impacts. Location-wise, we'll look at important differences between peripheral fat, subcutaneous fat, and visceral fat; color-wise, we'll look at white fat versus brown fat.

Belly fat (also called abdominal fat or visceral fat). An apron of fat, our *omentum* (Latin for "apron"), wraps protectively around our intestines. The omentum is an active part of our immune system, full of lymph clusters, fighting invasive cells. Belly fat is protective at the right size.[10] But if it grows too large, this is the fat that is most dangerous to health.[11]

Belly fat gives us what some call the "apple" shape. Picture a stereotypical cowboy, lean and fit all his life, who after middle age still has the wiry frame but now looks like he has a basketball under his shirt.

Peripheral fat (in the limbs, breasts, butt, and hips) and **subcutaneous fat** (under the skin) are less likely to lead to health risks. One reason exercise is so beneficial is that it relocates fat away from the abdomen to these healthier locations.

Fat also differs in type (color). The more mitochondria in the cell, the darker it looks. Mitochondria are the powerhouses of a cell, where our cells burn food for energy.

White fat stores energy.

Brown fat, with lots of mitochondria, burns energy. Brown fat pulls BG and lipids out of the blood. It keeps us warm, and *increases our sensitivity to insulin*. People with more brown fat have lower fasting BG. New research is exploring how we might increase brown fat to fight diabetes.[12]

"**People with higher levels of brown fat in their bodies have better blood sugar control, higher insulin sensitivity** and a better metabolism for burning fat stores. [New research] suggests that, because of brown fat's ability to better regulate blood sugar, this could be a potential medical weapon against diabetes," reports University of Texas Medical Branch[13] (my emphasis).

Exercise, and also cold exposure, may help our body make more brown fat.[14]

LET'S TALK ABOUT SEX

Or at least about the three main sex hormones: estrogen, progesterone, and testosterone. I grew up associating estrogen and progesterone only with women, and testosterone with men. I was surprised to learn that, while women have more estrogen and progesterone, and men have more testosterone, **both men and women have, and need, all three hormones.** And each of these hormones is *built from cholesterol.*

Fat, in its sweet spot, helps us procreate. In women, too little *or* too much fat interferes with menstruation and increases risk of miscarriage. In men, too little fat can lead to loss of libido and loss of sperm health, while too much fat can lead to erectile dysfunction.

We all need **estrogen** to have strong bones. Men produce estrogen in their adrenal glands and testes. From puberty to menopause, women produce estrogen mainly in our ovaries. When menopause turns off the faucet for women, most of our estrogen is now produced by—surprise!—our fat.

Fat produces estrogen, and estrogen builds fat, but estrogen steers fat toward healthier locations—breasts, butt, hips, et cetera—instead of the belly. When men are given estrogen as part of a medical treatment, they gain body fat overall, *even when their caloric intake stays constant.* They gain this body fat in non-belly locations.

The additional fat women carry does not make us less healthy than men. "Women have more well-behaved fat. In other words, it's doing a better job of clearing fats out of the blood," explains Dr. Michael Jensen, a physician at Minnesota's Mayo Clinic who studies the differences in fat storage between men and women.[15]

AGING AND FAT

As we age, our fat mass peaks. Between fifty and sixty, we are typically at our heaviest and have the most difficulty keeping fat in check. Many who were thin since childhood suddenly struggle with weight.

Declines in hormones in late-middle-aged women can increase our appetite, reduce fat burning, and redistribute fat to our belly. Since fat produces estrogen, as our spare tire expands, our estrogen may decline less than our progesterone, resulting in *estrogen dominance,* which can result in sleep problems, irritability, depression, sugar cravings, and increased appetite; some describe it as like being premenstrual . . . for years.

In both women and men, aging can lower **testosterone,** and this can decrease our muscle mass and our energy, and slow our metabolism. While we tend to think of testosterone as a male hormone, *there is more of it in a woman's body than estrogen* at most times of the month, especially after menopause. Exercise fights the aging effect: Exercise can increase testosterone, adrenaline, and other energizing, metabolism-boosting hormones.

In our seventies and beyond, we typically lose fat, not in a healthy way but in a fat-failing-to-perform-its-functions way. Fat-the-organ can shrink, dumping stored fat-the-molecule. This dumped fat can cause higher cholesterol or hardened arteries or pile up in organs or in weird places (*ectopic fat*), potentially weakening bones, decreasing muscle strength, increasing risk of diabetes, or harming the liver, kidneys, or pancreas.[16]

SO MANY HORMONES ON THE PLAYING FIELD

The Secret Life of Fat shares the story of Layla, who when just one year old developed an enormous appetite and became an obsessive eater. Layla was obese even as a toddler, constantly pleading, howling, and crying for more food. As a child she broke into locked cabinets, forced open a locked freezer to eat frozen fish, and dug through garbage, if she could get access to it, for scraps and rinds.

Doctors eventually figured out that Layla had an unusual genetic condition—she did not produce the hormone leptin. They decided to try leptin injections. "Within four days," said her doctor, "she was eating a quarter compared to what she was normally eating. She went from being a completely focused eating machine to being a normal kid."[17]

Thank you, fat, for making the hormone leptin so we can realize we are full.

And thank you, fat, for making the hormone **adiponectin**, which reroutes our fat to healthier locations, and pulls ceramides out of our blood (in blood, ceramides are a major risk factor for heart disease, insulin resistance, and inflammation).[18]

Some hormones clean our blood (adiponectin). Some burn fat, saying, *Burn, baby, burn* (adrenaline, thyroid hormones, growth hormone, estrogen, testosterone, and progesterone). Others say, *Let's build some nice comfy fat for a rainy day* (insulin and cortisol).

Growth hormone lets kids grow, and continues to be important in adults, helping us build lean tissue and burn fat, and may be part of the reason that intermittent fasting (IF) helps some people lose weight—for some, a longer overnight break from eating appears to release more growth hormone.

Hunger is a hormone . . . or actually a pile of them. Hunger is our brain taking a vote: listening to dozens of *I'm full* hormones (such as leptin) and a pile of *I'm famished* hormones (ghrelin and others) and deciding who wins. In part 4 of this book, we delve more deeply into hunger.

Because hunger and fat are so hormonal, stress and exercise have a big effect; as do good sleep, healthy fiber, and hydration.

STRESS AND FAT

I used to feel frustrated when people pointed out the well-documented research linking stress with fat and linking stress with diabetes. Were these folks blaming the victim, piling on guilt to those caught in a difficult situation?

Eventually the real message sank in. We can't delete the bad things that happen to us. But we can look stress in the eye and work with it, disarming the bomb of its toxic effects. *How we deal with and channel our stress affects whether we build fat or burn fat* (chapter 14).

Paralyzing or energizing? **Cortisol** and **adrenaline** are both stress hormones, yet they have opposite effects. *I feel trapped* cortisol builds fat, and *Run-run-run!* adrenaline burns fat. We could call adrenaline stress, or we could call it energy. A lot depends on whether we have *action* to channel the challenge into.

EXERCISE

Stress, blah, blah, blah, exercise, blah, blah, blah—too much talk of exercise once made me angry and defensive. I thought exercise meant calorie math at the gym, exercycling away yesterday's cookies-n-dreams splurge.

Nope. Much more important: Getting active, hitting the fresh air, is how we enlist our powerful crew of hormones to work toward health.

Being active is, if not a silver bullet, at least a *sine qua non*: "that without which there is nothing." Enjoying activities—be they tai chi, touch football, walking the dog, basketball, pickleball, walking a few blocks on a lunch break, gardening, hip-hop, bicycling, beach strolling, double dutch, or swing dancing—increases growth hormone, adiponectin, adrenaline, and testosterone, giving us more energy throughout the day, burning more calories, and routing our fat to healthier locations.

In addition to burning up stored energy, exercise builds muscle, increases brown fat, burns white fat, strengthens bones, increases metabolism, helps prevent dementia and osteoporosis, and releases hormones that give us energy, strength, drive, and confidence. For those of us working to manage or lower weight, **95 *percent of successful weight losers incorporate exercise.***

Dr. Hamdy, Joslin Diabetes Center's medical director, says: "[A] 7% weight loss can improve insulin sensitivity by 57%. That is the equivalent of two medications for diabetes management at maximum dose . . . [Through exercise] we have helped so many people [reduce] medications . . . [or] get off of their medications altogether."[19]

Fat-the-organ saves our life, daily. Thanks, fat. Unfortunately, fat-the-organ can become a helicopter parent. I had to learn to love my fat; and then I had to learn to set clear boundaries with this helicopter parent, because I was tired of living in its basement.

KEY TAKEAWAYS

1. Fat is an organ, controlling our appetite and influencing our thoughts, moods, immune system and more. Through hormones, fat constantly chats with our brain, pancreas, and other organs.

2. We can't survive without fat. Fat stores energy, strengthens bones, is part of our immune system, and allows us to think.

3. Body fat is wonderful unless it gains too much power. If this organ overpowers our other systems, our health can spiral down.

4. We have more than one type of fat in our body: different types have different colors, different functions, and different locations.

5. Yes, *it really is harder* for some people to alter their weight than for others. Genetics, age, sex, and more affect fat-the-organ.

6. While our genetics are powerful, an active lifestyle is equally powerful.

Expect Change

7. Supporting and moderating fat-the-organ gets harder as we age, and aging will be rougher if we lose control of fat-the-organ.

You're in Charge

8. To maintain a healthful weight lower than a past weight, we may no longer be able to simply listen to our body—we may have to consciously override the body's messages.

9. Being active burns up stored energy, and also does so much more: builds muscle, strengthens bones, increases metabolism, transforms our fat to healthier types in different locations, helps prevent dementia and osteoporosis, and releases hormones that give us energy, strength, drive, and confidence.

10. Whatever genetic tendency we get handed, or highest weight we've had, we can stay healthy and happy through life choices and the many cards in our hand, including healthful hydration, fiber, stress management, and good sleep.

11. When cultivating and managing our fat, we triumph like a gardener, starting fresh each day. Motivation, exercise, and persistence are the three magic beans.

○ ○ ○

11 TEND THE INNER GARDEN

Our Microbiome Battles Inflammation

The healthy and diverse microbes living in our gut provide
numerous benefits to our health.
> —Dr. Tai Guo, University of Georgia[1]

Many autoimmune and inflammatory diseases . . . have a
"gut origin" . . . [including] type 1 diabetes . . . and type 2
diabetes.
> —Dr. Yu-Anne Yap, School of Biomedical Sciences,
> Monash University[2]

OUR MICROBIOME—THE MANY FRIENDLY MICROBES EACH HUMAN
body hosts—is an ecosystem of thousands of species and trillions of
individuals.*

There is a trifecta at work in our body. Three key body systems interact, each of them constantly affecting the others: body fat (fat-the-organ),
inflammation, and our microbiome.

I used to roll my eyes when people tossed around such words. Was this
dreamed up by people wearing crystals dangling from aluminum foil hats?
Nope: The enormous medical importance of inflammation and of the
microbiome is cutting-edge medical research.[3]

---

* In this book, I'll use *microbiome* to mean the inhabitants of our digestive system only (I'm
not discussing the tiny friends on our skin and elsewhere—that's a different book).

CHRONIC INFLAMMATION

Chapter 6 briefly introduced inflammation. Short-term inflammation is a healer in the body, helping to fight infection. But *chronic* (long-term) inflammation inflicts all kinds of harm.[4]

Inflammation worsens diabetes—all types[5]—and diabetes worsens inflammation; it's a cycle.[6] Inflammation is a trigger for many autoimmune diseases, including T1 and LADA; and it also worsens insulin resistance. So inflammation strikes LADA from both directions.

Inflammation is in a similar vicious cycle with cancer, heart disease, dementia, arthritis, asthma, gum disease, leaky bowel syndrome, and more. Like a fire that's never put out, inflammation creeps through our body, igniting or aggravating so many deadly modern diseases that Harvard Medical School calls it "one of the four horsemen of the medical apocalypse."[7]

CHRONIC INFLAMMATION CAN BE TRIGGERED BY SOMETHING IN OUR environment: a pollutant, allergen, or food sensitivity.[8] Or a dysfunction within our own body, such as fat-the-organ growing too large, can trigger chronic inflammation.

When we are healthy, the wall of our gut is strong and protective. Our microbiome (the tiny friends we'll meet below) plays a key role in keeping the gut wall healthy. When our microbiome gets out of whack, our gut wall can leak, allowing things into our bloodstream that weren't meant to be there, triggering or amplifying inflammation.

"All of us adults have some level of chronic inflammation slowly waging a war of attrition on tissues and organs," says *Harvard Health Letter*. "But if it's turned up a notch or two, chronic inflammation can wear away at the body so that the damage is devastating."[9]

Inflammation produces molecules (such as TNF-α) that can interfere with insulin and can raise blood levels of BG and triglycerides.

"TNF-α seems to increase the liver's production of glucose and triglycerides and interfere with insulin," *Harvard Health Letter* explains. "Moreover, insulin has anti-inflammatory effects of its own. Thus inflammation not only sets the stage for insulin resistance but accelerates as insulin resistance sets in, which may further hasten the onset of diabetes."[10]

HOW DO WE FIGHT BACK AGAINST CHRONIC INFLAMMATION?

Chronic inflammation is long-term, like dust settling on furniture. The ways to push back are straightforward, but they are not a one-and-done. (Every dang week with the dusting, right?) We fight chronic inflammation with:

- Joyful activity (sometimes called exercise).
- Managing stress through healthful outlets.
- Healthy fat-the-organ, healthy weight.
- Avoiding inflammatory chemicals (chapter 18).
- Reducing inflammatory foods and enjoying anti-inflammatory foods (chapter 18).
- Having a healthy microbiome.

o o o

WHAT IS THE (GUT) MICROBIOME?

Our gut is a garden, blossoming with flora. We contain multitudes. We're home sweet home to trillions of friendly munchkins, our microbiome. Our microbiome feeds us, it doctors us (boosts our immune system), and (when healthy) it keeps the wall of our gut shipshape and strong. "We've got to get ourselves back to the garden," sang Joni Mitchell.

Our microbiome functions like an organ, sending hormonal messengers to communicate with our brain and immune system. Pound for pound, our microbiome is about the weight of our brain. Since the microbiome profoundly affects our mood and behavior, some call our it our second brain. As science studies what it now calls our *microbiome-gut-brain axis*, we are learning that a healthier microbiome can change behavior patterns, improve social interactions, alleviate anxiety and depression, and restore oxytocin.[11] The gut is not only a garden—it's a smart garden.

How big is our microbiome and what is it made of?

Our gut plays host to about forty trillion cells, give or take, which can include a thousand species of helpful bacteria along with many other types of microbes, such as co-evolved archaea, fungi, and viruses. There are as many helper cells in our gut microbiome as there are human cells in our body. The genome of your personal microbiome is about a hundred times larger than your human genome.

Where does our microbiome come from?

Genetics have surprisingly little influence on our microbiome—in this case, it's almost all environment. Our birth journey anoints us with a starter microbiome, and the foods and environment of our first three years of life hugely shape our microbiome. A surprising recent finding is that our microbiome becomes fairly stable after age three. Our personal microbiome may be almost as unique as our fingerprints.[12]

What does our microbiome do for us?

These little tenants are not mere invisible roommates—they play an enormous role in our health and happiness. Along with promoting our mental health, our microbiome boosts our digestion, energy, strength, stamina, and metabolism; helps us synthesize vitamins and essential fatty acids; and helps us metabolize drugs and defend against toxins. A healthy microbiome keeps the gut wall tight, protecting us against chronic inflammation. This garden digests foods we could not digest without it, and affects how much energy we get from our food, and what percentage of our food turns into fat.[13]

Because it influences how much of each bite of food turns into fat, our microbiome is tightly linked to fat-the-organ. A research team at the University of Chicago writes, "The gut microbiome can classify individuals as lean or obese with over 90% accuracy . . . and the abundance of [particular microbes] within the human gut . . . [is] negatively correlated with BMI . . . [and] can induce weight loss when experimentally fed to mice."[14]

What is *dysbiosis* of the microbiome?

Dysbiosis means an unhealthy change to our microbiota, such as a loss of key helpers, lower diversity, or an imbalance in amounts of different helpers. Negative changes to our microbiome impact our nervous system and our ability to fight disease, and can trigger or worsen a wide array of illnesses, from inflammatory bowel disease to cancer to depression. Dysbiosis can allow our gut wall to leak, increasing inflammation and opening the doors to autoimmune attack on organs like our pancreas. About 10 percent of variations in our immune response can be directly attributed to our microbiome.[15] "It is clear," writes Dr. Stefano Bibbò, "that the human microbiota hold a pivotal role in health and in disease."[16]

How does the microbiome impact LADA?

Improving microbiome health is an area of cutting-edge research in diabetes today. Specific changes to our microbiome may be diagnostic markers for diabetes.[17] Our microbiome directly impacts our control of our blood sugars, our level of inflammation, and our body fat.[18] An unhealthy microbiome can trigger autoimmune diabetes (LADA or T1).[19]

"Changes in the microbiota in type 1 diabetes occur before symptoms develop, and are not just a side effect of the disease," writes Dr. Hamilton-Williams.[20]

The T2 microbiome is low in bacteria that produces butyrate, a short-chain fatty acid (SCFA) that supports proper functioning of our beta cells, reduces inflammation, strengthens the gut wall, and helps glucose control.[21] One recent study found that patients with LADA were even more deficient in these protective SCFA-producing bacteria than T1 or T2.[22]

It's a spiraling loop: Negative changes to our microbiome raise our risk of LADA, and poorly controlled LADA pushes our microbiome toward an unhealthy state.[23]

If the garden in our gut gets out of whack, this hits a LADA from both sides: both triggering/worsening our autoimmune attack, and also worsening insulin resistance, weight gain, and chronic inflammation. Getting hit from both sides might sound like a raw deal, but it does mean that when we improve the health of our microbiome, we hit back in both directions, and perhaps can even slow our rate of progression toward the insulin cliff.[24] *A healthier gut reduces our risk of diabetes, and allows us to more easily manage diabetes, and to be healthy with diabetes.*[25]

When we talk about metformin in the upcoming chapter, we'll see that one of its beneficial effects is improving the garden in our gut.[26]

Can we change our microbiome?

Yes. Changing our food choices can profoundly change our microbiome in ways that improve blood sugar control. Making a significant dietary improvement can lead to profound change in our microbiome within days.[27] Research shows that exercise, healthful sleep, and stress management can also improve our microbiome health.[28]

"The gut microbiota represents a tool of great therapeutic potential," writes Dr. Marisol Aguirre of the Netherlands' Maastricht University.[29]

Will changes to microbiome health be long-lasting?

We each have a surprisingly unique and surprisingly stable microbiome signature.[30] Experimental treatments including diet, exercise, and even fecal transplants will dramatically alter our microbiome — but if the treatment is only temporary, the change will likely be as well, and the microbiome will tend to drift back to that person's "normal." As Dr. Gilbert puts it: "The original microbiota and structure re-emerge when the original conditions resume."[31]

This doesn't mean we can't change; it means that our tools for a healthy microbiome are *lifelong* tools. Healthy life, lifelong tools, is a theme we'll see again and again in this book.

Among microbes, who's good? Who's bad?

No simple answers yet, but we're getting closer. Scientists have spent recent decades just taking roll call: counting, classifying, and describing who's in there, mapping the microbiome's diversity, worldwide trends, and variation by genetics and disease state.[32] Similar to the Human Genome Project, the National Microbiome Initiative launched in 2016 unified microbiome description.

"Human microbiome investigations have now reached a critical inflection point," writes Dr. Jack Gilbert of the University of Chicago's Microbiome Center. We are right on the cusp, he says, of transitioning from describing patterns to understanding interactions and developing medical interventions.[33]

Meanwhile, you and I don't have to wait. We can begin making our microbiome healthier today. In part 3 of this book, we'll learn about simple, straightforward choices in foods, vitamins, activity, sleep quality, and stress management that can profoundly heal our microbiome. As the garden in our gut heals, it will reward us by reducing chronic inflammation, easing weight management, improving our blood sugar control, pampering our beta cells, and perhaps even slowing our autoimmune attack.

HOW DO WE TEND THIS GARDEN?

Like any gardener, we want to weed out bad strains, and to seed, fertilize, and nurture good strains.

- Prebiotics are food for our garden.
- Probiotics are seeds for our garden.

Prebiotic is just a fancy word for fiber. And fiber is simply the ultimate slow carb, a sugar stack bundled in such a complicated way that your human organs say, *I can't break this apart*, but your friendly flora say, *No problem, we can*. Fiber doesn't just swish through your gut like a broom and poop out the other end. Fiber feeds your flora.[34]

Yes, celery comes instantly to mind, with those dang strings that stick in the teeth. But fiber can be smaller: small to us, big to our trillion inner besties. For great sources of fiber think: whole nuts, whole seeds, whole fruits, whole vegetables (particularly the stem, leaf, and flower veggies), legumes, and whole grains. Yes, shop the farmers market, or the edge of the supermarket. Yes, put foods that look like themselves, foods Great-Grandma would recognize, into your shopping bag. It's really that simple.

Probiotics are live bacteria, live little minion helpers. Many types of probiotics are already naturally within our foods. To add probiotics to your diet, try yogurt with live cultures, kimchi, pickles (pickled asparagus on that white-tablecloth night, or zesty dills with your Super Bowl burger), kombucha, refrigerated sauerkraut, and similar foods.

Your probiotic food *should say* KEEP REFRIGERATED. If not, the bacteria might be there, but not alive. Dead seeds won't do much for your garden.

VITAMIN D HELPS OUR GARDEN

Vitamin D deficiency is one of the known environmental triggers for LADA and other types of diabetes (chapter 7). Upcoming chapter 12 explains how vitamin D protects and assists our beta cells, fights chronic inflammation, reverses insulin resistance, and helps BG control. These benefits are strongly linked to the fact that vitamin D promotes a healthy microbiome. When we have sufficient vitamin D, our gut wall is stronger and healthier, we have a healthier balance of minions in our microbiome, and the microbiome-immune interaction tips toward health.[35] Chapter 12 will look more deeply at vitamin D, discussing dosages and more.

KEY TAKEAWAYS

1. Show the trifecta—fat, inflammation, and the microbiome— some love. While this helps anyone's health, it is particularly important with diabetes (all forms).

2. Cultivating a healthy microbiome improves energy level and mood along with physical health, and impacts how much of our food turns to fat. Enjoy:
   › Plenty of fiber.
   › Plenty of fermented foods.
   › Sufficient vitamin D.

3. To fight chronic inflammation:
   › Enjoy joyful activity (sometimes called exercise).
   › Manage stress through healthful outlets.
   › Enjoy omega-3 foods (chapter 17) and other anti-inflammatory foods (chapter 18).

- Reduce exposure to inflammatory chemicals (chapter 18).
- Encourage/shift/maintain body weight and fat-the-organ toward health.
- Tend your garden—support your microbiome.

o o o

GOOD NEWS OR BAD NEWS?

Is the trifecta—the close interrelationships among body fat, chronic inflammation, and our microbiome—good news or bad news? Hard to say, but one takeaway is: *Anything we do that helps one of these will help all of them.*

We're steadily building the tools in our toolbox. We now know why fiber (prebiotics), probiotics, other healthful foods, and exercise are so important. The next few chapters will add more tools: medications (especially metformin, insulin, and vitamin D), stress management, and healthful sleep. Together these tools can build a healthy gut, calm inflammation, manage weight to our personal goal, protect us from BG spikes and valleys, and protect and pamper our beta cells. With this full and varied toolbox, we can be healthy with LADA (or other forms of diabetes).

It may feel almost frustrating to be told that such cliché things as fiber and restful sleep are scientifically proven to be hugely important. Yada, yada, whatever, give me a challenge, give me something new: Tell me to eat worms, tell me to climb Everest, tell me about the magic pill! (Embarrassingly, this was me in early days.)

But consider: If you can accept that "eating healthy" is important with LADA, surely sleeping healthy, playing and frolicking healthy, and chillaxing healthy could be equally key.

12 THE SKINNY ON MEDS

[For LADA] insulin treatment . . . can sustain residual beta
cell function . . . [but] sulfonylurea may hasten insulin
dependency and should not be used.
    —Dr. Paolo Pozzilli, Director of Endocrinology &
    Diabetes, U. Campus Bio-Medico, Rome[1]

WE LADAS ARE HIGHLY VARIABLE IN OUR GENETICS, IN HOW MUCH
insulin resistance we have, and in how our disease acts and progresses; and
each LADA's situation changes over time. A medication that's helpful to
one LADA may not be the right choice for a second LADA. A medication
that won't help a LADA at one point in her life could be helpful later. We
each, together with our doctor, needs to dig deeper than the simple label
LADA and understand exactly which mountain we're standing on—at this
moment—to know our best treatment.

This chapter will look at a few oral medications, and the following chapter will look at insulin. I won't dive super-deep into meds because I'm no
doctor, and because so much might change just in the time it takes this book
to come to print, but I can share key big picture thoughts.

WE'LL LEARN WHY

  › What's helpful to one LADA may not help every LADA at
    every point on her journey.
  › The vast majority of LADAs will benefit from metformin
    and vitamin D.
  › Sulfonylureas are not recommended for LADA.

> ＊ Most LADAs should begin insulin much earlier than is cur-
>   rently the norm.
> ＊ There are many names on the long shopping list of medications
>   to reduce insulin resistance (T2 meds). Exercise can do as much
>   or more for us than many of them. (Not that meds-versus-
>   exercise is an either/or choice—we can do both.)
> ＊ Not all meds are created equal. It's a fairly low bar to be more
>   effective than a placebo and an improvement over uncontrolled
>   diabetes: the current standard for approving a medication.
> ＊ **This is not medical advice. Bring any questions to your
>   doctor.**

o o o

METFORMIN (GLUCOPHAGE)

Metformin* is the go-to first drug for a T2. But is it helpful for LADA? Yes,
almost always. And that's a relatively new discovery, as we learn more about
how metformin acts.

Outdated ways of thinking are still out there, so three different endocrinologists gave me three different answers when I asked: Would metformin help
me?

"No," said Dr. Hawaii.

"Unknown," said Dr. Chicago.

"It may well be helpful," said Fabulous Dr. Five, "and there's almost no
risk: Let's try it and evaluate whether it's helpful *for you*."

Metformin has been around for decades, is considered very safe, and is
available in an extended-release (XR) form that for most people eliminates
side effects.

Metformin reduces insulin resistance (helps insulin be more effective in
our body).[2] Back before we knew that metformin has other important benefits
in addition, many doctors assumed metformin was only helpful for T2—an
outdated idea.

Metformin calms the liver, which is extremely helpful to those of us
who no longer produce much insulin, as explained in chapter 9. "The

---

* Metformin is the generic name. Brand names include Glucophage.

main antidiabetic effect of this drug is to decrease hepatic [liver] glucose production," writes endocrinologist Benoit Viollet[3] (my emphasis).

A third helpful effect of metformin is a healthier gut: It gives us a friendlier crew of microbes and increases our gut's goblet cells, which absorb nutrients.[4] Metformin has also been shown to reduce inflammation, improve our lipid profiles, and perhaps reduce cancer risk.[5]

As Dr. Yevheniia Kyriachenko writes in the *World Journal of Diabetes*:

> Metformin is . . . currently the drug of choice recommended by the American Diabetes Association and the European Association for the Study of Diabetes. Metformin has blood glucose-lowering and insulin sensitizing effects and inhibits liver glucose production . . . and rais[es] plasma levels of GLP-1 . . . patients treated with metformin can experience improvement in their lipid levels [and] attenuation of chronic low-grade tissue inflammation.[6]

Should we continue taking metformin after we begin insulin? In a word: yes. Even "classic" T1s are increasingly prescribed metformin along with insulin because it calms the liver; research shows metformin helps T1s maintain their healthiest weight and improves their BG control.[7]

I didn't know about this research when I began insulin, so I wondered: Should I keep taking metformin? Let's experiment, Dr. Five suggested. We tried it both ways, and found that when I took my daily metformin, I could use less insulin to achieve the same BG control.

A false worry that metformin might reduce vitamin D[8] has been put to rest by the latest research.[9]

LADAs online joke about "met-fart-min" and worry about gassiness and bloating. It's true that, just like "beans, beans, the musical fruit" and other healthy fiber, when we hit the garden in our gut with something new (even good-new), we can have short-term symptoms until our gut catches up to the change. Most people find that extended-release metformin solves the problem, or that the gassiness goes away after several weeks; some remark that reducing carbs as they began metformin solved the "fart problem" for them.

SULFONYLUREAS

"Sulfonylureas may hasten insulin dependency and should not be used as first-line therapy for patients with LADA," writes Dr. Pozzilli.[10] Sulfonylureas include glyburide (brand names include DiaBeta and Glynase), glipizide (Glucotrol), glimepiride (Amaryl), and more. Drugs in this group force the pancreas to secrete more insulin. They are often still prescribed to T2s, so if you are a LADA originally misdiagnosed as T2, double-check with your doctor that none of your medications are sulfonylureas. Sulfonylureas overwork a LADA's weakened beta cells and burn them out more quickly.[11]

INCRETINS AND DPP-4 INHIBITORS

In an upcoming chapter on hunger, we'll spend more time with the helpful hormone I call "*Glip*" (GLP-1, glucagon-like peptide-1). Produced when we eat nourishing food, Glip helps us feel well-fed and happy, heals the garden in our gut, reduces inflammation, protects beta cells, increases insulin production, and tells the liver not to dump sugar.[12] Wow! Glip is a star player on a LADA's team. But we lose Glip as we lose beta cells.

In the natural cycles of our body, Glip is broken down by an enzyme called DPP-4 (dipeptidyl peptidase-4).

Two types of drugs were recently created: *mimetics* that mimic our natural Glip, and *inhibitors* that slow the breakdown of our natural Glip. Both types of drugs are relatively new and may have both pros and cons.

Mimetics. Incretin mimetics mimic GLP-1. They include exenatide, lixisenatide, dulaglutide, albiglutide, and liraglutide.[*]

Inhibitors. DPP-4 inhibitors, also called *gliptins*, slow the breakdown of our natural GLP-1. They include sitagliptin, vildagliptin, saxagliptin, alogliptin, and linagliptin.[†]

---

* Trade names include Bydureon, Byetta, Lyxumia, Trulicity, Tanzeum, Eperzan, Victoza, and more.

† Trade names include Januvia, Janumet, Galvus, Onglyza, Kombiglyze, Nesina, Kazano, Oseni, Tradjenta, Glyxambi, Jentadueto, and more.

Early short-term studies on LADA patients confirmed that sitagliptin preserved beta cell function.[13] But some doctors have concerns about potential side effects.

GLP-1 mimetics increase the risk of thyroid cancer. Gliptins now carry an FDA warning of possible "severe and disabling" joint pain. Both mimetics and gliptins increase the risk of pancreatitis,[14] and they have a long list of other potential side effects, including allergic, gastrointestinal, or mood reactions.

"The use of GLP-1 [mimetics] and DPP-4 inhibitors has been widely incorporated . . . However . . . the long-term safety profile of their use has yet to be determined," Dr. Lillian Smith wrote in 2016.[15]

In the upcoming Carb-craft section, we'll look at how to promote our own naturally produced GLP-1 through diet and lifestyle: by enjoying leafy greens, fiber, and protein; and by reducing inflammation and moderating our BG spikes.

THIAZOLIDINEDIONES

Reasons to be excited about TZs (Thiazolidinediones such as rosiglitazone/Avandia and pioglitazone/Actos) include anti-inflammatory effects and the improvement of insulin sensitivity. Reasons to be less excited are risks of heart failure, weight gain, and bone fractures.[16] Avandia is now banned in Europe due to risk of heart failure.

VITAMIN D

Vitamin D is a hormone our bodies make when we have sunshine on our skin. Having too little vitamin D increases risk of many autoimmune diseases, including autoimmune diabetes, and can harm the garden in our gut and increase inflammation.[17]

Dozens of studies have found that supplementing vitamin D lowered risk of diabetes and reversed insulin resistance.[18] "Vitamin D decreases insulin resistance, severity of T2D, prediabetes, metabolic syndrome, inflammation, and autoimmunity . . . [in] a large number of observational studies," writes endocrinologist Sunil Wimalawansa.[19]

Dr. Po Sing Leung explains, "Vitamin D might have dual anti-diabetic influences: (1) modulation of [liver] glucose and lipid metabolism; and (2) promotion of pancreatic islet function and survival . . . vitamin D supplementation may represent a promising, cost-effective **preventative *and* therapeutic** agent for the management of . . . insulin resistance and diabetes"[20] (my emphasis).

There has even been a study *on LADA* and vitamin D, which found that vitamin D preserved beta cells, maintained insulin production longer, and made blood sugar control easier.[21] Other studies found that taking vitamin D reduced T1 risk in children; or that when mothers took vitamin D during pregnancy or while breastfeeding, their children were less likely to develop T1.[22]

Researchers in Quebec found that vitamin D helped beta cells meet insulin demand (as measured by something called the *disposition index*), while also improving the body's insulin sensitivity. They concluded that vitamin D may pamper beta cells and *prevent or reverse early stages of autoimmune diabetes.*[23]

Supplementing vitamin D *along with probiotics* may be even more effective.[24] "Our review documented improvement in insulin sensitivity, antioxidative patterns, and dyslipidemia markers with co-supplementation of vitamin D and probiotics," writes Dr. Myriam Abboud.[25]

According to endocrinologist Lorena Wright of UW Medicine's Diabetes Care Center, being *low* on vitamin D increases diabetes's risks, but if our vitamin D is already where it should be, further supplementation may not help (although the *normal* supplementation dose is also unlikely to harm).

For many of us, ten to thirty minutes a day of (sunscreen-free) time in good direct sunlight provides all the vitamin D we need.

In parts of the world like Washington State, where I live, many people become low on vitamin D every winter, because our latitude makes the winter sun less powerful and because of frequent cloudiness in winter. Anywhere in the world, those who stay indoors a great deal, or must never expose their skin without sunscreen, may also become low on vitamin D. For most adults, says Dr. Wright, taking one or two thousand standard units daily of a reputable vitamin D brand has possible benefits and few risks—but do **check with your own doctor** about risks for your particular situation, or medication interactions.[26]

NATURE'S PILL: EXERCISE

Reducing insulin resistance is one of the many things *exercise* does for us. Every time we exercise, we are not only burning up the BG in our blood at that moment, we are adding new "locks" to our cells, helping our insulin be more effective.

As we saw in chapter 10, exercise, moderate weight loss, or both, can be *as effective as medication* in lowering insulin resistance. Through exercise, says Dr. Hamdy, medical director of the Joslin Diabetes Center, "we have helped so many people [reduce] medications . . . [or] get off of their medications altogether."[27]

There are **many other** meds out there for diabetes; discuss with your doctor whether any may be right for you.

This brief thumbnail is not an exhaustive look at diabetes medications. ***Bring any medication question to your doctor.***

1. Not all meds are created equal. If you have questions, ask.
2. Metformin: gold star. Metformin quiets our liver, makes our limited insulin more effective, and has a potpourri of other positive effects. Metformin is increasingly being prescribed to classic T1s and remains helpful when we begin supplementing insulin.
3. Vitamin D: gold star. It has many benefits and, at a reasonable dose, few risks: Check your particular situation with your doctor.
4. Sulfonylureas: frowny face. These might push a LADA off the insulin cliff faster.
5. Finding the doctor who is both well versed in LADA and shares your philosophy and outlook is crucial for guidance on medications and other questions.

o o o

When "patients with LADA . . . are incorrectly diagnosed with type 2 diabetes," writes Professor Katherine O'Neal, doctors may "suspect non-adherence, and enforce further lifestyle modifications when, **in actuality, these patients are in need of insulin therapy**"[28] (my emphasis).

When should we begin insulin? Some doctors say: immediately.

13 EMBRACING INSULIN

*Patients with autoimmune diabetes should be **insulin-treated
as early as possible*** [my emphasis].
  —Dr. Gunnar Stenström, Kungsbacka Hospital,
  Sweden[1]

*Clinical trials highlight the importance of an **early initiation
of insulin therapy in LADA** regardless of presence of some
endogenous insulin secretion . . . to improve metabolic control
while protecting beta-cell function* [my emphasis].
  —Dr. Paolo Pozzilli, Director of Endocrinology &
  Diabetes, U. Campus Bio-Medico, Rome[2]

I'VE WORKED AND PLAYED IN THE WILDERNESS MOST OF MY LIFE, AND am pretty calm around sharks, rattlesnakes, ticks, and tarantulas. While kayaking, I've come around a bend in a narrow channel to discover that my only route downstream will drift me, frozen statue-still, past a huge Alaskan brown bear nibbling sedges on the bank. I've waded Carolina swamps between cypress dripping with Spanish moss where alligators, poisonous cottonmouths, and brain-eating amoebas lurk. When in *anyone's* home, I try to respect their customs and culture—especially when a slip-up could kill me. Majestic carnivores, floating 'gators, hairy spiders, scurrilous microbes: I treat them all with deferential respect.

But insulin? Now, that *scared* me. Screw up, and it's like standing in a burning building, two steps from the wide-open door to freedom, yet your brain can't tell you to take those two steps; you might die staring slack-jawed at the open doorway. The deadly BG lows we risk once we begin insulin are scary in part because there's such a simple solution—*eat that granola bar in your pocket, you silly goose*—but the condition can fog your brain to where you don't take the simple action to save your own life.

Insulin is an unusual medication: It's very powerful; it's dangerous if mis-dosed; and dosing is complicated, a moving target affected by many factors, a decision most users need to carefully think through multiple times a day.

Not to mention: Insulin is expensive, is time-consuming, involves poking ourselves with needles or wearing a machine, and might push us toward weight gain—a fraught issue with diabetes. Insulin comes with baggage—the need to carry around supplies, monitors, glucose, yada yada yada. It makes our private health concerns visible to every stranger: We literally wear our diabetes on our sleeve—perhaps in the form of a medical ID or CGM (continuous glucose monitor).

The thought of beginning insulin made me feel vulnerable . . . to my own mistakes, and to common travel mishaps like lost luggage or a bag stolen from a beach. In some parts of the world, where insulin is difficult to get, losing my bag could transform from annoying to life-threatening.

When I was first diagnosed, I was determined to manage my LADA just through food and exercise. And I made that work . . . for a while. But the majority of LADAs will not be able to make this work for their entire life (assuming it's pleasingly long). Chapter 19 shares some of the frustrations and challenges of trying to manage by non-insulin tools alone in an ever-shrinking food space. If we cling too long and stubbornly (something I can speak to from experience), we risk driving ourselves and loved ones bananas, yet no longer controlling our BG as well as before: harming our health and racing toward our insulin cliff more quickly.

There are many wonderful ways to push back on LADA, to slow it or even slightly reverse it. Even so, for most, LADA will be the disease we can't fully outmuscle, can't outrun. It's best to expect to depend upon supplementing insulin, sooner or later.

Studies show that many with diabetes wait up to four years too long to start insulin, harming their health.[3] I understand the hesitancy. I've been there.

But I was surprised. It actually is *not* as scary as brain-eating amoebas. When I finally took the plunge, I found that it's more like driving a car. When you learned to drive, did you have to sit through a blood-gushing driver's ed movie? I did, and the movie scared me—my imagination snowballed. But today when I slide into my driver's seat, I'm more worried about my shopping list than about being decapitated; driving feels easy and normal, not scary. Insulin: same.

WHEN SHOULD WE START?

Most LADAs should start insulin earlier than we do.

Some start immediately. Starting early can keep more beta cells alive, and keep us healthier. "The rationale for early initiation of insulin is based on evidence demonstrating **multifaceted benefits**, including . . . facilitating 'beta-cell rest,' and preserving beta-cell mass and function, while also improving insulin sensitivity . . . **early initiation of insulin therapy may . . . positively alter the course of disease progression**" (my emphasis), writes Dr. Owens of Swansea University's Diabetes Research Group,[4] echoing many others.[5]

Counterpoint: Some prefer to get practiced and knowledgeable with their other tools first, before jumping into insulin's learning curve. That's what I did, although by accident, not design, during my long wait for a proper diagnosis and a doctor who really "got" LADA. With hindsight, this did make it easier to experiment to find my best metformin dose, and to let carb-counting and Carb-craft (part 3) become muscle memory, before adding the layer of constantly monitoring and finessing my insulin needs. While waiting several months worked well for me, that's partly luck; if I were back at the beginning, and deciding now, I'd probably start insulin sooner than I did.

Ultimately this will be a very individual decision made in consultation with your doctor.

How long will our insulin honeymoon be? If only we had an answer to this crucial but currently unanswerable question: How long until we run out of insulin?

We'll talk more about the honeymoon dilemma in chapter 19. Like other *How long have I got, Doc?* questions, our desperation for an answer does not mean the doc has one; there are mysteries between here and there.

That said, our numbers, types, and levels of antibodies, and our fasting or stimulated C-peptide (chapter 4), can give us a very imprecise hint.[6] Some researchers recommend that LADAs with higher levels of antibodies start insulin immediately.[7] One panel of experts suggests LADAs be divided into treatment scenarios based on C-peptide levels: those with lower levels beginning insulin immediately along with all the other cards in a LADA's hand (diet, exercise, metformin, et cetera); and those with higher levels of C-peptide beginning just with our non-insulin tools, while watching carefully for the appropriate time to begin insulin.[8]

Fear of needles. For many, insulin hesitancy stems from a fear of needles. Here's the thing: Insulin needles are as different from the other needles we've dealt with in doctors' offices as iPhones are from 1960s rotary landlines. The honking needles that collect our blood samples or vaccinate us have to move significant quantities, and have to poke down into blood vessels surrounded by nerves. But insulin is dosed with tiny needles that only need to get barely through your skin, and can avoid nerves and be literally painless. Sure, cramming a rotary phone into your pocket wouldn't be comfortable, but slipping a cell phone into your pocket is painless—and injecting insulin can be, too.

Fear of weight gain. There are heartbreaking stories of serious self-harm through deliberate insulin underuse, sometimes motivated by fear of weight gain. But does supplementing insulin *actually*, necessarily, lead to weight gain?

It's true that when we are falling off the insulin cliff (becoming unable to make our own insulin), we often are losing weight. Extreme lack of insulin means our body can't properly utilize our food: We literally "piss away" sugar while our muscles melt and we feel weak and exhausted (chapter 3). When this is happening our blood is filled with ketones (emergency fuel) *and* with the sugar our cells can't take up. This combination of very high ketones and very high blood sugar makes our blood acidic and puts us at risk of deadly ketoacidosis. This is not a weight loss plan, peoples!

It has been clearly shown that the best way to rev our metabolism and burn fat is to build muscle, build brown fat, and increase activity. When we gain muscle, we burn more fat just sitting around breathing. But we can't build muscle if food can't enter our cells.

It's true that high insulin can tip our body toward making fat—but high BG does so to an even greater degree! An insulin dose that is high enough to be *effective will give better health and build less fat* than an insulin dose that struggles to keep up (see chapter 6 discussion of "persistently elevated" insulin).

Underdosing insulin causes more weight gain than correctly dosing insulin. *Deliberately underdosing insulin will push your BG high, causing all kinds of harm* (chapter 6), *but will not lead to weight loss—that's a myth.*

When we do these three things simultaneously:
  ➤ moderate carbs,
  ➤ match insulin to carbs, and
  ➤ be active,

this is the best path to a healthy weight.

o o o

Bottom line: We'll gain so much benefit if we begin injecting insulin while we still make a bit of our own. Beginning insulin while we still have working beta cells will pamper and preserve our beta cells, keep food flowing to our muscles, make supplementing insulin safer and easier, and postpone our insulin cliff (the complete loss of our own insulin). The closer we suspect our insulin cliff may be, the more urgent it becomes to begin insulin now.

Exceptions: A doctor may recommend avoiding/delaying insulin in certain situations such as for patients with limited decision-making ability.

USING INSULIN IS SO MUCH EASIER TODAY—THANKS, TECHNOLOGY

In 1985, college student Gary Scheiner didn't know why he was "skinny as a clothes hanger."[9] Gary couldn't tighten his belt enough to keep his pants from falling down, often became extremely low-energy, and knew the location of every restroom in Houston. One day, watching an episode of *M*A*S*H* where a helicopter pilot has diabetes, Gary thought: *Huh . . . that sounds really familiar.*

Diagnosed with help from his TV, today Gary is a diabetes educator, author, and exercise physiologist. He laughingly describes the diabetes technology of the '80s, from "mini guillotines" where a pendulum fired at your finger to draw blood, to BG test strips that gave a color instead of a number, to a brick-size glucometer weighing a pound.

Back in the bad old days, Gary was told to plan his activities and food to match a rigid insulin regime. Today he lives much more freely, spontaneously joining in on last-minute pickup basketball or Chinese takeout— because he knows how to adjust his insulin.

For most people, the best case is when **our insulin supports *our* choices**; not when we feel we must eat to meet our insulin.

GETTING STARTED: DECISIONS, DECISIONS

When we begin insulin, we face a slew of choices. Wear a CGM (see chapter 8) and, if so what type? Syringe, pen, or pump? Basal, bolus, or both? What's up with all the types of insulin: regular, intermediate, mixed, and so on? Does switching brands matter?

We'll want to weigh and discuss each question with our medical team in terms of:

- Quality of BG control.
- Risk of dangerous lows.
- Daily effort.
- Flexibility to tailor to our schedule/lifestyle.
- Cost/insurance coverage.

Table 2 offers a brief summary of insulin types. Each is discussed in more detail below.

TABLE 2. Types of Insulin

Insulin Choices

Action:	Bolus	Basal		
	Rapid-acting. Meets the BG wave of a meal.	Slow-release. Meets the constant basal drip of BG from our liver.		
Era:	**Historic**	**Old-School**	**Modern**	
	Insulin from animals. No longer used.	Includes *Regular*, *Intermediate*, *NPH*, and *Mixed*. Less effective (most patients have worse control of highs and greater risk of lows) but for some the only option due to cost, insurance, or other factors.	*Analog* insulins. More effective, more expensive, better timed to meet meal peaks. Not available to all.	
Delivery:	**Inhaled**	**Syringe**	**Pen**	**Pump**
	Less precise dosing and less precise glycemic control. Older forms discontinued due to health concerns; some have health concerns about current forms.	Less user-friendly than a pen.	User-friendly, painless. Some pens dose to the half unit. Some users have one pen for rapid (bolus) and one for slow-release (basal); others dose only one form.	Worn continuously (can be removed for short periods). Continuously injects rapid insulin. Set to a best-guess regime, which user adjusts and fine-tunes.

Basal Insulin? Bolus Insulin? Or Both?

Our liver is constantly drizzling a small amount of background sugar into our blood (chapter 9). A healthy pancreas matches this with a steady drip of insulin to carry this sugar into hungry cells. This constant drizzle, *basal insulin,* makes up 40 to 50 percent of our daily insulin.

Other times glucose piles into our blood in a slug—maybe we ate a stegosaurus pizza, or were attacked by an irate bookstore customer. ("Why isn't this out in paperback yet?!") In response, the pancreas wants to pump out a big slug of insulin, ***bolus insulin.***

Modern analog *basal* insulins release very slowly, without a sharp peak, like a timed-release medicine. Modern analog *bolus* insulins begin to affect BG fifteen to twenty minutes after injection, have their peak effect at one hour, less effect after two hours, and little after six hours.

Some people begin with both: injecting basal once or twice a day, and injecting bolus to meet a meal or major stress. Others begin with basal only; and still others begin with bolus only.

Basal only. Some who still make their own insulin, and are just easing a toe into the insulin supplementation waters, begin with just a basal injection to add a little extra insulin to their system throughout the day. This doesn't allow precision dosing and optimal BG control, and it can complicate spontaneous exercising, so it's not my cup of tea, but some prefer it.

Rapid only. I use rapid (bolus) only. Rapid is more similar to our own insulin. It doesn't linger in the body for hours, possibly complicating things like spontaneous exercise. When I saw that pumps use rapid only, I thought: *Using a pen, I'll be my own pump.* This has worked well for me for nearly four years because I still make enough insulin to get through the night. If you can't last the night with your own insulin, you'll need to either (a) inject both basal and bolus; or (b) wear a pump.

Rapid and basal. My friends who are fully off the cliff (T1s and LADAs whose honeymoons have ended) either use a pump or carry two pens: one with basal, one with rapid. The two-pen folks are becoming less common as pump wearability and usability continually improve.

Old or New?

Older types of insulin (including *Regular, Intermediate, NPH,* and *Mixed*) are rarely prescribed now in the US, because **modern analog insulins do a better job** of meeting demand, and autoimmune diabetics who use these modern insulins have better blood sugar control.[10]

Modern analog *basal* insulins are less likely than older forms to cause a dangerous low, because they release more slowly and steadily. Modern analog *bolus* insulins do a better job than older forms of meeting the BG rise of a meal, because they act more quickly.

Regrettably, although older forms are less effective at controlling highs and have a greater risk of dangerous lows, they are less expensive, and may be the only form of insulin available to people with inadequate access to health insurance or health care.

Inhaled Insulin?

A decade ago, the advice on inhaled was simple: Don't do it. But as new types of inhaled insulin come on the market, this question is worth another look.

Inhaled insulin may cause cough and a reduction in lung function[11] (which may be temporary[12]); for this reason inhaled insulin is not recommended for smokers, ex-smokers, asthmatics, or others with specific lung vulnerabilites.[13] Inhaled insulin is delivered in four-unit doses (although some users feel they can finesse this), so dosing is less fine-tuned than with all other methods (which typically dose by the unit or half unit). Perhaps this is why research has found *less precise glycemic control* with inhaled insulin.[14]

Inhaled only delivers rapid insulin, so some use two systems: injecting long-acting insulin, then inhaling meal insulin. Some are excited that inhaled's effects begin and end more quickly, but the difference is small (five to ten minutes);[15] and because of lower dosing precision, blood sugar control is worse with inhaled.[16]

Dr. Nasser Mikhail, an endocrinologist at UCLA Medical Center, writes that inhaled insulin "is slightly less effective [than injected and] . . . its use is limited by high incidence of cough . . . and lack of long-term safety data."[17]

If you're tempted because a leftover fear of needles lingers in our society like the smell of boiled cabbage—free your mind. Today's technology makes injecting insulin easy and painless: definitely as easy as huffing or swallowing your medicine.

Syringe, Pen, or Pump?

Which fits best with your lifestyle: to wear and manage a pump that releases a near-constant stream of insulin into your system, or to give yourself multiple daily injections? In choosing your insulin delivery system, consider its accuracy, convenience, and flexibility. There are many brands of pumps, CGMs, and pens, and a full comparison is beyond the scope of this book; consult your doctor.

Insulin Pens

If you decide against a pump, I recommend a pen over a syringe. Most find pens much quicker, simpler, more mistake-proof, and more transportable than a syringe and vial. Once the cartridge is in the pen and a clean needle attached, simply dial in your dose and press a button. Pens that dose as finely as half units are ideal for LADA. Experienced injectors describe sitting in a restaurant with friends and injecting "under the table" without their friends even noticing.

I find my pen portable, simple, and quick. (Easily backpack-able.) Because my doctor prescribed the shortest (four to eight millimeter) and slimmest (thirty to thirty-two gauge) needles, I was stunned to find I could barely feel the needle going in. (Like electrical wire, needle gauges go by the fascinating upside-down logic whereby the bigger number is the smaller gauge.)

The goal is to inject into the layer of fat just under the skin; not into muscle, because that would change the action of the insulin. Needles too thick or too long can cause bruising, unnecessary pain, or accidental injection into muscle.

Today's needles are so tiny that injecting insulin hurts way less than the finger poke to test your BG. I promise. When I do it right, it is literally painless.

Insulin Pumps

Insulin pumps and continuous glucose monitors* are not the same thing (although as we go to press they are beginning to be integrated). A pump continuously injects tiny amounts of insulin into your blood. A CGM continuously monitors the BG level in your blood. You can use a CGM but not wear a pump, or vice versa. However, they are often used together.

A pump is about the size of a pack of cards. Some are worn in a pocket or pouch and connect via tubing to a needle in your body. Others are little pods that attach directly to your body. Most pumps are waterproof. Many

---

* Chapter 8 gives an overview of CGMs.

pumps can be removed for a few hours for showering, swimming, group sex bacchanals, or on other whims. Pumps can be especially helpful to children, teens, younger adults, and athletes.[18]

With a pump, the insulin delivered can be pre-programmed with a best guess at your unique needs and schedule; then this best guess can be adjusted on the fly for any schedule change or for stress, fever, exercise, or other surprises.

Features to consider in selecting a pump include readability, wearability, alarms, water resistance, output/displays, volume of insulin held, delivery increments (smallest and largest), and of course, whether a given brand is covered by your insurance. Or, most important of all for patients of a certain age: whether the decorative cover choices include "My Little Pony."

INSULIN CARE

Purchasing Insulin

> ⇢ Check the expiration date.
> ⇢ Check the strength. While U-100 is a standard strength in the US, U-40 is common overseas. Other strengths you may encounter include U-200, U-300, and U-500. A bigger number means a more concentrated (more powerful) drug.

Care and Keeping

> ⇢ Once opened, insulin expires in a month; the vial/cartridge should then be discarded.
> ⇢ Refrigerate *stored* insulin (your extra, unopened vials/cartridges) to protect it from deterioration.
> ⇢ A vial in use should *not* be refrigerated because it is more comfortable to inject room-temperature insulin.
> ⇢ Protect insulin from direct sunlight and from temperatures above eighty-five degrees Fahrenheit or below thirty-four degrees Fahrenheit.
> ⇢ Travelers and backpackers will find lightweight, water-activated reusable temperature-protection cases, such as FRIO, available in many sizes.

The Best Delivery System for You

- Will depend on many personal factors and should be decided together with your doctor.
- Will depend on whether you still make enough insulin to last the night.
- **Pump:** Often favored by youth and athletes. The technology is constantly improving. High cost makes insurance essential.
- **Pen:** Portable, simple. Carry in purse or pocket and inject as needed. Recommended: a half-unit-capable pen with four-millimeter, thirty-two-gauge needles.
- **Syringe and vial:** Less user-friendly than a pen.
- **Inhaled:** Dosed to the lungs, instead of to just below the skin. Currently does not allow the same precision when dosing. Today's inhaled options may be improved over older forms of inhaled, but safety questions remain.

o o o

HOW DO CARBS, PROTEIN, AND FAT AFFECT OUR INSULIN DOSE?

Your doctor or diabetes educator should explain how to calculate insulin for each meal—a calculation that will depend on your age, weight, sex, type of insulin, and many other factors, along with carbs, protein, and fat—so I can't get very specific here.

Many of us dose a little differently in the morning than later in the day (because of dawn effect; chapter 9). Recent stress, recent exercise, or planned upcoming exercise might also affect our dose decision.

Carbs

The key to dosing insulin is accurately estimating how many carbs you are about to eat, and injecting the correct amount to meet that. "The more accurate you are at carb counting, the better you will be able to control your blood sugar," say diabetes educators.[19]

Protein

When we eat *few* carbs, our liver takes protein from our meal and manufactures sugar from it. When a meal has abundant carbs, we don't need to consider the effect of protein, because our liver doesn't then turn protein into sugar. So if your meal is carby, match insulin to carbs. If your meal is low-carb, count carbs and add a protein factor.

Fat

Fat slows the release of glucose into the blood, spreading out and lowering our BG peak. So two meals that are otherwise the same but have very different fat contents may need different insulin protocols.

TIMING

Best case, we inject about fifteen minutes before eating, but in practice . . . life happens.

I'm that person who will wander into a host's kitchen, preview what's in the pots and pans, and ask what's in the casserole. I'll mentally plate this food in my imagination and estimate the carbs on my envisioned plate. Then I try to inject five minutes before we sit down at the table (since the food isn't in my mouth the moment I sit down).

And if the garlic mashed potatoes are so delicious I need a second helping, my insulin pen is right in my pocket, and I inject for the second helping while saying "please pass the potatoes"—I don't fret about injection timing.

Sometimes we just can't know our meal until a plate is set before us. When I inject after the plate's set before me, my insulin won't meet my BG peak quite as well, but it's usually acceptable. In a social setting, I prefer to err on the side of later injection rather than risk injecting too soon . . . since one never knows when a blessing will go long, a server will drop a plate . . . It's so awkward if I have to start stuffing candy in my mouth while friends share heartfelt gratitudes around the holiday table.

CALCULATING THE RIGHT INSULIN DOSE FOR YOUR CARBS ALWAYS IN-volves a bit of guesswork, because many things are always pushing on our BG (chapter 9). The lower your carbs in a given meal, the smaller the margin of error. "If you eat too many carbohydrates," says Dr. Morstein, "it will be nearly impossible to have stable, low glucose numbers without having [dangerous lows] as a regular occurrence."[20]

WHAT ELSE AFFECTS OUR INSULIN?

We all have daily rhythms to our hormones, energy, and blood sugars. Even in an insulin-normal person, BG varies over the day, typically highest when he wakes, and lowest right when sensible countries have siestas; or, in the US, just in time to fall asleep during 1:00 p.m. chemistry class.[21]

Puberty, growth spurts, being premenstrual (having high estrogen in the days before menstruation), or running a fever can all *increase* the need for insulin.

Improving our diet, getting good sleep, meditating/controlling stress, losing weight, increasing insulin sensitivity through exercise or medication, and improving our microbiome can all *reduce* insulin requirements.

THOUGHTS FOR ATHLETES

Too much sugar in the blood can cause fatigue and limit aerobic capacity because it limits our blood cells' capacity to pick up oxygen and carry it to the muscles. High BG can also cause muscle stiffness, make strains and pulls more likely, and increase likelihood of dehydration and cramping. Athletes perform best when blood sugar is in the 80 to 140 range.

Different types of exercise affect my BG differently. A two-hour bike ride or steady jog *lowers* my BG steadily and consistently. Even exercise as modest as being on my feet all day at the bookstore shelving books and helping customers reduces my lunchtime insulin dose.

I was surprised at first when heavy exertions, like pushing heavy wheelbarrows, or a high-energy muscle-building workout, *raised* my BG. Makes sense, though—in the long steady jog, our body is burning energy and adding "locks" to hungry cells (lowering insulin resistance). In the intense muscle challenge, our body says: *Sudden big energy demand happening— liver, please toss sugar into the blood right now!*

If I know I'm going for a bike ride after lunch, I take less insulin at lunch. If I spontaneously exercise right after lunch and didn't reduce my lunchtime dose because I didn't know I'd exercise shortly afterward, I typically eat a small fast-carb snack just before the exercise, such as a few slices of apple. And of course, anytime I exercise (or go anywhere) I have a portable, fast-carb snack like dried fruit or a granola bar in my pocket.

Gary Scheiner writes about his experience with exercise and insulin:

> After being diagnosed with diabetes my passion for staying in shape soared to a whole new level . . . Unfortunately, a serious low blood sugar often followed the emotional high I got from exercise . . .
>
> Perhaps the greatest breakthrough . . . was my decision . . . to try an insulin pump . . . For the first time in almost ten years I could sleep past 8 am without having my blood sugar skyrocket. I could delay my lunch without bottoming out. And best of all was that I could work out to my heart's content without going low in the middle of the night. In fact, I haven't had a single severe low blood sugar since I started on the pump more than 15 years ago . . .
>
> Personally, I've found CGM to be the best thing . . . the alerts have saved me from many highs and lows. Perhaps the best thing about them is that they provide context to glucose values. Knowing you're 100 is one thing; knowing that you're 100 and dropping or rising quickly is another.
>
> I was officially sold on CGM when I completed my first ten-mile run . . . I ran the entire course with my CGM receiver in my fist . . . My control was immaculate, and I finished the race without having to stop once.[22]

AN INSULIN REGIME IS NEVER ONE-AND-DONE

The more involved and hands-on we are with insulin, the better our BG control.[23]

"Getting on insulin" is not a one-and-done. We typically start with a low dose and titrate up very slowly, waiting three to five days between each increase, because it takes several days for insulin to reach its full effect in the body. It may take a month or more before our insulin regime is fully in place.

It's not about instant perfection, it's about improvement. Each day is an experiment. With the help of our journal (chapter 9) we make small, sensible adjustments, and our control will gradually improve.

"Using insulin requires being calm, patient, and attentive. It can take weeks, and sometimes months, until a full protocol is figured out," says Dr. Morstein. Make one small change at a time, and watch the effect of a change over more than one day, meal, or scenario. "Patients need to know that there is always some 'winging it' when using insulin," adds Morstein, "and educated guessing is common . . . *educated guessing in a step-by-step process is effective and safe*"[24] (my emphasis).

STAYING SAFE

For most LADAs, beginning insulin means crossing a significant mental divide. We step forward both into better health (lower big-picture risks) and also into a new risk of sudden dangerous BG lows—the kind that might leave us standing in the flames, gawping at the open doorway. That's a vulnerable thought, especially for solo adventurers. Through technology, and by reaching out to friends, family, and sometimes strangers, insulin users build a safety net.

Most insulin users always carry glucose tablets. (Or a juice box, piece of fruit, energy bar, or tiny box of raisins.) Most own, teach friends and family how to use, and replace yearly, a glucagon kit. Most wear a medic alert: There are bracelets, dog tags, shoelace tags, sports-type wristbands—some have even had TYPE ONE DIABETIC tattooed on a wrist.

There is a natural resistance to wearing a diabetes ID. Often, we don't want to feel defined by our disease, or prejudged by people we're just meeting. On the other hand, death is pretty permanent.

KEY TAKEAWAYS

1. Many LADAs wait too long to begin insulin. Ideally, we begin supplementing insulin while still making a bit of our own.
2. Done wisely, supplementing insulin does not condemn us to weight gain; by helping build muscle, it can make reaching our ideal weight easier.

3. Insulin goals: have excellent BG control, reduce both peaks and lows, minimize weight gain, minimize daily effort and expense, and choose technologies that fit our lifestyle.

4. Starting insulin does not mean we stop using our other tools such as exercise, metformin, vitamin D, carb counting, and meal spacing (chapter 16). Insulin supplementation works best when it's one of many cards in our hand.

You're in Charge

5. You'll be asked to make a lot of choices when you begin insulin. Think of it like choosing which you'd prefer to drive: pickup or convertible, Cadillac or Kia? None of them do everything perfectly, but which one best suits *you*?

6. For most, using insulin requires some educated guessing. Educated guessing in a supported step-by-step process is effective and safe.

7. The more involved and hands-on we are with insulin, the better our BG control, health, and energy.

Expect Change

8. With LADA we expect to end up fully dependent on insulin eventually. Beginning insulin while we still make some of our own lets us start in a safer situation, with some native insulin to cushion our lows and highs.

Demand Change

9. Both in the US and across the globe, access to insulin is extremely precarious for many, due to availability or to expense. Every year our children die due to lack of insulin access. Chapter 24 gives a small glimpse into the crisis and rising solutions.

o o o

Beginning insulin once scared me more than a grizzly, cottonmouth, and brain-eating amoeba all rolled into one: It made me feel vulnerable. But as I spend more time with insulin, it begins to look less like a brain-eating amoeba and more like a powerful river: worthy of respect, yet more friend than foe.

Insulin made my world bigger again. Restaurants, birthday parties, and Thanksgiving are a lot more fun now. While climbing Aasgard Pass, swimming Colchuck Lake, and dancing to the Paperboys are still as fun as ever. Who knew?

Insulin, says Supreme Court Justice Sotomayor, "is the medicine that saves my life every day."[25]

14 MIND THE MIND

Soothing Stress and Building Support

*[There is] a significant co-morbidity of diabesity with . . .
depression. Importantly, not only is the prevalence of mood
disorders elevated in patients with type 2 diabetes, depressed
patients are also more prone to develop diabetes.*
    —Dr. Aitak Farzi, Medical University of Graz, Austria[1]

He who finds no way to rest cannot long survive the battle.
    —James Baldwin

THE CHILDREN'S BOOK *JUST ASK* BY SUPREME COURT JUSTICE SONIA Sotomayor features children with conditions from diabetes to Tourette's. In an interview with Trevor Noah, Sonia explains how the title was born. In a restaurant one evening, Sonia went into the restroom to give herself an insulin shot, and as she was injecting, a stranger entered the restroom. After dinner, as Sonia was leaving the restaurant, she passed the stranger's table and overheard her tell a companion: "She's a drug addict." Sonia said:

And I stopped. And the first emotion I felt was shame. I was mortified. And then, I thought about it for a second, and I turned around and marched back to the woman and said: "I'm not a drug addict. I'm a diabetic. And that shot you saw me take is the medicine that saves my life every day, insulin. And if you don't understand when someone's doing something different than you expect, just ask. Don't presume the worst in people." And I walked away.[2]

All her life, since age seven, Sonia had hidden her diabetes, even from friends. "I was embarrassed by my condition . . . I thought my friends would make fun of it, and so I hid it," she says. But as an adult she had a life-changing moment. She was hosting a gathering of close friends, "people who I know adore and love me, and who take care of me in every situation. And all of a sudden, I fell asleep on my bed. And they thought I was asleep. But really I was in a sugar low. I was semi-unconscious . . . Well, my friends didn't know what was happening. Because I had never told them [I had diabetes]. And **so I almost died in a room full of people who loved me**" (my emphasis).

From that day on, Sonia decided to never again hide her condition. "Not only because it was dangerous for me, but because if something had happened to me, and my friends were there, they would never be able to forgive themselves . . . I think it was a kindness to me and . . . to my friends where I then chose to become open about my condition."

IN THE EARLY DAYS, I DIDN'T CHOOSE TO TELL EVERYONE ON THE street, or everyone who sat down at my table, that I had LADA. I was still figuring out what LADA meant and how to handle it, and I didn't want to have to fend off a barrage of well-meaning interrogation. I didn't want "diabetes" to be the first thing every new person I met knew about me. I was just plain tired of talking about diabetes, especially when it was so new that talking about it revved up my anxiety, loss, confusion, and depression.

While I didn't want to have to "out" my diabetes to every random person, I also hated appearing a picky eater—"Excuse me, what's in this?" I wanted to be flexible, gracious, and adventurous, game for whatever was set on the table, be that lutefisk or gefilte fish, caviar or chitlins, mopane worms, fried okra, chocolate-covered ants, guinea pig, haggis, or spotted dick. We give others a gift when we embrace their food.

In my experience it almost never works to keep the diabetes disclosure to one sentence.

"I gave up drinking," my friend says, and others instantly grasp that this may be a sensitive topic and don't insist on details.

"No bread," I say, "thanks." If I add "because I have diabetes" I often find myself sucked down into the quagmire of a conversation I'd rather not have. Bringing up diabetes seems to inevitably prompt questions; and if I don't answer those questions, I'm rude, and why did I bring it up at all then?

As Justice Sotomayor reflected, the decision whether to reveal our diabetes can feel fraught. I waited to "out" my diabetes until I felt confident and informed, so that hurtful questions (or seemingly endless ones) didn't knock me off course.

LADA AND STRESS

Research shows that stress makes us sick, raising our risk of diabetes, inflammation, heart attack, and other serious illnesses.[3] And research shows that stress makes us gain weight,[4] releasing hormones whose job is to build us a nice cushy safety zone. Further research shows that inflammation and the microbiome—part of a tightly knit trifecta (chapter 11)—are tightly linked to mental health, with the power to either worsen or alleviate depression and anxiety.[5]

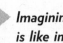

Imagining you can manage your diabetes yet ignore stress is like imagining you can manage diabetes without thinking about your food.

OUR AUTOMATIC STRESS RESPONSE IS LIGHTNING-QUICK, TRIGGERING faster than we can consciously think; that's how we survive. It sets off physiological changes, including the liver dumping sugar into our blood.

While stress triggers in a blink, it dissipates slowly. We need downtime with stress turned off to clean away the physical residues in our body—the tension in our muscles, and the stress hormones and high BG in our bloodstream.

In LADA, our limited insulin is a three-year-old chasing chickens: We take longer to clear away high BG after stress triggers a spike, so we suffer the effects of chronic elevated stress more acutely than most people.

In ancient times, people didn't trip over a grizzly's paw every eight minutes, and we had good downtime between stresses. In the modern era, many of our physical, emotional, and mental ills are due to the fact that our body isn't throwing the stress switch to "off" often enough or long enough.

Stress allows hypervigilance, which lets us survive battle. After prolonged hypervigilance, many struggle with PTSD: Their body no longer reliably turns off its threat response.

At the right level and frequency, stress can be energizing, making us more successful and happier. The wrong kind of stress PTSD's us. Much of the difference between good stress and bad depends on how we perceive the stress—on our inner narrative.

Teaching stress management to CEOs, the military, or the police, author davidji never uses the word *meditation*. He talks to them about "tactical breathing." Passing along ancient wisdoms, he uses language his listeners will accept.

No one lives a life without stress, says davidji, who calls stress "universal . . . contagious [and] relentless." "Stress is how we respond when our needs are not met."[6]

We want to bring our whole brain into our stress response so we can ride stress's energizing surge, keep our response appropriate to the situation, and turn our response off when the coast is clear. Whether we call it *tactical breathing* or *meditation*, managing stress is about creating a micropause, so that a consciously chosen response can replace the automatic one. Consciously breathing deeply and slowly is a simple yet powerful way to reduce stress.

As neuroscientist Dr. Bolte reminds us, an emotion that lasts longer than ninety seconds is one we are retriggering with our inner narrative.[7]

There are a bazillion breathing, chanting, and similar techniques for managing stress, more than can fit in this book—I'd need a whole bookstore! Here are two techniques many find helpful:

Box Breathing

Count to four as you breathe in. Count to four as your hold that breath. Count to four as you breathe out. Count to four as you pause between breaths. In-hold-out-hold. Notably, used by Navy SEALs.

Mantra

Mantra literally means "mind-tool." Repeat (out loud or mentally) any calming or motivating word or phrase, letting it block out negative self-talk. Examples of mantras include "Yes I can," "I am enough," and "Breathing in, I smile. Breathing out, I let it go."

o o o

In addition to responding differently when stress attacks, we may wish to practice deep relaxation daily or weekly, clearing our mind and our stress molecules at a more profound level. We might meditate in a yoga pose, or in a comfy chair, or while walking. We might use common things that could irritate us, like each red light that halts us while driving, or each telemarketing call during dinner, as a *mindfulness bell*: a reminder to take three deep, relaxing breaths.

Perhaps on some evening when we've decided to form a new habit (for me, a habit that doesn't revolve around opening my freezer), we might sit or lie in a comfortable position for ten minutes, breathing deeply and calmly, and consciously relaxing our muscles. We think about each muscle group one by one. *Resting, breathing deeply, I relax my toes . . . I relax the arch of my foot . . . I relax my ankles . . . I relax my calves . . .*

I asked one friend if she meditated and she said, "Sort of. I pray. I go out into the garden in the evening, and watch the day fade and the stars come out, and talk over my day with God. My mind feels so much cleaner and quieter afterward."

This is science: Research has shown that peaceful breathing and other relaxation techniques lower levels of stress hormones, clear stress symptoms from our bodies, help us eat healthfully, and *reduce our incidence of many diseases* including diabetes.[8]

"Meditation is neither shutting things out nor off. It is seeing things clearly, and deliberately positioning yourself differently in relationship to them," says Jon Kabat-Zinn.

Radically changing our food identity is a stress; counting calories is a stress; watching others eat things we'd love to be eating, but are avoiding for the sake of our brain, eyes, and loved ones, is a stress; managing a chronic disease is a stress. If we decide to see these as mountain-size impediments, they may crush us; if we see them as challenges, we can crush them.

LIKE OTHER ASPECTS OF CARB-CRAFT AND DIABETIC HEALTH, CHAN-neling stress in more healthful ways is the art of gentle persistence: Beginning again. And again. Successful people think mistakes can teach, and that resilience and perseverance are what keep us in the game.

My friend Ginger has likened gentle persistence to the way you need to blow on embers to revive a fire. If you blow too ferociously, you blow the flame out. If you blow weakly, in the wrong place, or stop too soon: also no good. You have to be steady and focused, and blow with effort but not obsession and drama. With gentle persistence, the flame comes to life.

A few favorite resources for quieting the stress chickens:

> * Thich Nhat Hanh, *Peace Is Every Step.*
> * Brené Brown, *Daring Greatly.*
> * Pema Chödrön, *Living Beautifully with Uncertainty and Change.*
> * James Baraz and Shoshana Alexander, *Awakening Joy.*

o o o

WHEN WE LACK SUPPORT, WE CAN BUILD IT

At a party, the hostess who has just been urging me to eat more scalloped potatoes, to try the sweet-and-sour rice, and not to miss the homemade sourdough, begins to pass me a plate of homemade fudge. As I start to reach for the plate, she jerks it roughly away.

"Oh, sorry," she says. "You can't eat this."

NO MATTER HOW HELPFULLY INTENDED, WHEN SOMEONE PUTS MY eating under a microscope, it can be triggering. As I realized when I burst out laughing reading an online LADA forum.

A LADA had asked the group: What do *you* say when someone asks, "Are you sure you can eat this?"

My favorite replies:

- I'll do my best. At what point would you like an update?
- Are you sure you should ask that?
- I'm going to give it a go. I'll let you know how it comes out.
- Yes. Thank you. (Full stop. Eye contact.)

As my friend Maggie, who had to endure idiotic comments about her "free boob job" when she had breast cancer, puts it: "Sometimes it's fun to think about what we *might* say in reply. Even if what we ultimately say out loud is kinder."

IF YOU'RE LOOKING TO SUPPORT A LOVED ONE WITH DIABETES, RE-member that in the weeks and months after their diagnosis, they are likely on a journey through grief. Look to them for guidance. Remember that trying to *diet for* someone is not support. Pity is not support. Unsolicited advice is not support, and often reveals what we *don't* know about the other person's situation. Links to resources can be support, if offered in the right manner.

In general: Try not to make us feel more anxious and self-conscious about food than we already do.

Speaking just for myself, here's what I found helpful:

- Don't judge what your friend eats. You don't know what the past week has held for her food-wise or stress-wise. She may be rewarding herself for doing great. She may "need" this right now in some way not clear to you. If she has *asked* you to do or say something partic-ular in regard to her food, great. Otherwise, shut up.
- It's hard living under a low-carb ceiling. Don't make it harder. If your friend decides there's nothing he can eat at the taco stand, don't take offense. He's not slamming your culture.

- Listen when he wants to talk about diabetes. Don't keep asking when he doesn't want to talk about diabetes. We all need a life that's bigger than our disease.
- Include options that don't revolve around food. Say, "Do you want to meet for coffee tomorrow or shall we walk the park loop?"
- Don't assume. Listen and love. If you're wondering how you can help, say, "How can I help?"

As Brené Brown reminds us in a hilarious YouTube about the difference between empathy and sympathy, if you're looking to support someone, beware of statements that begin: "Well, *at least* . . ."

Guilty. This used to be me. I suppose it's natural to wish to comfort others, but perhaps I sometimes did this to take away my own discomfort: I tried to say something positive about any situation.

"Oh, your three grandchildren were run over by a bullet train? Well, *at least* it was quick."

Next time *at least* pops into my head, maybe I'll just say instead: "I'm so sorry." And then listen. And take my cues from the person who's hurting.

SAFETY NET

We're in control when we're cooking at home. When I go out, I like to have a safety net.

- Concealed carry. I travel with a safe protein, such as nuts, in purse or pocket.
- I avoid being served by others. When I say, "Just half that much please," they somehow think they are doing me a favor by giving me more.
- I give more thought to what I bring to potlucks instead of a last-minute swing by the store for chips or a pie to fly. I bring something healthful, substantial, and with enough protein that, should it be the only thing I can eat at the potluck, will give me a safe, satisfying serving.

- I don't go hungry to social events. My inner mockingbird tells me I'm a weirdo for eating before going to a potluck. But it puts me in a healthier space, a space that's more about people and less about food.

YOUR MOST IMPORTANT SUPPORTER: A DOCTOR WHO "GETS" YOU

For me, it was a struggle learning to advocate for myself in today's medical system. If you are a diagnosed diabetic, of any type, stripe, or flavor, never apologize for working to be your healthiest. Your questions and concerns are as valid as anyone's. Don't let yourself be dismissed as one of "the worried well" if you're a partial success story, and have worked hard to earn a healthy A1c—yet *still need help*.

Your doctor doesn't have to win the Miss Congeniality award as long as she really gets you—and really gets LADA.

With one in three Americans likely to have diabetes by 2050 according to the CDC, the strain on our system looms. With diabetes, doctors face an avalanche of need, an enormous spectrum of variability, ever-new treatments and ever-changing nutrition wisdom.

Our doctor has to focus first on preventing horrible complications— kidney failure, blindness, stroke. This may not leave her a lot of time to discuss *living well* with diabetes. If I had fifteen minutes to bring someone up to speed on diabetes, I'd probably have a bit of a script, too. In her allotted minutes, the doctor is supposed to carefully digest our long printout of lab results and—often knowing little about our culture, priorities, and activities—prescribe medications, explain side effects, try to field questions about costs (do I look like Siri?), and then explain everything in this book, including a crash course on how radically our understanding of nutrition has changed in the past decade.

Not every doctor is equally knowledgeable about nutrition. *Time* notes that as recently as 2015, only a third of US medical schools offered the recommended twenty-five hours of nutrition curriculum; and that when med school graduates were given a basic nutritional quiz by an international medical journal in 2016, the average graduate got half of the questions wrong—as *Time* put it, "a failing grade."[9]

Doctors are trying to meet us where we are. If we don't tell them anything about ourselves, their most on-average-correct assumption is that *we* are average, and eat the SAD standard American diet. If you want your doctor to see you differently, you have to speak up.

A BIGGER LIFE

I can get stuck in the idea that my illness is a weakness, something I "should be doing better at." My support network is a huge part of my mental health. Pushing myself farther out into the world, farther out of my comfort zone, helps too. As I make my world fuller and complicated by larger issues, I focus less on the contents of my refrigerator.

"The knowledge comes to me that I have space within me for a second, timeless, larger life," wrote Rainer Maria Rilke.

A new tavern opened in town, and I stopped in with Jayson (yes, the friend whose heart attack launched my diagnosis—thanks, Jayson). After watching me flounder trying to order a drink that didn't have too many carbs, Jayson asked for an empty glass, poured me a third of his beer, and said, as he slid it across the table, "Jackie, you need to stop stressing about food, stop stressing about family, and get out of town for a while."

Touché. Sometimes friends remind us of what we already know.

A few weeks later, puppy and I point the car south. I've got a tent, sleeping bag, skis, swimsuit, Ava's hot springs guide, six thousand dog toys—everything but a plan.

At dusk in Snow Canyon, the full moon rolls along the curves of petrified dunes as a canyon wren duets with the throaty whispers of an owl. In Utah, I hike slot canyons, sleep in a female hogan, and am served a café's special of the day—keto salad—by polygamist wives in crisp white bonnets. In Oregon, as I soak in Cougar Hot Springs, aging high school sweethearts regale me with stories of friends' jailbreaks.

In Claire's Café, tucked among the saguaros and spiky century plants of the Santa Catalinas, every inch of the walls covered with local art for sale, this cartoon is taped to the register:

> A couple, menu open, asks their waitress: "We don't eat meat, fish, eggs, or gluten. What do you recommend?"
> The waitress answers: "A taxi."

Wearing a wonderful hat dangling crocheted flowers (it looks like something out of *Go, Dog, Go*), Claire sits down at my table, introduces me to poets that wander in, tells me about her life in New York City, pours me more coffee, and then is off to join friends at the next table as I head out to hike along the Arizona trail.

"Life is great and good and fascinating and eternal, and if you dwell so much on yourself and flounder and fluff about, you miss the mighty eternal current that is life," wrote Etty Hillesum.

KEY TAKEAWAYS

1. With LADA, the effects of stress are as important as the effects of food or exercise.
2. Stress is an automatic hormonal response. Following stress, other hormones, including insulin, help us rebalance. Just as we now consciously manage our insulin when we eat, we also now need to adjust insulin for stress.
3. Create a micropause between the stressful event and your response. Breathe. Choose. You can't be in charge of everything, but you can be in charge of yourself.
4. What will *your* safety net be for social eating situations?
5. You deserve a doctor who can hear you and communicate well with you. Believe in yourself, advocate for yourself.
6. Ask for support. Let friends and loved ones know:
   > Please don't scrutinize or judge my eating. Don't try to eat "for" me.
   > Please don't assume. Listen and love.
   > "At least" can lead a conversation wrong. You may imagine you are comforting me, but may instead be minimizing or dismissing my experience, and that can hurt.

o o o

PART II | SUMMARY

Our doctor is a crucial guide and our best supporter, but whether we are healthy with LADA is up to us. Many have to become proactive just to get correctly diagnosed, or to find a doctor who *gets* LADA. As we fine-tune our BG goals and other health goals, we become even more involved. And each and every day, whether we meet those goals rests on our shoulders.

Food, stress, fever, sleep quality, and other factors constantly push on our BG. Matching carbs to insulin is not rocket science, but it's not third-grade flash cards, either.

LADA interweaves with many of our body systems. On the downside, that means a learning curve; but on the upside, it means we have many tools for health; or as some think if it, many different cards in our hand. Cards from brown fat to vitamin D, from building our natural GLP-1 to destressing with favorite friends.

"Hand me a pill so I can keep running myself into the ground," some days sounded easier than treating myself like a person I love. But good sleep, stress reduction, joyous activity—many of the same things that pamper *us* also pamper our beta cells. Well, darn it. Now we *have* to treat ourselves well. For the kids or grandkids: to make it to their graduations. For our spouse: to make it to that special anniversary. For our horse, gerbil, dog, cat, or poker partner. Or even, who knows, for ourself.

"There is one consolation in being sick; and that is the possibility that you may recover to a better state than you were ever in before," wrote Henry David Thoreau.

CHECKLIST FOR HEALTH

❐ You've gotten comfortable with a technology to test your BG, and have begun your journal. You know why occasional strange readings might occur and understand the need for repetition.

❏ You have a list of your top three questions to answer with your BG meter.

❏ You've set a *time in range* goal. (Or, if you don't have a CGM, you've set a goal for maximum and minimum BG and have a testing plan designed to reveal highs and lows.)

❏ You've tasted fermented foods, you've found some you like, and they are in your fridge right now.

❏ You've increased your activity level by 15 percent (unless you were already a super-athlete), choosing activities that are fun and realistically fit your schedule.

❏ You have a support network and a self-compassionate stress management plan that is not fictional or something you'll do "when you have time."

❏ You're determined to pamper your beta cells, reduce inflammation, and gently bring your BG into excellent range.

❏ You've gained enough insight to bring informed questions to your doctor about insulin, metformin, vitamin D, and possibly other medications.

○ ○ ○

Now, with a tool belt bristling with these tools, we're ready to return to the question of food, no longer wailing "What can I eat?" but instead asking: "How do I enjoy the flavors and foods I love in a way that supports and protects my health?"

PART III

JOYFUL CARB-CRAFT

15 MY JOURNEY TO CRAFTY

From Clueless to Confident

*The low-carb diet is **the** diet for diabetes.*
—Dr. Mona Morstein[1]

"LET'S HAVE A COZY GIRLFRIENDS' BREAKFAST!" WENDY GROUP-TEXTS. "O'Grady's?"

When I discovered Sunday breakfast out, it felt like one of life's great occasional treats—really, you can go out for *breakfast*? I add my enthusiastic yes! to the flurry of thumbs-up emojis.

But as I slide the phone back into my pocket, that old *What can I eat?* that's always on repeat cranks up the volume.

It's been five weeks since my d-bomb (diagnosis): enough time and practice with my glucometer to be startled time and again when foods I "knew" were "healthy" rocketed my BG up into the danger zone. Foods from favorite "healthy" cafés: a salmon-veggie wrap; half a whole-grain bagel; a bowl of vegetable soup with small green salad—these meals had blasted my BG out of my safe zone. I'm feeling twitchy and gun-shy.

I've added lots of "don'ts" to my list, but very few "dos." I'm eating things I'm bored with (for breakfast: eggs . . . almonds . . . lettuce . . . actually, that's all I've got so far). Meanwhile I'm devoting a lot of mental energy to not-eating foods I love (pancakes, muffins, bagels, waffles, granola, oatmeal, hash browns—yikes, if I get going on *this* list I'll never stop).

But I love Wendy, and haven't seen her since her recent move—I'm not going to miss a chance to spend time with her. And I have lead time! I click on O'Grady's website and pore over their menu. Most items are a clear no. But here's a roasted pepper and mushroom omelet—sounds delicious.

ON O'GRADY'S PAVING-STONE PATIO, A WATERFALL MURMURS AND rosy-headed finches twitter in the aspens. Scents of chai, cinnamon, warm crostini, and fresh-baked muffins swirl as Wendy in her dozen silver rings, a lock of dark hair falling across her eyes, pulls us each into a hug. While the others open their menus, I push mine aside, lean back, and smile. I can give all my attention to my friends because my food situation is completely solved.

Until I order.

The waitress frowns. "We don't have that today."

"Oh. It was on your online menu."

"The *online* menu, well, we don't offer everything there every day."

"Okay, what omelets do you have today?"

"No omelets today. But the brioche French toast is to die for."

She has no idea that in my case this is literally true. (And I'm tempted anyway.)

Now everyone else has ordered and I'm scrabbling through the menu.

A biscuit breakfast sandwich—I love biscuits! I mean I used to. Banana pancakes, loco moco, grilled naan, breakfast croissant, maple-pecan waffles . . . they whisper my name, but nope, nope, nope—they're all on the no-fly list. I just want it to end.

Under "sides" I see: eggs.

The waitress nods. "Biscuits, naan, toast, or homefries with that?"

"No thanks."

"A side salad?"

Oh, what a great idea. "Yes please." I smile. *Something* has been salvaged.

Which is how I came to pay $13.50 for two scrambled eggs and a pile of plain iceberg lettuce on a day I was mightily tired of both.

It felt a bit like going to a vindaloo restaurant rotating atop a skyscraper and ordering PBJ off the kids' menu. You can do it, but why?

Restaurant fear. Would I ever fully enjoy a meal out again? Was the relaxing celebration of Sunday breakfast out as lost to me as waffles drowned in Vermont maple syrup and piled high with strawberries and freshly whipped cream? Could we just meet at the park next time?

I left delighted to have seen my friends, but at the same time deep down I felt dissatisfied, irritable; drooly as a dog who had a steak waved under her nose, then jerked away.

Quite the privileged problem, I scolded myself. Still, I felt teased by the space itself and all the old memories it held for me, by the smell of maple cookies, blueberry scones, and fresh-ground coffee, the laughter of the other diners, the old wooden tables, the tinkle of copper wind chimes in the aspens.

It would be another year before I would learn how brain chemistry, food, and memory intertwine; and how people, places, sights, smells, and sounds can trigger us when we're trying to change what we eat (chapter 21). A little bell of recognition would go off when I read that research. O'Grady's came to symbolize for me the way our brains can mess with us when we're trying to change how we eat.

TAKE TWO: CHERRY BLOSSOM FESTIVAL

One year after the O'Grady's debacle, I'm exploring Seattle with friends. We've just taken the light rail back from the Cherry Blossom Festival and are walking up to Jet City Improv to buy tickets. We have an hour until the show starts, haven't had dinner . . .

"Look," says Noah, "across the street."

He points to a hole-in-the-wall noodle restaurant, bright red-and-gold Chinese lettering painted on the windows. It's packed with customers and cheerfully noisy.

"I'm game for anything," I say. Because that's who I *want* to be. Even though: It's a *noodle* restaurant. And noodles are straight-up carbs, and I'm at this point matching carbs and insulin just by reducing the carbs I eat. A bowl of noodles is definitely on my no-fly list.

As we approach the counter to scan the menu, I'm relaxed. If there's nothing on the menu I can eat, I'll enjoy the atmosphere, my friends, and some jasmine tea . . . and there's a bag of almonds in my purse I can eat in the theater while others munch popcorn. If I'm hungry after the show, I'll figure something out later.

Never mind; here under side dishes is something translated, beneath the Chinese characters, simply as "broccoli." Broccoli-what, I wonder? Well, I'll give it a try. If it turns out to be something I can't eat, I'll give it away to my friends.

It turns out to be exactly as advertised: simply broccoli, in a fragrant broth flecked with chili. It turns out to be satisfying, spicy, and scrumptious.

While Noah, who recently traveled in China with his school, enthusiastically compares pulled noodles to shaved noodles, waving his chopsticks like imaginary knives, everyone offers me a few bites from their piled-high noodle bowls. My BG would hit the stratosphere if I ate a whole bowl, but I'm loving these delicious samplings! This hole-in-the-wall eatery becomes a highlight of our Seattle visit.

Apparently #itgetsbetter.

Give Carb-craft a little time to sink in: Once it becomes muscle memory, you'll once again move through the world having fun and eating delicious food.

What Is Carb-Craft?

1. Carbs are not "bad." A carbohydrate is simply any food that isn't a protein or fat. This includes most of the food energy in spinach, cauliflower, blueberries, pomegranates, and other healthy foods—it includes most of the food energy on the planet.
2. That said, there are many kinds of carbs. Upcoming chapters will help sort them out.
3. Our body used to run on autopilot, seamlessly matching our insulin with our carbs. With LADA, we now do this consciously. That's Carb-craft.
4. **Cut the carbs, keep the joy.**

o o o

16 CARB-CRAFT FUNDAMENTALS

Fiber, Fasting, Glycemic Index, Snacking, Martha, and More

*Priorities are reduction in **refined** grains, starches, sugars, and [**processed**] meats . . . increasing intakes of fruits, vegetables, nuts, yogurt, fish, vegetable oils, and whole grains; [and] sleeping at least 7–8 hours nightly [my emphasis].*
   —Dr. Dariush Mozaffarian, dean of the School of Nutrition at Tufts University[1]

CORONAVIRUS THREW GROCERY SHOPPING INTO A BRAVE NEW WORLD. We suddenly valued junk mail, because toilet paper disappeared off store shelves. Waiting in enormous checkout lines snaking down aisles, strangers furtively played "I'll show you mine if you show me yours."

In a Safeway where the canned goods aisle, the potato bin, and the frozen meat display were all eerily empty, I overheard one fellow mutter to his neighbor: "I heard you can still get chicken at the King Soopers on Broadway . . . what have you heard about potatoes?"

I was wondering about potatoes too, but in a more existential way. Still in line, having finished both Tolstoy novels I'd brought, I picked up a checkout magazine: a *Time* special edition on nutrition. "Mini-meals or Three Squares?" the cover teased, along with "What About Fat?," "Food and Your Mood," and my favorite, "Is Your Dog a Vegan?"

Time reminded me that eating can be complicated for anyone. (Except my puppy. Her food test: If it's not moving, eat it. If it's moving: Even better!) And I was chasing my tail a bit, too. Because *healthful for us insulin cherishers is different* than for the insulin-affluent. Here's the checkout-stand "skinny" *just for us*.

To Carb-craft means to stop being a follower of mysterious decrees (*Never eat purple foods!*) and to understand underlying reasons, empowering us to tailor big-picture rules to our own body, culture, and joy.

Since the broccoli, carrots, and daikon in the vegetable aisle don't have nutrition labels, we'll want a big-picture understanding of what's in different types of foods and why.

PLANTS VERSUS ANIMALS

Plants

Of the three things to eat—carbohydrate, protein, and fat—plant-based foods are most often a mixture of all three. It's hard to get protein or fat from a whole plant food without getting a solid serving of carbohydrates as well.

Animals

Animals munch plants and digest them into protein and fat. There are no carbs in a simple animal-based food (although there might be in the final dish; carbs might be added during cooking/prep). Animal-based foods, whether meat, dairy, or egg, are a mixture of protein and fat. A few animal-based foods are nearly pure fat (butter, whipping cream).

If You're Going to Cut Carbs...

Since the only things to eat are carbs, protein, and fat, if we want to cut carbs—what's left? I didn't even need all the fingers on one hand to figure that one out.

Bummer, I thought, *that's not who I want to be.*

I'd been eating largely meat-free meals my whole adult life. I loved thin-crust arugula-and-chanterelle pizza, and Thai ginger eggplant drizzled with spicy peanut sauce. Would I now need to instead eat big slabs of meat, heavy with cloying fat?

Good news: Whether you love or avoid meat, Carb-craft offers mouthwatering options. When pondering plant-based or animal-based, there's a lot more to weigh than the total number of carbs, including religious, ethical, heritage, ecological, and other pros and cons, as we'll discuss further in chapter 18. For now, know that Carb-craft is inclusive of options from vegan to keto, from halal to kosher, from gluten-free to paleo to pescatarian and more.

Carb-craft is **balancing carbs with insulin while eating healthful foods,** and there are many ways to do that.

FRUITS AND VEGETABLES

What do we even mean by these two words? A grocer means one thing, and a botanist means something different. *Vegetables* is a sloppy, inexact term for edible leaves, stems, and roots, as well as certain flowers (broccoli, artichokes) and certain fruits (seed "packages," like tomatoes, peppers, cucumbers, avocados).

Stems and Leaves

Stems and leaves (collards, spinach, bok choy) are where plants capture energy, spinning sunlight into gold. Stems and leaves tend to be rich sources of vitamins and fiber with relatively few carbs.

Roots

Roots are where overwintering plants store food: like a root cellar. Just as my grandma Dot stashed her homemade persimmon preserves in the cellar, plants store sugar and starch in roots (potatoes, beets, cassava, jicama). Root vegetables are typically packed with carbs, and many are also great sources of vitamins and fiber.

Seeds

Like my Polish immigrant great-great-grands, most plants dote on the next generation. Seeds (beans, quinoa, almonds, flax, coconuts) typically hold a plant's highest concentration of protein and fat, along with a big bankroll of carbs. This is why seeds—notably corn, beans, rice, and wheat—are the foods that built most of the world's large, city-dwelling civilizations, and the foods that many plant-based eaters depend on for protein and fat.

Fruits

Fruits are a package around seeds to entice animals. They are the little temptations plants wave to domesticate us animals. When you eat a strawberry or raspberry, you've been beguiled into carrying seeds far and wide, inside you, and back in the day you deposited those seeds in a new field along with a nice dose of fertilizer. Fruits are generally sugar plus colorants and perfumes that are often healthful vitamins and antioxidants. A few fruits tend more toward fat than sweet (avocados, olives), since animals like fat, too.

Bottom Line

Stems and leaves offer fiber and vitamins with few carbs; root veggies are often packed with carbs; seeds are the plant kingdom's kings of protein and fat; and fruits are tempting little "desserts" frosted with healthful nutrients. The foods that grocers call vegetables—especially the stem and leaf type— are the foundation of my meals with Carb-craft; while the foods grocers call fruits are my special treats: the cherry on top.

IS FIBER GOOD?

Yes, absolutely.

Our health depends, to an astonishing degree, on the health and diversity of the garden in our gut—the friendly microbes we all carry naturally—and fiber is food for this garden (chapter 11).

The best way to get fiber is from a whole food: cauliflower, raw carrot, nuts, mushroom, edamame—practically any vegetable—or an appropriately sized serving of fruit, grain, or legume (apple slice, rice, beans, oatmeal). I avoid spooning my fiber out as a powdered supplement; many of these products have a surprising amount of sweetener, or other unhelpful additives. Fiber supplements can be valuable for some, but a salad is usually better.

Does fiber make us fart? Only temporarily, while there's a mismatch between fertilizer (fiber) and flora (microbes). As soon as the flora catches up to the new level of fertilizer, even beans-beans-the-musical-fruit will pass on through without a toot. (Unless you're old, like me—then expect alpenhorn farts even if you eat nothing but manna and bathe in rose-petal rainwater.)

When Counting Carbs: Don't Count Fiber

Fiber is not only fun, it's free! When you check the nutrition label to see how many carbs a food has, you get to *subtract fiber* from total carbs (this bit of math gives you *net carbs*). Fiber is technically a carb, so it must be included there on the label, but it doesn't count because it doesn't feed *you*, it feeds your flora.

Net carbs feed you. Fiber feeds your garden. The two added together equal the *total carbs* found on a nutrition label.

UNPROCESSED VERSUS ULTRA-PROCESSED

One of the clearest messages of modern food research is just how harmful to health today's "convenience foods" and ultra-processed foods can be.

An *un*processed food is one that looks like itself: an ear of corn, a basket of okra, an egg in its shell, a halibut steak. *Processed meats* include things like lunch meat, sausage, and hot dogs. *Processed plants* include highly "refined" grains.

Processed Meats

Several older, less careful studies sometimes seemed to show that red meat was not healthful. But the latest, more careful research—where the study distinguished between processed and unprocessed meats—found that these are vastly different, health-wise. Many health risks previously attributed to meat—including risks of diabetes, heart disease, and cancer—now seem to be linked to processed meats, not to all meats.[2] Dr. Josefin Löfvenborg, author of a 2021 study, writes: "Consumption of *processed but not unprocessed* red meat may increase the risk of LADA"[3] (my emphasis).

Processed Grains

A century ago, manufacturers discovered that "refining" flour (removing the bran and germ, which contain many of the healthful components) gives a longer shelf life and also makes the carb faster, which gives our brain a zingier pleasure rush, and makes our brain say: *Let's eat more of that!*

Enrichment just means adding back in, in the form of synthetic analogs, some of what was removed—some of the iron and B vitamins, anyway, although not all the phytochemicals and antioxidants.

Fortification means adding nutritional supplements that were never there: letting Wonder Bread and Cap'n Crunch be your vitamin pill. For example, the FDA mandates adding folic acid to many grain products. Natural folate is in leafy greens, but since America wasn't eating enough of those, the FDA said: Let us eat cake—and also bread-like-fluff colored brown and decorated with oatmeal flecks—injected with folic acid. Folic acid supplies folate but may have other health effects, so if you are after folate, there are better ways to get it. (On the other hand: Does everyone today have access to leafy greens?)

No Standard Definition

Different people mean different things by the term *processed*. Some prefer the word *ultra-processed* to point out foods that have been engineered in laboratories—foods we typically can't touch or smell at purchase and must choose based only on their pretty packages.

With ultra-processed foods, writes Dr. David Kessler, former dean of Yale's medical school, "The food processing industry has destroyed the inherent structure of food. . . . Ultra-processed foods are designed to be irresistible and to prompt overconsumption. . . . they short-circuit our digestive systems."[4]

It's important to make a clear distinction between engineered foods and traditional foods.[5] In this book, when I refer to processed food, I am *not* including traditionally smoked meats, pemmicans, artisanal forms of cheese, beer, jam, wine, or kombucha, or traditionally prepared fermented foods such as yogurt, tempeh, or pickles.

RAW OR COOKED?

Research on ancient humans shows that our large brains evolved thanks to cooking—for which I sincerely apologize to any among us who have given birth. Cooking can make the energy from food more available; protect against parasites and diseases; and sometimes deactivate unfriendly plant compounds like lectins.

When fruits or other delicate foods are cooked, this can reduce their nutrients and fiber. But in other foods, nutrients become more available after cooking (for example, yams). Most mushrooms, beans, and grains are more healthful when cooked (or, in the case of grains, sprouted).

Cooking begins breaking down our food, making its energy more available. Cooking breaks the starches in plant-based foods into shorter "trains" (chapter 3) and sometimes all the way into sugars,* which is why a sweet potato does taste sweet—after it's cooked. Often, cooking increases the number of digestible carbs, and makes those carbs faster. This is why when I eat foods like carrots or zucchini, *I can enjoy a larger portion of raw than cooked without spiking my BG.*

Different cooking methods break down starches to a different degree. So *how* it's cooked (lightly sautéed beets versus slow-simmered-for-hours borscht) affects how fast a root vegetable or other starchy food will be. Grinding up a food like almonds into flour and baking the flour makes its carbs faster than in the whole raw nut.

A good rule of thumb for LADA: If humans typically cook it to eat it (potatoes, oats, pinto beans), a LADA will likely have to pay close attention to portion size.

CARB SPEED AND GLYCEMIC INDEX

In chapter 8 we talked about carb speed and about how a fast carb (juice, fruit) spikes BG high and fast, while a slower carb (brown rice, barley) makes the BG wave roll up slowly, then stay up at that broader peak longer. Either fast or slow carbs can give you significant time in the red (above your safe BG range). To predict the BG picture a food will create, we need to think about both the wave's *size* (made by carb amount) and its *shape* (made by carb speed) (chapter 9).

 For any food, the *details* of *your* preferred recipe matter.

Adding fat tends to slow the release of sugars into your blood. For example, full-fat yogurt is less spiky than nonfat yogurt

---

* Recall that a sugar is just the shortest starch, the littlest Lego block.

(assuming the amount of sweetener is the same). Whole-grain pizza dough releases its sugars more slowly than dough from refined (white) flour, and if there's fat-containing cheese on the pizza, the BG rise will be further delayed and flattened, and linger longer. Plain tofu has a relatively small BG impact, but tofu is often served in a sauce (often sweetened or including fast carbs), so the finished dish might give a BG spike.

o o o

Glycemic index (GI) is one way to measure carb speed. When the food industry began to create never-before-seen types of food—ultra-processed foods—we began to see foods with ultra-high GIs: faster carbs than nature had ever produced. America's rise in T2 diabetes closely parallels the rise of refined carbs in our diet.[6]

Research shows that if you give everyone in a group a milkshake, and the milkshakes are identical except that in half of them the carbs are ultra-processed (high-GI), the people who sip the high-GI milkshakes get sugar rushes, hunger jags, cravings, mood swings—and beg for another serving. The lower-GI group, on the other hand, has more stable blood sugars and is less excited about the shake.[7] Studies like this confirm what *ultra-processed ultra-high-GI* foods do to us: They profoundly mess with us, physically and mentally.

A food doesn't have to be ultra-processed to have high GI. Any sweet food, whether it's a sweet version of matcha tea or kombucha, a standard soda, or a homemade oatmeal cookie, can be high GI. When sweetened and ultra-processed are combined in a food, GI can explode over the top.

WHEN I WAS DIAGNOSED, DIABETICS WERE BOMBARDED WITH ADVICE to eat according to GI. The GI books, blogs, and articles seemed so sure of themselves that I jumped right on board. I made a list of the GIs of my common foods to carry in my wallet. (Yep, I'm that nerd.) Based on GI, I vowed: papaya no, plums yes. Acorn squash no, Hubbard squash yes. Oat milk no, soy milk yes. Couscous no, quinoa yes. It was confusing, but I was a believer.

Until, that is, I did my own test-test-test.

I'm not saying GI has no value. GI can point out the difference between a Cinnabon and a tangerine (although . . . so can common sense). The very lowest-GI foods *are the same group* as the low-carb group of foods—our old friends: stems, leaves, and animal-based foods (celery, lettuce, eggs).

In between lettuce and cake is a vast muddle in the middle, where some have suggested we should worry about the GI difference between corn tortillas versus wheat tortillas, injera versus chapatis, or papayas versus plums. Test-test-test revealed that *for me* as a person with little insulin, and *probably for most LADAs*, the GI differences of natural/traditional foods are not worth our mental effort. Although the GI numbers are different for black beans versus chickpeas, bananas versus kiwi, and grits versus oatmeal, I discovered that, for me, these differences were not worth stressing about—what I did need to know was *the number of carbs* of these foods I was eating.

Both the size and shape of a BG wave are important, but size (amount) is typically the much bigger factor.

"Studies show that the total amount of carbohydrate in food is generally a stronger predictor of blood glucose response than the GI [glycemic index]. Based on the research, for most people with diabetes, the best tool for managing blood glucose is carbohydrate counting," says the Mayo Clinic website.

Yes, GI is the reason a doughnut spikes my BG faster and higher than a whole-grain bagel—but I didn't need to carry a GI card in my wallet to figure that one out. Feel free to enjoy oat milk; feel free to enjoy corn tortillas if you prefer them to flour tortillas; just count carbs.

At Barb's birthday party, where her pastry-prodigy-son has baked her favorite cake, I enjoy the heck out of that seven-layer handcrafted delicacy! Also, I slowly savor a smaller serving than I used to take; increase my insulin dose per carb; and know that I'll live with a higher BG peak that day and will need to watch carefully for a post-party low.

As Fabulous Dr. Five says: "If you love cake, eat cake. Just don't eat cake every day."

IS SNACKING GOOD?

Not with diabetes. Which completely surprised me!

When I was pregnant (back in the Pleistocene), I was urged to snack. String cheese. Peanut butter crackers. I became a grazer, a bowl of almonds on my desk. Type, nibble, type, nibble, all day long. If I'd had a healthy pancreas, this might have been fine. But with a pancreas that struggled to keep up, this was a very unhealthy food habit.

Spacing meals at least four hours apart is the most widespread and least disagreed-with advice for diabetes, all types.[8] Spacing our meals allows each new BG wave to begin from a low stable trough instead of from high choppy froth. Also, our wacky liver tosses a little BG into our blood *every* time we put food, even one almond, in our mouth.

Spacing meals at least four hours apart has a deliciously wicked side effect: I had to *add* calories to my meals so they'd carry me for four hours. Nice! I began sloshing on extra calories the way I once heaped whipped cream onto hot chocolate.

Timing is everything, it turns out, in our relationship with food, too.

INTERMITTENT FASTING?

Fasting? *Yikes, one step too far over the woo-woo line*, I thought, hiking along behind Ava and other friends who couldn't stop chattering about fasting as we trekked through avalanche lilies and delicate windflowers up breezy Icicle Ridge. Luckily I was at the back of the line and could roll my eyes to my heart's content.

Too bad for me, my friends' positive experiences are backed up by solid science.

Fasting, writes Dr. Andrea Di Francesco of the National Institutes of Health, may: "exert a therapeutic, antidiabetic effect by fostering **regeneration of pancreatic beta cells** and restoring insulin secretion" (my emphasis).[9] There is now extensive research showing that, in addition to possibly regenerating beta cells, intermittent fasting (IF) also improves insulin sensitivity, BG control, and fasting BG, and makes weight loss easier with less hunger.[10]

These benefits may be due to what researcher Dr. Stephen Anton calls "flipping the metabolic switch." The metabolic switch flips when we use up the BG from recent meals and then the backup sugars stored in our liver, and flip to burning fat for fuel; for many, this happens about twelve hours after our latest meal.* Repeated flipping of this switch appears helpful to those with diabetes.[11]

People may mean different things when they say intermittent fasting, such as:

- Spacing meals by several hours; not snacking.
- Extending the overnight break from eating.
- Not-eating one day a week, not-eating for three consecutive days each month, et cetera.

I'm sorry to report that having an unfashionably early dinner (or no dinner) seems to have better health effects than skipping breakfast.[12] Lengthening our overnight food break while eating a solid breakfast can ease weight loss and reduce hunger.[13] Even when weight loss is not desired, extending the overnight break from eating can improve health by increasing our growth hormone, helping build muscle,[14] and improving "insulin sensitivity, beta cell responsiveness, [and] blood pressure."[15]

For longer fasts, to get the benefits without the pain, some suggest a fasting mimicking diet (FMD): eating just a little food that has few or no carbs. Some exciting but very preliminary evidence for *beta cell regeneration* involves repeated FMD cycles.[16] In a study at MIT, "results indicate that a FMD promotes the reprogramming of pancreatic cells to restore insulin generation in islets from T1D . . . and reverse[s] both T1D and T2D [in mice] . . . periodic cycles of a prolonged FMD is . . . ready to be tested [on humans] . . . for the treatment of both T1D and T2D."[17]

We should take care not to become dehydrated, dizzy, or malnourished when fasting, and fasting may not be right for pregnancy, children, the frail elderly, or those prone to certain eating disorders.[18]

---

* Burning fat for fuel is called ketosis. Going into ketosis through fasting **does not** put us at risk for ketoacidosis, which is entirely different—see chapter 6.

Fasting is a word that for years made me flinch. Fasting used to make me Stupid, Grumpy, and Sleepy: I could have been *three* of Snow White's dwarfs. I didn't yet know I was a sugar addict—I just knew that fasting made me ravenous, shaky, jangled, and brain-dead. I assumed it must be like that for everyone else too . . . *whaaat??! It's not?* In part 4 of this book we'll learn more about what food does to our brain, and why my difficulties with fasting were a common, but *not a necessary*, response. I would never have believed this back then but: resting our digestive system *doesn't have to be painful.*

Endurance athlete and fitness educator Mark Sisson explains that our carb consumption affects how we experience fasting. "If you are a heavy carb eater . . . fasting will be hard . . . Once you are in [low-carb mode] you can prolong the fasting time."[19]

Fasting is one card of many in our hand, and it's fine to leave this one on the table—for now, or forever. At the beginning of my journey, fasting felt brutal, but after I became a Carb-crafter, I was stunned to discover that fasting was no longer painful or scary, and at times was even energizing. Research shows that (once we stop being one of Snow White's dwarfs) fasting can promote mental sharpness.[20]

Bottom line: Many patterns/durations of fasting seem to boost insulin sensitivity, pamper or even rejuvenate beta cells, and ease weight loss, as long as they flip the switch back and forth, pulling our body across that metabolic threshold. "Once the metabolic switch occurs, both the tolerability and sustainability of IF regimens are greatly increased," writes Dr. Anton.[21] Just as folks training for marathons build rest days into their schedule, which help them get stronger faster, it may be helpful to build rest periods into our food consumption. But we are all different: test-test-test, do what works for you, and keep in mind that what works for you may change over time.

IS THE CALORIE DEAD?

As articles with catchy titles like "Death of the Calorie"[22] point out, calories can be inaccurate, overemphasized, and misleading. There is a growing consensus that **thinking of weight gain as calories in versus calories out can be unreliable and harmful.**[23]

An alternative way to understand weight gain, called the carbohydrate-insulin model, explains that when our blood sugar goes high this triggers fat creation, increases hunger, and (long-term) slows our metabolic rate.

As we saw in chapter 10, two different people will build different amounts of fat from the same amount of calories; and we build more fat if our BG goes high, or if our insulin never takes a rest and stays persistently high. Eating *low-quality* food (particularly ultra-processed foods—these spike BG for most people), ramps up food cravings and triggers unhealthy body-system loops that can progress over time into many health problems, including developing diabetes.

There may be two paths to weight gain. One path, too-high quantity, is real but has been overemphasized. The second path, too-low *quality*, is becoming better understood as we learn how low-quality foods trigger food cravings that urge overeating as *a symptom, not the underlying cause.*[24]

As Dr. Camacho of the Heidelberg Institute of Public Health explains, struggling against excess weight "results from particular dietary composi- tions closely linked to modern [highly processed] food habits . . . Under a constantly high presence of insulin, the body constantly stores fat but does not use it as a source for energy . . . [and we] become constantly hungry . . . In this situation, [overeating] would actually be **the symptom** of obesity and overweight . . . If we really want to succeed in tackling the obesity epidemic, we must stop treating its symptoms, and start treating its causes instead"[25] (my emphasis).

Obviously, the quantity/energy we eat remains relevant. But to over- emphasize calories or obsess down to the last digit can—for me, and for many—do more harm than good. I'll continue to use the word *calorie* in this book as a shorthand for quantity/energy, but perhaps you'll find a better way to think about quantity.

Tuft University's dean of nutrition writes: "Of course total calories matter **in the short term**, which is why people can initially lose weight on nearly **any** type of diet" (emphases mine); but, he adds, for long-term health, we want to focus on diet **quality**: a healthful balance of foods.[26]

Bottom line: Low-quality ultra-processed foods can leave us paradoxi- cally "stuffed and starved," as Raj Patel noted,[27] spinning our body systems in an unhealthy direction, spiking food cravings, and pushing us to over- eat quantity because we're lacking quality. Avoiding colorful cartons when shopping and instead picking up foods that look like themselves goes a long way toward solving this, and is often not more expensive; what it may cost is *time* in the kitchen (so this is particularly challenging for those who lack housing).

NOW I NEED TO . . . ADD CALORIES?

To my great surprise, when I limited carbohydrates, I struggled, at first, to take in *enough* calories.

Beans, rice, yogurt, hummus—many of the meal mainstays I'd depended on for years were, I was so sad to discover, only peripherally in my safe space when I worked to control BG entirely through diet and exercise (before I began supplementing insulin). I hit my carb limit with these foods at very small serving sizes, before I'd gotten much protein or calories.

Pure protein (animal protein) is carb-free, but there's only so much a person wants to eat. While two scrambled eggs give me all the protein I need for breakfast (more on recommended protein amounts on page 176), they only give me 140 calories, and I need twice that many calories to go four hours well fueled and full of energy. (*Your* calorie needs will depend on your age, sex, activity level, and more.) Similarly, one chicken breast, one burger, or six ounces of fish give me all the protein I need for a meal—but not enough calories.

If we try to—not intermittently but full-time—cut calories too drastically, our body slams on the brakes on our metabolism and pumps us full of hunger hormones; if we trigger this starvation mode, both long-term health and weight management become harder.

I found myself counting calories to *add* calories. Guess I better throw an extra handful of sunflower seeds on that salad, or an extra slurp of creamy dressing, or add avocado slices, or sardines, or olives, or drink a glass of milk or a cashew milk smoothie. Adios, deprivation: Toss on more, more, more!

EAT MINDFULLY

A friend I'll call Jeff wished to reduce weight and had long struggled to do so, but then had an epiphany, lost over a hundred pounds, and maintains his desired weight today. Jeff explained, over a relaxed, delicious dinner: "I used to eat for many reasons; for social and emotional reasons. Now, when I stop feeling actual physical hunger, I put down my fork and do not eat one bite more."

Part 4 will explore the many types of hunger. For some of us, hunger cues become lost or misaligned; and some of us lack the privilege to choose the timing and amount of our meals. But for many, Jeff's joyful new relationship to food and to his body is worth considering. His example supports me as I take a quiet moment to reflect deeply: Am I feeling that powerful urge because I'm hungry . . . or to please someone else . . . or because I'm angry, sad, relieved, celebrating, exhausted, bored, lonely, or anxious?

If eating is a habitual response to something other than hunger, we can explore habit-changing strategies to find what works *for us*: chewing gum, cranking the tunes, a peaceful walk, a hot bath, a conversation with a friend, break dancing, a check-in with a sponsor, meditation, five minutes of stretching or strength training, journaling, basketball, a sauna, an escapist romance novel, ten minutes of relaxing in a comfy chair, tai chi, a foot massage.

Today I try not to eat the way I used to: with the fridge door open, or in the car on the way to work, muttering "late, late, late." I try not to eat when I'm rushed, distracted, or multi-tasking. I try to notice my food, and to allow eating to be a happy time.

If you were fixing dinner for someone (else) you loved, would you find the time?

I know, easier said than done. For now, even holding the intention, saying it out loud, is a great start.

EVOCATIVE SMELLS, PRETTY DISHES, MOOD MUSIC

"That Martha Stewart stuff doesn't matter to me," I growled.

I was wrong, of course. Scientifically provably wrong. People who eat off small, pretty dishes, eat fragrant foods, and have a pleasing acoustic environment while eating, eat less and enjoy their food more. Yes, there are scientists who took the time to study this; and no I *don't* think their job is more fun than mine.

"Who has time for that?" I kvetched. Then I sat down to binge-watch Netflix.

Okay, fine . . . since it's science. I treated myself to a few lovely dishes, adding some much smaller, and much larger, artisan bowls. In the tiny forest-green bowl, fruit and yogurt sprinkled with walnuts mounds gracefully, instead of being a puny lump down in a crater. A broad, open serving bowl with an elegant etching of leaves became my salad bowl as my salads became meal-size. This stuff mattered more than I wanted to admit.

Healthy doesn't mean rocking skinny jeans. Healthy means healthy: mind, body, and soul. Treat yourself like a person you love. Serve yourself well.

THE OTHER SECRET: GO PLAY

Joyful activity, "nature's pill," revs our metabolism, pumps up energizing hormones, burns fat, and reduces insulin resistance.

At the time I was diagnosed, I was caught in a negative feedback loop. So tired all the time! I felt so draggy and low-energy, I was hardly getting outside at all. It was like having the flu . . . for months . . . sure, I'll get out there . . . tomorrow.

Diagnosis was a little electric jolt that shocked me into reacquainting myself with my favorite physical activities. Every dang day no matter what. Fresh snow fell, covering the tastee-freeze slush, and I swished down glistening hills and up wandering mountain roads under trees so snow-feathered, a California friend Facebooked: "OMG! So beautiful! Can't be real! You photo-shopped this!"

The Hebrew word *dayenu* roughly translates: "this alone would have been enough." Many things changed for the better in my life with my diagnosis, but if only this had changed—the change from *Gee I really ought to* to actually getting outside every day—*dayenu*.

HOW SHOULD WE ALLOCATE AMONG THE THREE THINGS TO EAT?

Given that the only things to eat are carb, protein, and fat, does it matter how we allocate among these?

Protein

Getting enough protein is important, but it should not be our only food energy. We want to be Goldilocks with protein—either too much or too little is not good for us.

The guidelines for a healthful upper limit to protein intake have recently been revised upward. Active people, athletes, those pregnant or breastfeeding, and people over sixty are now advised to eat substantially more protein than the old RDA guideline of 0.8 gram protein per kilogram of body weight per day. Based on the latest research, many of us want to eat between 1.2 and 2 grams of protein per kilogram per day.[28] And it's preferable to have protein in each meal, rather than a big wad at dinner.[29]

Carbs

Reducing highly refined or processed carbs helps anyone's health, and is particularly important with diabetes. For healthful carbs like whole grains and legumes (such as brown rice and black beans), a "normal"-size serving will give most LADAs a BG spike. Most LADAs, to eat *any* type of digestible carb, must limit portion size, supplement insulin, or both.

Fat

Annnd . . . now my brain is panicking. If I'm limiting carbs and protein, what am I supposed to eat—air? Because all my life I've heard that fat is bad! The next chapter considers this million-dollar question: Should we eat fat?

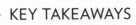

KEY TAKEAWAYS

1. Our body has always run by matching carbs and insulin. Carb-craft is a set of tools for doing this consciously, effectively, and with kindness and joy.

2. In every person, insulin needs to balance with carbs; when we have diabetes, this balancing act becomes easier when we eat fewer carbs.

3. Freely enjoy leaf, stem, and flower foods; moderate your serving sizes of roots, fruits, and grains. Be Goldilocks with protein, and aim for a bit of protein in most meals.

4. Avoid or minimize processed meats and ultra-processed carbs.

5. Understand carb speed but bear in mind that for natural—not ultra-processed—foods, number of carbs has a bigger effect than carb speed.

6. Both glycemic index and calorie counting were previously overemphasized compared with simply mindfully eating a rainbow of high-quality foods.

7. Fiber—from real food—is fabulous. When reading a nutrition label, subtract fiber carbs from total carbs to get net carbs.

8. Don't graze all day. Rest your digestive system. When you've gotten comfortable limiting carbs, try "flipping the switch" from time to time.

9. Eating nutrient-dense, high-quality foods helps us be happy with lighter portions.

10. What if you deserved to enjoy eating? What if you made your environment comfortable, even delightful, while eating? What if you treated yourself like someone you love?

11. It's about food . . . and it's about more than food. It's about life. Activity. Energy. Joy.

o o o

17 SHOULD WE EAT FAT?

Advice to reduce saturated fat in the diet without regard
*to nuances . . . could actually **increase** people's risk of*
[heart disease] . . . [if] saturated fats are replaced with
refined carbohydrates [my emphasis].
    —Dr. James DiNicolantonio of Saint Luke's
    Mid America Heart Institute[1]

*Conventional **low-fat diets are inferior to all higher-fat***
***comparisons** including ketogenic diets* [my emphasis].
    —Dr. David Ludwig, Harvard Medical School[2]

TODAY I AM HONORING JUNE FROM JUNEAU: A STRONG, WARM, GENEROUS woman with a lilting laugh. I didn't know my mother-in-law June well until after her heart attack. Because she had no medical insurance, she didn't get full care, and spent the rest of her life out of breath after a dozen steps and largely limited to where we pushed her in a wheelchair. From her wheelchair she planted public flower beds, fundraised for public art, spearheaded a recycling program, lobbied for bear-safe dumpsters, and volunteered tirelessly with the Humane Society.

June's heart attack was her ice bucket moment: She radically changed her eating habits to what we were told *then* was healthy: zero fat. And during the years she lived with us, we ate the same.

Like many people, I've steeped in a long history of believing "fat is bad." And now I want to limit carbs and be Goldilocks with protein (chapter 16) . . . and there are only three things to eat . . . okay this *is* third-grade flash cards! And they are not adding up.

Should we eat fat?

CHAPTER 10 EXPLORED HOW THE FAT IN OUR BODY IS AN ESSENTIAL organ, part of our immune system, a literal lifesaver—thank you, fat! However if fat-the-organ becomes unbalanced, it can spin into a loop with chronic inflammation and insulin resistance that can damage our health.

It's confusing that we use the same word, *fat*, to talk about something much smaller: molecules with specific structures/shapes, found in our food and body.* Just as with fat-the-organ, we *cannot survive* without fat-the-molecule. Cholesterol, triglycerides, and other fats perform key roles: We must have them to build our cell walls and many essential vitamins and key hormones—and they literally allow us to think. While the wise body can build for itself nearly all our needed fats, there a few (called *essential fats*) we must get through our diet—if we don't eat these we can develop vitamin deficiency, depression, low energy, low estrogen and testosterone, harm our eyes and brain, have dry hair and loose teeth, and more.

Because we could not survive without cholesterol, our liver carefully controls the level of cholesterol in our body. ***Our liver makes almost all of our cholesterol.*** If we eat less cholesterol, our liver will simply manufacture more.

While too little fat-the-molecule in our body is bad, having too much can also be a problem: We don't want too-high levels in our blood, our organs (like liver, pancreas, or kidneys), or random weird places (*ectopic fat*). We don't want too much cholesterol in our blood—yet it's our own liver that decides how much is there. What's up with that?

Of course we've already seen that our liver, amazing ninja-powerhouse though it is, is vulnerable to being fooled or overwhelmed. To take care of our heart, we must take care of our liver. This is the reason the increased risk of NAFLD (nonalcoholic fatty liver disease), caused by insulin resistance or by fat-the-organ becoming unbalanced, is such a big deal.

---

* Some of these molecules essential to human life are technically lipids and others are fats, but for ease I will refer to all of them as fats.

Meanwhile it's natural to ask: If too much fat-the-molecule *in our body* is bad, is fat-the-molecule *in our food* good or bad?

THE "OLD NEWS" ABOUT FAT WAS FLAWED

Fifty years ago, many wondered if bad levels of fat in the human body came from "bad fat" in our diet. Journalists like Ian Leslie have recapped this half century to explain how a small amount of bad science got over-hyped, while more balanced science was ignored, as study after study showed that *food fat—dietary fat—is not the bad guy* in cholesterol levels or heart disease.

"There is no significant evidence for concluding that dietary saturated fat is associated with an increased risk of . . . coronary heart disease and cardiovascular disease," writes Ian Leslie, yet this idea "somehow held up unsupported for nearly half a century . . . rejected by several comprehensive evidence reviews, even as it staggers on, zombie-like, in our dietary guidelines and medical advice."[3]

Current research makes clear that dietary fat is not the bad guy. For example, a 2017 international collaboration led by Dr. Dehghan, studying 135,000 people in eighteen countries for many years, concluded: "High carbohydrate intake was associated with higher risk of total mortality, whereas total fat and individual types of fat were related to *lower* total mortality. Total fat and types of fat were not associated with cardiovascular disease, [heart attack], or cardiovascular disease mortality . . . [and] saturated fat [reduced the risk of] stroke. Global **dietary guidelines should be reconsidered** in light of these findings"[4] (my emphasis).

In a medical journal article subtitled "50 Years of Confusion," Dr. Norman Temple of Athabasca University writes that a great deal of research has accumulated "since 1990 inform[ing] us that the role of SFA (saturated fat) in the causation of CHD [heart disease] has been much exaggerated." Fats are not the bad guy, says Dr. Temple; it is when fats are replaced with refined carbohydrates and sugars that our risk of heart disease increases.[5]

Many, many other recent studies confirm these findings.[6] "The recommendation to limit dietary saturated fatty acid (SFA) intake has persisted despite mounting evidence to the contrary . . . recent meta-analyses . . .

found no beneficial effects of reducing SFA intake on cardiovascular disease . . . [or] mortality," writes Dr. Arne Astrup of the University of Copenhagen.[7]

RESEARCHERS WERE STILL TRYING TO LAY THE BAD-FAT ZOMBIE TO rest when a new wave of confusion came along. In the early 2010s, several researchers reported that dietary fat seemed to cause insulin resistance—in laboratory rodents. Popular culture began to ping with the idea that fat-the-food might cause insulin resistance. But as this question was investigated further, scientists found that while this is true for mice and rats force-fed through feeding tubes until they were obese, *it is not true for humans*.[8]

But not all "internet experts" are up to date. Yesterday's news—the half century of flawed research, and then the rodent studies—keeps getting re-churned in some forums. When it comes to dietary fat's connection to diabetes, insulin resistance, and heart disease, expect to see some outdated, overturned information still floating around on the internet.

WHAT ABOUT *SATURATED* FATS? DO DIFFERENT *TYPES* OF DIETARY FAT HAVE DIFFERENT HEALTH EFFECTS?

The short answer: While some fats are better, few are bad. Fats in processed meats are bad for your health[9] and that's about it.*

Table 3 compares saturated, monounsaturated, and polyunsaturated fats. Saturated fats are *not all the same*: **many saturated fats are heart-neutral, and some improve diabetes health**.[10] As Dr. Béatrice Morio of the University of Lyon and many other researchers point out: Specific saturated fats can vary greatly in their biological characteristics and health effects.[11] Polyunsaturated fats are the heart stars, the most heart-healthful fats, especially the polyunsaturated fats that are also omega-3. Monounsaturated fats are generally good. Many fats decrease the risk of stroke, including some types of saturated fats.[12]

---

* Artificial trans fats, also bad, have now been banned from food in the US.

TABLE 3. Terms We Use When We Talk About Fat

Cholesterol	Essential building block.	Essential to build cells and certain key hormones and vitamins. Our liver is the cholesterol king, making most of our cholesterol and determining how much is in our blood.
Triglyceride	A glycerol backbone with three fatty acid tails. Since there are many types of fatty acids, there are many types of triglycerides.	Having enough of the right kinds is key to our health; having too much in our blood is bad. Triglycerides store unused calories and provide energy. Most of the food fats we eat are triglycerides: Our gut breaks these apart into their tiny building blocks (fatty acids) and reassembles them into the triglycerides we want and need.
Fatty acid	The building blocks (Lego bricks) we assemble into fats (triglycerides). A fatty acid is a particular type of chain of carbon molecules.	Common ways to group fatty acids include by their length; by their bonds; as omega-3 or omega-6; and by whether we must eat them to have them in our body (essential fatty acids) or can instead manufacture them ourselves.
Saturated fatty acid (SFA)	No double bonds.	Examples: butter, yogurt, other dairy, human milk. Individual SFAs vary, but as a group they are heart-neutral, and many improve diabetes health.
Monounsaturated fatty acid (MUFA)	One double bond.	Examples: almonds, avocados, olive oil. If healthfully extracted, **generally heart-healthy** or heart-neutral.
Polyunsaturated fatty acid (PUFA)	Two or more double bonds.	Examples: fish and fish oils, walnuts, pine nuts, and flax. Many plant foods are a mixture of MUFA, PUFA, and SFA; so it becomes about percentages and how the oil is extracted. When eaten in a whole food or extracted by a healthful process, PUFAs are **very heart-healthy** fats. O-3s, O-6s, and our essential fatty acids are all PUFAs.

Dr. Ulrika Ericson at Sweden's Lund University studied nearly twenty-seven thousand people for fourteen years, and found that those who ate high-fat dairy (cheese, full-fat milk, yogurt, and cream) had *less* risk of diabetes than those who ate lower-fat dairy products.[13] Other studies confirm that on average across a large population, full-fat dairy (1) protects against diabetes, and (2) improves the health of those who have diabetes.[14]

In 2016, three different research groups on different continents undertook comprehensive reviews of the published research on dietary fat and human health. In sum they reviewed hundreds of studies, both observational and experimental, including very large studies such as the Seven Countries Study and others that followed thousands of participants for decades. All three reviews cleared total dietary fat, as well as each major type of dietary fat (saturated, monounsaturated, and polyunsaturated), from blame.[15] All three agreed that "dietary cholesterol is not a . . . concern . . . [and] **diets higher in healthful fats . . . *reduce* risk of cardiovascular disease and diabetes**"[16] (my emphasis).

While science has cleared fat's name, there is a bad guy in heart disease. Dr. DiNicolantonio explains that diets high in *refined* carbs and sugars are bad for our hearts. Such diets not only raise BG and insulin levels and trigger insulin resistance and leptin resistance; they also harm our liver (increase NAFLD risk) and "cause a 3-fold increased risk of death due to cardiovascular disease." He concludes: "**Dietary guidelines should shift focus away from reducing saturated fat . . . [and focus] on reducing intake of concentrated sugars**"[17] (my emphasis).

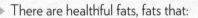

There are healthful fats, fats that:

> - Lower diabetes risks.
> - Reduce insulin resistance.
> - Control or reduce cholesterol and triglycerides levels in our blood.
> - Promote heart health.

> Our solution to the seemingly brain-breaking only-three-things-to-eat dilemma is:

> Keep carbs low, keep protein moderate, and increase healthful fats.

o o o

EMBRACING FAT-THE-MOLECULE

Many Americans — "dieters" especially — eat, as I once did, too few healthful fats.[18] A splash of healthful fat is a perfect way to add calories without carbs to a meal, keep BG calm, and quench hunger.

Fats from plant foods, fish, dairy, and eggs can improve our BG control and our health with LADA, while lowering our risks of heart

disease and stroke. And the fats in *un*processed meats can make managing our LADA easier, with no risk to heart health.

Polyunsaturated fats (found mainly in plants) and healthful fish have the most health benefit for our hearts; and the latest research finds that high-fat dairy is excellent for diabetes and good for our hearts; while eggs, dark chocolate, and unprocessed meats are fine (neutral for heart health, helpful for diabetes). As Dr. Astrup of the University of Copenhagen explains: "Whole-fat dairy, unprocessed meat, and dark chocolate are SFA-rich foods . . . that are not associated with increased risk of CVD [cardiovascular disease]."[19]

The healthiest fats occur naturally in whole foods: particularly certain fish, grains, and other seeds (including coconuts, avocados, and olives). Many pure extracted fats (oils) are also healthful.

The fats to avoid are the ones in processed meats, those mixed with ultra-processed carbs, or oils extracted through an unhealthy process.

Bottom line: If you're eating lots of foods that look like themselves, you're doing great for your LADA. Enjoy healthful fats, and for the sake of your heart, tip toward plant, fish, or dairy fats.

TABLE 4. Whole Foods Containing Fats and Their Effects on LADA and CVD (Cardiovascular Disease)

In Our Diet	For LADA Health	For CVD Health
Ultra-processed carbs	bad	bad
Sweetened foods and drinks	bad	bad
Cholesterol	neutral	neutral
Fat in general (total fat)	good (usually)	depends on details
Saturated fats	depends on details	depends on details
Monosaturated fats	good	good
Polyunsaturated fats	good	excellent
Fiber	good	excellent
Processed meat	bad	bad
Unprocessed meat	good	neutral
Eggs	good	neutral
Dairy, Fish	good	good

Whole grains and legumes	small amounts are good	good
Olives, coconut, nuts, avocado	good	good
Omega-3 foods	good	excellent
Inflammation-fighting foods	good	good
Increased activity (exercise)	excellent	excellent

neutral = no reason to avoid

Table four assumes that all foods discussed were produced and processed in a healthful way.

WHAT'S AN OMEGA?

Polyunsaturated fats come in two flavors: omega-3 and omega-6 (O-3 and O-6). Historically we ate somewhat equal amounts of the two, and we want to return toward that healthful balance. Today, almost all Americans eat too little O-3, and five to thirty times more O-6. An O-3/O-6 imbalance can raise our blood pressure and increase our risk for insulin resistance, weight gain, inflammation, cancer, heart attack, stroke, and depression.

Omega-6s (olive oil, tofu, sunflower seeds, almond butter) aren't bad, except when they crowd out the O-3s (salmon, walnuts, chia seeds) most of us want to eat more of. Too much O-6 can block our O-3s from being metabolized, blocking their anti-inflammatory benefits.

Increasing our omega-3s "prevent[s] beta cell destruction and insulin resistance. It also enhances insulin secretion, reduction in lipid profiles, and glucose," writes Dr. Habtamu Baynes.[20] O-3s are especially important during pregnancy, for building the baby's brain.[21] O-3s are also *anti-inflammatory* and can reduce our risk of heart disease and cancer, lower blood pressure, lower triglycerides, and improve our lipid profiles.[22]

"The benefits of omega-3 fats from fatty fish and . . . from plant sources like flaxseeds and walnuts are well known," summarizes *Harvard Health Letter*. "[Omega-3s] help protect the heart . . . They ease inflammation. They inhibit the formation of dangerous clots in the bloodstream. They also lower levels of triglycerides."[23]

The best sources of omega-3s are:

- Particular species of fish, if healthful (wild from unpolluted waters), have the highest levels of healthful O-3s: salmon, herring, mackerel, and sardines.
- High-quality fish oils.
- Walnuts, flaxseeds, and chia seeds. Yes, the walnut stands far above other tree nuts as an O-3 source.

Smaller but significant O-3 sources include:

- Leafy greens.
- Grass-fed milk. Studies show that the O-3 levels in meat and dairy can be extremely different in pastured versus feedlot animals.[24]

The benefits of eating uncontaminated healthful species of fish are based on rock-solid science. And fish oils—if made by a healthful process from healthful fish and kept refrigerated—can be the next best thing. In addition to protecting our heart, fish oils and other O-3s can help us build muscle, and also help LADAs **preserve beta cells, reverse insulin resistance, decrease inflammation, and improve BG control.**[25]

ARE KETO AND OTHER LOW-CARB-HIGH-FAT DIETS HELPFUL?

Yes. Any low-carb-high-fat diet, of which keto is one type, is ideal when we have diabetes.

Replacing carbs with healthful fats can improve BG control, A1c, insulin sensitivity, fatty liver, triglycerides, lipid panels, and other cardiovascular markers—sometimes to the point of allowing patients with diabetes to reduce medications[26]—while a low-fat diet may do the opposite. Research finds that **people with more saturated fat in their diet have less saturated fat in their body *when they reduce carbohydrates*.**[27] In line with high BG's harm to memory and cognition (chapter 6), there is some evidence that keto helps reverse memory loss.[28] Higher-fat diets have also been shown to suppress hunger compared with other diets.[29] As we saw in chapter 16, periodically flipping the switch into fat-burning mode has many health benefits, including protecting and possibly rejuvenating beta cells.

A recent study of T1s (adults and children) found that low-carb-high-fat diets gave excellent BG control with few highs or lows, improved cardiovascular profiles, and were not difficult or unpleasant: Participants reported high satisfaction.[30] "Ketogenic diets appear to be more effective than low-fat diets for treatment of obesity and diabetes," writes Dr. Ludwig, "and can be considered a first-line approach for obesity and diabetes."[31]

Keto advocates love to talk about putting the body into healthy ketosis, and ketosis is safe with diabetes: It's different from deadly ketoacidosis (chapter 6). One caution: I've seen keto misused when people add lots of fat to their diet and still eat lots of carbs. *That's* not healthy!

Many recent studies show that for all types of diabetes, reputable low-carb-high-fat diets such as keto are safe and health promoting.[32] For diabetes, writes Dr. Eric Westman of Duke University Medical Center, "The ketogenic diet is an effective alternative that relies less on medication, and may even be a preferable option when medications are not [reliably] available."[33]

A keto approach built from healthful whole foods is great; but keto is not mandatory. Any diet that moderates carbs, minimizes highly processed carbs and processed meats, is Goldilocks with protein, and is high in fiber and nutritious plants, nuts, and oils, is ideal for LADA (and for most of us).

IF WE HAVE A HEART-HEALTH GOAL

I had to begin by *unlearning* things that weren't true. Eating low-cholesterol, or low-fat, or low-saturated-fat: *none of these* improve our cholesterol profile or lipid panel. (Sorry, June.) And cholesterol levels get worse if we eat sugars or highly processed carbs in place of fat.

For heart health, healthful fats help, especially healthful kinds of fish, and whole plants that naturally contain fat (walnuts, flax).

How can we reduce cholesterol levels in our body? Four things are typically recommended today:

- Getting more active is usually the number one recommendation and has been proven to do a great job reducing cholesterol in the blood.

- If fat-the-organ has gotten out of balance, losing even five to twenty pounds can improve cholesterol levels.
- Reducing fatty liver (through weight loss or other means) helps the liver up its game.[34]
- Reducing inflammation improves cholesterol panels: omega-3 rich foods help with this, and other anti-inflammatory foods may also.[35]

KEY TAKEAWAYS

1. Fat-the-molecule allows us to build cells and create key hormones, and literally allows us to think. Cholesterol and triglycerides are not bad, they are essential: Just as with BG, what's bad is when they go too high.

2. Our body builds its own cholesterol. Our cholesterol levels rise not in response to eating fat, but in response to eating sugar and ultra-processed carbs.

3. For both diabetes and heart health, processed meats are the main food to avoid.

4. Healthful fish, eggs, and full-fat dairy are good choices, as well as nuts, avocados, olives, and other plant-based fat-rich foods.

5. It's great to get our fats from whole foods. Oils can be extracted in a healthful or an unhealthful way; finding healthful oils requires a bit more label reading.

6. While polyunsaturated fats are the heart-health rock stars, many monounsaturated fats (like olive oil) are also great choices, and many saturated fats (like eggs, full-fat yogurt, and cheese) improve our diabetes health with no risk to our heart.

7. We want to eat roughly equal amounts of omega-3s and omega-6s. For most today, this means adding O-3s.

8. Reducing carbs and increasing healthful fats is ideal with LADA and can be **as effective as medication** in controlling blood sugars. (Not that we have to choose between healthful eating and medications—many of us have the privilege to do both.)

Which Are the Best Fats to Eat?

1. Polyunsaturated fats are best (if extracted in a healthful way).
2. Monounsaturated fats are good (ditto).
3. Saturated fats are not all the same. There are many types. Saturated fats in different foods can be very different: good, bad, or neutral.
   - → Bad: processed meats.
   - → Neutral: eggs and unprocessed meats.
   - → Good: plant-based fats (nuts, avocado, olive, coconut, grains, dark chocolate), fish, and dairy.

o   o   o

18 PROS AND CONS OF SPECIFIC FOODS AND DIETS

You are a story fed by generations.
—Joy Harjo[1]

WE MAY HAVE HERITAGE CONNECTIONS, FOND MEMORIES, RANDOM preferences, or moral, ethical, or religious reasons to eat, or to not eat, particular foods. If you avoid a food for a non-health reason, no problem. There are no required foods in Carb-craft—only healthy balance. Carb-craft is compatible with virtually any inclusion or exclusion—kosher, halal, plant-based, keto, paleo, meat lovers, and more: It's a framework you can tailor to the foods you already love or choose.

This chapter focuses on *health* pros and cons relevant to LADA and assumes you have read chapter 17 on healthful fats. It's important to recognize that a person could have an allergy to *any* food: This chapter will assume you are not allergic to the food being discussed—but if you are, don't eat it! Obviously. This discussion also assumes you've chosen a version of the food that is not highly processed, sweetened, or chemically contaminated.

Stem/leaf/flower veggies are the stars, the centerpieces of a LADA meal. Healthful fish, dairy, eggs, meats, mushrooms, nuts, or insects offer excellent protein and healthful fats. Avocado, coconut, and olives add healthful fats. Grains, legumes, root veggies, and fruits add good vitamins, but as we've seen, a LADA-size serving of these is on the petite side and often a sidenote of a LADA meal. Appendix A gives a summary—pros, cons, and verdict—for each major food type.

CHOOSING HEALTHFUL FISH

Seafood/fish is a great source of protein, chock-full of vitamins and minerals, and certain species are our very best source of omega-3s (chapter 17). Studies show that eating fish is good for your brain and helps treat depression. Eating wild salmon twice a week lowers blood pressure, triglycerides, and risk of heart attack and stroke, and is an official recommendation of the American Heart Association.[2]

But the bigger and older the fish, the more mercury it's likely to contain. Mercury is released into the air from coal plants and other sources, settles onto water, is eaten by plankton, and bops up the food chain, becoming more concentrated each time a big fish eats a little fish.[3] All fifty US states have mercury-related fish advisories.[4]

So **eat small fish** because they aren't at the top of the food chain, accumulating the mercury their food's-food's-food ate. Tuna and swordfish suffer from being at the top of the food chain and should be eaten only rarely. But two thumbs-up for sardines, herring, mackerel, wild trout, anchovies, squid, and wild salmon.

Avoid farmed salmon, because like other factory meats they are fed weird stuff, are intensely crowded, become sick as a result, and are pumped full of antibiotics. Research on the nutritional value of farmed salmon shows that, like other cheap meats, they've lost a lot of their nutritional value, on top of being bad for the environment. Also avoid farmed shrimp. Some species of fish and seafood can be farmed in a sustainable and environmentally friendly way: You can find up-to-date apps or lists online.

Lobsters—along with scallops, shrimp, crab, sole, tilapia, flounder, cod, and snapper—are relatively low in omega-3.[5] This doesn't make them bad for you, but I'm sorry to say sardines are more healthful.

High-quality **fish oils**—those made by a healthful process from healthful fish and kept refrigerated—can be the next best thing to high-O-3 wild fish. Reputable fish oils are packed with omega-3s, which have many health benefits with diabetes, and for most people (chapter 17).

GRAINS AND LEGUMES

Are grains the evil Darth Vader of foods? Nope.

Whole grains (brown rice, oat groats, quinoa, wheat berries) have very similar health benefits to legumes (black beans, chickpeas, lentils). Grains and legumes provide lots of protein, fiber, iron, vitamins, minerals, and essential fatty acids, along with antioxidants and other healthful phytochemicals.

The lectins in *uncooked* grains or beans can give you quite the tummy-ache if, for example, you chomp on raw dry kidney beans. But most of the lectins in grains and legumes are deactivated by soaking, sprouting, or cooking. If you use traditional recipes/methods (boil your rice; soak, rinse, and cook your beans; sprout your alfalfa seeds), these foods will be nutritious and healthful for most people.

About 8 percent of Americans must avoid gluten or sometimes all grain (see "Gluten" below). But for the rest of us who don't have this sensitivity, moderate amounts of whole grains are healthful. That said, it is easy to cross the line from a healthful amount of grain to too much. I now understand that prediagnosis, I ate far too much grain. Comfort food, convenience food, affordable food: it was just so easy. For breakfast: granola or toast. For lunch: a sandwich, a soup loaded with pasta, or a rice bowl. At dinner, my heavy hitter was often pasta, bread, rice, or another grain.

I eat lots of vegetables! I said indignantly. But my acculturation said: Vegetables are a *side* dish. My habits were grain-heavy—and this was so engrained, I couldn't see it clearly. Not until I began my food journal and really noticed what I ate.

While for most of us, grains aren't bad, two (related) problems in America today are: (1) Grains are the food most likely to be junked up and overprocessed; and (2) grains are likely to be overrepresented in our diet—overeaten to the point of pushing other healthful alternatives off the menu.

Gluten

Because of my beloved cousin with celiac, I applaud the gluten-free foods on grocery shelves. Arriving in Port Townsend for a family reunion, Dad and I dash into the grocery and grab gluten-free brownies and a watermelon. But I don't eat (er, try not to eat) the gluten-free brownies we bring to the potluck. Because unless we are one of the 8 percent with celiac, glu-ten sensitivity, or a wheat allergy, ***store-bought gluten-free products may be worse for us*** than the alternative.[6]

Gluten is a protein found in wheat, rye, barley, triticale, brewer's yeast, malt, and a few other sources. Most whole foods do not contain gluten. But many processed grains (like rolled oats) or grain products (like crack-ers) can become contaminated with small amounts of gluten — enough to be harmful to those with celiac disease. And gluten can sneak into almost any food found in a can, box, or restaurant takeout, because it's often in rice syrup, soy sauce, soup thickeners, and more. Gluten can even slip into things like medicine and lip balm.[7]

In gluten-free (GF) baked goods like breads, crackers, and brownies, wheat may be "refined" even more than normal, or refined potato or rice starch may be substituted for wheat. Gluten-free foods have often been made less nutritious — they can lack fiber, iron, zinc, niacin, thiamine, riboflavin, calcium, vitamin B_{12}, and phosphorus[8] — and their carbs have typically been made even simpler, faster, and more likely to spike BG.

While this applies to those handy grocery shelf products, my cousin's *homemade* gluten-free baked goods are very healthful.

So if you haven't dug into the details of an item's creation, and don't have a gluten sensitivity, you're more likely to win the coin toss by assum-ing that GF is worse for you, both nutritionally and in terms of spiking blood sugar.

How do we know if we are in the gluten-sensitive group? This is an important question, because there is a genetic link between autoimmune diabetes and celiac disease.[9] Both are linked to genes in the HLA region[10] (chapter 7). Genetics loads the gun, but in this case environment dith-ers over whether to pull the trigger: While one in three Americans has the genes for celiac, only one in one hundred is diagnosed with the dis-ease.[11] If a person has autoimmune diabetes, the odds that they have also been diagnosed with celiac rise from one in one hundred to eight in one hundred.[12] With LADA we should give thought to, and speak to a doctor about, whether to be screened for celiac disease.[13]

Celiac is lifelong, and those with celiac must avoid even a speck of gluten. Wheat allergy, on the other hand, is sometimes outgrown. And gluten *sensitivity*, which has symptoms very much like celiac, may possibly

TABLE 5. Three Types of Reaction to Gluten

	Celiac Disease (CD)	Non-Celiac Gluten Sensitivity (GS)	Wheat Allergy (WA)
Genetically linked to autoimmune diabetes?	Yes	No	No
Prevalence	1 in 100 overall in the US, but 8 in 100 autoimmune diabetics in the US	6 in 100 in the US	0.5 in 100 in the US
Cause	Autoimmune response (our body attacks our own cells as if they are invaders)	Irritation/harm to gut; underlying cause uncertain	Immune response: Our body fights the wheat proteins as if they are invaders
Diagnosis	Presence of autoantibodies	Absence of celiac disease, but similar symptoms	Allergy test (skin, blood, or oral challenge)
GI symptoms	Diarrhea or constipation, vomiting, bloating, pain	Similar to celiac	Stomach cramp, nausea, vomiting
Other symptoms and risks	Headaches, fatigue, itchy skin, joint pain, acid reflux, mouth ulcers, seizures; may lead to malnutrition, osteoporosis, or stunted growth	Many similar symptoms to celiac except that seizures and mouth ulcers are unlikely, and evidence of long-term health impacts is lacking	Headache, congestion, rash, difficulty breathing, anaphylaxis
Will it go away someday?	No	Maybe	Maybe
Gluten avoidance	Lifelong and complete	Reducing or avoiding gluten for a time is sufficient for many	Consult an allergy specialist; wheat avoidance may not need to be lifelong

offer more leeway for eating small amounts of gluten; but at this moment, as we go to press, gluten sensitivity is less well understood than the other two wheat reactions.

Lectins

Lectins are found not only in grains and legumes, but also in seeds, tree nuts, peanuts, tomatoes, and soy—in virtually any plant/mushroom food. Over five hundred different lectins have been described from plants alone (and many more in mushrooms and other sources). The huge variety of lectins are highly variable in their health effects. Some lectins increase inflammation, but others decrease it. Some lectins are antiviral, fight cancer, improve diabetes health, or have other positive health effects in humans.[14]

For many foods, soaking, sprouting, or cooking deactivates their lectins, but in a few foods (for example, tomatoes) significant lectins remain after cooking. Understanding the health effects of lectins is a huge topic and is a case-by-case question for each whole food; I don't recommend a knee-jerk reaction against all lectins.

TREE NUTS AND SEEDS

Nuts and seeds are very healthful for most of us,[15] as long as we don't eat too-large quantities, and are a mainstay for many Carb-crafters who wish to eat a largely plant-based diet. Consider buying your nuts and seeds in bulk, raw, because commercial roasting can make them less healthy. Home roasting, or soaking-then-roasting nuts, can retain the nutrients while making them even more delicious.

"I can't eat nuts—they cause kidney stones!" said a man in my diabetes class. I brought the nut-versus-kidney-stone question to a doctor well versed on the subject. It turns out that other pro-kidney dietary changes can have a bigger impact than giving up nuts; and different nut types vary greatly in their oxalate content.

As Dr. Maury Hafermann explained to me, some doctors, in an attempt to keep things simple, may tell a patient something like, "Stop eating nuts." But in fact, said Dr. Hafermann, there are a lot of subtleties, and *people with kidney stone concerns often can still eat some nuts*, by being careful of total oxalate and consuming dietary calcium or calcium citrate at the same time. If this is a particular concern for you, check out the details in this footnote,* then have a conversation with your doctor or nutritionist—and ask them to give you the full story, not the one-liner.

PEANUTS AND SOY

These nut-like legumes provide good protein and are rich in antioxidants, folate, and vitamin E. Like wine and grape juice, they contain resveratrol, which seems to fight inflammation and reduce insulin resistance.[16]

Peanuts

Aflatoxin can grow on improperly stored peanuts, grains, and other foods, particularly in the tropics, and has become a global concern as food travels the world before it reaches our hands. The World Health Organization recommends buying grains and nuts grown locally when possible and buying only "reputable brands" of nut butters.[17] For this reason, and because many commercial peanut butters have unhealthy additives, and most of all because I love the taste, I buy peanut butter where you can push the button on a grind-it-yourself machine. Like fresh-ground coffee, it has much richer flavor.

---

* To avoid kidney stones, the most important thing you can do is to hydrate extensively: You're doing it right if your pee looks nearly clear. Since caffeine and alcohol are dehydrating, when you drink them, extra-compensate with even more water. There are different kinds of kidney stones; stones formed by too much oxalate are one common kind. Cutting back on salt and sugar can be even more helpful than reducing oxalate, so don't hydrate with soda. Also, entice your oxalate to exit by a different door, not through your kidneys (poop it out, don't pee it out). Citrate helps your oxalates exit by the correct door, so your doctor may recommend taking calcium citrate or magnesium citrate . . . or you can squeeze lime or lemon into all that water you're drinking. Low calcium can raise oxalate levels, so be sure you're not deficient in calcium. If despite all this you still need to limit oxalate, keep in mind that spinach and rhubarb have much higher oxalate than nuts. Coffee, black tea, figs, oranges, and chocolate all have oxalate (and only a monster would expect us to give up those!). Nuts low in oxalate include pistachios and chestnuts. Moderate: cashew, pecan, and peanut. Highest oxalate among nuts: almonds, Brazil nuts, and pine nuts. Excessive protein in your diet can produce urate, which can be a concern for a different kind of kidney stone. Consult with your doctor or nutritionist.

Soy

Some people avoid soybean oils, soy protein isolates, and some soy meat-substitutes as unhealthy; some fear that soy can mess with our metabolism, thyroid, and hormones.[18] Others believe the isoflavones in soy foods are beneficial to many, particularly with diabetes, and say soy foods increase serotonin, promote better sleep, may protect bone density, and may protect cardiovascular health.[19] I personally choose to enjoy moderate amounts of tofu, tempeh, edamame, and soy milk. Fermentation (tempeh, miso) makes nutrients more available in soy foods.[20] Ninety-five percent of soy grown in the US is GMO and high in pesticide content, so when I choose soy, I choose organic.

WHAT CAN I DRINK?

To hydrate is great—but what should we drink?

Not (or rarely) soda. Soda and other sugar-sweetened beverages have repeatedly been proven to increase our risk for insulin resistance and diabetes; and they have a stronger link to weight gain than any other food or beverage.[21] "Zero-calorie" sodas cause almost as much weight gain as regular soda, because they fool our body and amp up hunger hormones.[22]

One hundred percent fruit juice can contain more sugar than Pepsi or Coke.[23] I can't quite picture eating a pile of five oranges along with my coffee and pancakes . . . but back in the day, that's what I was doing when I drank a glass of orange juice with breakfast.

BYOB. When the girlfriends gather to watch *The Full Monty*, mixing drinks from the selection on the Ping-Pong table, no one even remarks as I sip my dry kombucha. I'm so glad I brought it. Each tiny bottle of Canadian Club mixer on the Ping-Pong table has more carbs than I allow myself in an entire meal.

The easiest recipe in the world: Drop a few tea bags in a jar of water and set it in the sun. Try sun tea iced or hot; try it like Thai iced tea with a swirl of cream. Toss a chunk of gingerroot in a pan of boiling water and in twenty minutes you have a spicy, healing beverage, tasty either hot or cold; I add a big squeeze of lemon. Ginger brewed with turmeric has a delicious color and even more health benefits. (Turmeric root is probably right next to the ginger in your grocery; chop off a chunk and toss it in along with the ginger.) There's a world of cucumber coolers, turmeric tang, green smoothies, lightly fruit-sweetened bubbly water, and low-carb kombuchas to be discovered and enjoyed.

Coffee, Tea, or Me?

Some diabetics find that coffee impacts their BG, and some find it does not. (Perhaps depending on the person, their caffeine tolerance, and the strength of the coffee.) A few studies suggest coffee and black tea may reduce risk of T2; other studies suggest they are not as good for autoimmune diabetes. So far, the research on diabetes and coffee / black tea is inconclusive.[24] People are very individual in their responses to coffee and black tea and may become more so with age.

Green tea, on the other hand, is thumbed-up fairly unanimously as being healthful and full of antioxidants.[25]

Alcohol: Go Straight and Dry

With a great deal of searching, you may find low-carb beers[26] or low-carb hard ciders . . . but don't expect them to taste like the normal brands, and good luck finding them in a typical bar. Many bartenders don't know the carb levels of their drinks, but may happily spout random numbers anyway, not knowing that there's genuine medical significance to their words.

Most nonalcoholic drinks in a bar are carbier than their alcoholic counterparts. Still, there's always unsweetened seltzer water with a twist of lime. (Yippee. Add it to the list with lettuce and eggs.)

If you want to get a buzz, straight shots of tequila, whiskey, vodka, gin, and the like are the lowest-carb way to get there. Dry wines are also a low-ish-carb choice.

Heavy consumption of alcohol raises risk of heart disease and weight gain, and has other negative health effects. Moderate consumption (such as one drink a day) can affect our health in many varied ways: Most doctors agree that alcohol should not be viewed as pro-health. Moderate consumption may lower risks of diabetes, heart disease, and stroke[27] (and this is as true for beer, spirits, and white wine as for that spotlight-hog, red wine). Alcohol may quiet or dumb down the liver: anecdotally, some insulin-users say they reduce their insulin dose slightly if they're having one drink with dinner, while significant drinking can set them up for dangerously deep low BG.

Alcohol does have calories even when it doesn't have carbs: "a pork chop in every glass," as one friend jokes.

Big picture: Most doctors say those who enjoy alcohol can do so in moderation without harming health—but if health is our only motivation, we may just want to go for that seltzer-and-lime. Always consider potential medication interactions and discuss them with a doctor.

TABLE 6. Beverage Chart

Beverage	Grams of Carbohydrate	Per
Distilled spirits (whiskey, tequila, rum, vodka)—straight, no mixer	essentially zero	
Mixed drinks	sugar bomb	
Virgin version of mixed drinks	sugar bomb	
Hard-to-find low-carb beer (Michelob Ultra, Bitburger Light)	under 4	12 oz bottle
Light beer	5–12	12 oz bottle
American beer	10–14	12 oz bottle
Good-tasting beer	13–15	12 oz bottle
Really good-tasting beer (including IPAs, stouts, and microbrews)	16–17	12 oz bottle
Nonalcoholic beer	14–18	12 oz bottle
Hard-to-find low-carb hard cider (Rhinegeist's Cidergeist; Seattle Cider Company's Dry Hard Cider)	3	12 oz bottle
Normal hard cider	12–30	12 oz bottle
Dry wine (red or white)	4–7	6 oz glass
Most wine	6–10	6 oz glass
Port	12	6 oz glass
Dessert wines	24–27	6 oz glass

Beverage	Grams of Carbohydrate	Per
Bailey's Irish Cream	11	1.5 oz jigger
Kahlúa	22	1.5 oz jigger
Hard-to-find dry kombucha (Lion Heart)	10	16 oz bottle
Typical kombucha	12–22	16 oz bottle
Gatorade	11	16 oz bottle
Mountain Dew	34 (43)	16 oz (20 oz)
Root beer, Coke, Pepsi, Dr Pepper	29–32 (37–40)	16 oz (20 oz)
7-Up	22 (27)	16 oz (20 oz)
Orange juice	26	8 oz
Apple juice	28	8 oz
Cranberry juice	31	8 oz
Pomegranate juice	33	8 oz

This chart lists beverage carbs but not total beverage calories; it is to help manage BG, not weight gain.

BREAKFAST: GO GLOBAL

"Everything you know about breakfast is wrong," quips one foodie book.[28]

Guilty as charged. Oatmeal is the ultimate healthy breakfast—I once mistakenly thought! And back in the day, my luxurious Sunday mornings began with pancakes heaped with fresh nectarine slices, or homemade banana pecan waffles. When I ate yogurt, it was honey vanilla, topped with granola—and my granola was mostly oats coated in some fancy-ass version of sugar.

We aren't the only country to love a morning croissant, pan dulce, youtiao, paczki, or mandazi. But popping my head up out of my bubble, I see that those of us who think breakfast flakes or sugar-frosted bombs are a normal way to start the day are the odd ones out. Thinking internationally can be a helpful way to break out of breakfast grain-gridlock.

In Korea, breakfast looks much like dinner, with tofu or cabbage soup, kimchi, fish, or beef. In India, you might breakfast on chutneys, sambaar (a veggie dal tamarind stew), poori masala (a spicy potato veggie dish), or idli (lentils and rice). Iranians breakfast on haleem, a rich lentil-meat stew. In Israel, shakshuka: baked eggs, onions, peppers, and tomato. In Egypt, ful medames (fava beans, parsley, and olive oil topped with tomatoes). Gallo pinto (rice and beans) in Costa Rica. Chilaquiles or huevos rancheros in Mexico. Roasted plantain with pork in Peru. Feijoada, a hearty bean-meat stew, in Brazil. Miso soup, pickled veggies, fish, and tamagoyaki (omelet) in Japan. An open-face sandwich layered with fish or cold cuts, cheese, mayonnaise, cucumber, and tomato in Sweden. Shredded pork and steamed egg in Vietnam. Beans, sausages, mushrooms, and tomatoes in England. A spread of meats, cheeses, eggs, tomatoes, cucumbers, peppers, and fruit in Germany; and a similar spread in Turkey, but with sucuk, a spicy Turkish sausage, and Turkish tea. Sure, a lot of these nationalities also toss in rice or bread—but we don't have to.

Veggie-centered meals applies to breakfasts, too. If you can wrap your head around eggs and hash browns . . . just fry up golden greens (your favorite mix of stem/leaf veggies, like bok choy, broccoli, kale, or cabbage) instead of potatoes to accompany your eggs. Stir-fries, scrambles, fry-ups, omelets, avocado bakes, tofu bakes, veggie custards, poached fish, veggie-meat-cheese smorgasbords, and, if you can think internationally enough, even soups, stews, and curries—there's no end to the variety of delicious veggie-centered breakfasts you can enjoy.

What do I miss most about my grainy breakfasts? The honest truth is: autopilot. In the old days I didn't even have to wake up to know what was for breakfast.

At first I was heartbroken to lose my every day go-to. Now I think: Maybe my food world just wasn't big enough.

ANTI-INFLAMMATORY DIET

The science of anti-inflammatory eating is young, so you'll find patchy and contradictory claims. Foods containing omega-3s are considered anti-inflammatory. Other foods commonly called anti-inflammatory include plants packed with bioactive polyphenols such as flavonols (onions, broccoli, tea, various fruits), flavones (parsley, celery, chamomile tea), flavanones (citrus fruits), flavanols (flavan-3-ols) such as catechins and procyanidins (cocoa, tea, apples, grapes, red wine), anthocyanidins (colored berries), isoflavones (soy), and others.[29] Some of the most-likely-to-be-nominated foods are listed in table 7.

If we're eating salmon and walnuts (or other omega-3 foods), citrus and berries, and a wide variety of whole fresh vegetables that look like themselves, we're already eating in a generally anti-inflammatory way.

Beyond that . . . it's complicated. Because many foods commonly called anti-inflammatory are also common allergens. And *an allergy is an inflammatory response*. About one in ten Americans has a food allergy.[30] *So for a significant number of people, one or more foods commonly called anti-inflammatory will in fact be inflammatory.*

The FDA requires labeling for the most common food allergens: milk, eggs, fish, shellfish, tree nuts,* peanuts, soy, and wheat. Also common are sensitivities to gluten (see the section earlier in this chapter) and to nightshades.† Even ginger, garlic, and turmeric, often held up as "perfect" anti-inflammatory foods, can be allergens for some.

"There is no single anti-inflammatory diet," writes health journalist Jenna Fletcher, "but a diet that includes plenty of fresh fruits and vegetables, whole grains, and healthful fats [and avoids added sugars and processed foods] may help manage inflammation."[31]

Bottom line: Good news: Foods commonly called anti-inflammatory overlap nicely with the LADA-healthy foods we've already discussed: berries, walnuts, greens, cauliflower, and (for those who eat fish) salmon and sardines.

TABLE 7. Top Anti-Inflammatory Foods and Related Sensitivities

Anti-inflammatory for most of us...	But could be inflammatory for those with:
Wild salmon, sardines, similar (see chapter 17)	fish allergy
Tree nuts, especially walnuts	tree nut allergy

---

* People with an allergy to one tree nut may or may not be allergic to many or all tree nuts. They may be allergic to almonds, walnuts, pecans, cashews, hazelnuts, and/or pistachios; must also avoid milks and flours made from their allergic nuts; and are sometimes allergic to Brazil nuts, macadamia nuts, coconut, and/or various seeds.

† Nightshades include potato, tomato, tomatillo, goji berry, eggplant, bell pepper, chili pepper, and paprika.

Flaxseeds and chia seeds	seed allergy
Tomatoes	nightshade sensitivity
Peppers (bell pepper, chili pepper)	nightshade sensitivity
Green tea	catechin sensitivity
Greens: kale, spinach, collards, nettle, chard, etc.	salicylate sensitivity
Crucifers: broccoli, cabbage, brussels sprouts, etc.	salicylate sensitivity
Blueberries, raspberries, blackberries, cherries	salicylate sensitivity
Turmeric	oxalate sensitivity or another sensitivity
Cinnamon	allergy/sensitivity rare but real
Ginger	allergy/sensitivity rare but real
Garlic	allergy/sensitivity rare but real
Olive oil	allergy/sensitivity rare but real

WE ARE WHAT OUR FOOD ATE

A truck spill in Wisconsin spewed hundreds of thousands of red Skittles across the highway—Skittles that had been on their way to feed cattle.[32] It's common to feed cattle Kool-Aid powder, potato chips, and other "food waste," including old Halloween candy, still in the wrapper.[33] Things legally and routinely fed to standardly raised livestock and poultry include poop ("recycled animal waste" in the biz), plastic ("polyethylene roughage replacement"), and pesticides and POPs (persistent organic pollutants).[34]

I've known in the back of my mind, for a long time now, that large-scale meat production was inhumane and highly polluting, but I kept that thought under lockdown. I didn't want to know the details. I'd be in the grocery store, and that fresh-looking, innocent-looking chicken was just so dang cheap . . . and I reached for it. Now I'm catching on to how expensive, in so many ways, it can be when our food makes us sick. Cheap-seeming food is just one more way social inequities play out: It's those of us eating paycheck-to-paycheck that are most likely to buy cheap food, with apparent savings up front, but huge costs down the line.

ADVERTISERS PLAY ANNOYING WORD GAMES. YOU HAVE TO LEARN THE language.

Grass-fed animals can have a healthier omega balance (chapter 17), but the words *grass-fed* have lost some meaning, because a grass-fed animal can still be "finished" for months in a feedlot, where it loses most of the benefits of being grass-fed. So look for *grass-fed, grass-finished*. Also look for: *Animal Welfare Approved, Certified Humane, Global Animal Partnership*, or *Food Alliance Certified*. Two thumbs-up if you see the logo of the American Grassfed Association (AGA), because this means the animal was born and raised in the US, was raised entirely on open grass pastures, was not harshly confined, and was not fed antibiotics or growth hormones.

On your egg carton: *Cage-free* does not mean crate-free. (Loophole!) *Natural* is meaningless (has no standard definition). *Free-range* and *cage-free* are meaningless. *Fresh* is meaningless. *Pure* is meaningless. *Gluten-free* is just silly.* *Vegetarian* is bogus since these birds are supposed to eat bugs. *Raised on shady porches* means crammed with forty thousand other chickens deep in their own dung and too tightly packed to turn around: In the biz those production sheds are called "porches."

If you're able, say yes to: *organic, pastured, grass-fed and grass-finished*, and local (as in, it names a place, and you know that place).

For eggs: *Antibiotic-free, arsenic-free, organic*, and *Certified Humane* are good. *Pastured* is best. Or your neighbor. Or your own backyard.

The health differences are scientifically documented. We'll be healthier if we're able to choose these things.

DOES "ORGANIC" PRODUCE REALLY MATTER?

I said I'm diabetic: Did you think I said "millionaire"?

I wish this *was* just elitist foolishness. But this hits us all, and especially the economically disadvantaged. It's not elitist to choose the swimming hole upstream of the factory outflow.

But I get it. When we look at organic produce and healthfully raised meats, and then at "standard" foods, it can feel like the old joke about

---

* All eggs are gluten-free unless contaminated during prep/cooking.

modern art and a kid's crayon endeavor—if they look so much alike, how can one be so much more expensive?

For over two decades the scientific community has clearly documented that a long shopping list of chemicals, many of which we may be exposed to on a daily basis, both increase our risk of diabetes and worsen our diabetic complications.[35] Dr. Schug of the National Institute of Environmental Health Sciences writes, "There is now compelling evidence linking . . . a variety of chemicals . . . [to] metabolic disturbances such as diabetes."[36]

Many of these chemicals are lumped into a category called EDCs—**endocrine disrupting chemicals**. (Oh, and with diabetes we go to our . . . endocrinologist.) While some of these toxins come from car exhaust, indoor air pollution, or our shampoos and beauty products, a *lot* of them enter us through our food and drink: agricultural residues on our food or plasticizers in food packaging.[37] "Endocrine disruptors can be found in many products including plastic bottles, metal food cans, detergents, flame retardants, food, toys, cosmetics, and pesticides," writes Dr. Oneyeol Yang, adding, "These increase risk of diabetes."[38]

Heartbreakingly, the economically disadvantaged bear the greatest burden from EDCs,[39] but few of us escape: When a random American takes a pee test, 98 percent of us pee out at least one of the toxic chemicals that raise our risk of diabetes.[40]

I still struggle to convince myself to pay for toxin-free food. Standing in that grocery aisle, I bet I look ridiculous, reaching one way, then stopping, then reaching the other way, then stopping . . .

For many, it's difficult, but **if you're able, buy organic, bulk, "naked" foods**: unpackaged (or minimally packaged) organic foods that look like themselves, that Great-Grandma would recognize.

MANY NAMED DIETS ARE LADA-FRIENDLY AND CARB-CRAFT COMPATIBLE

Table 8 compares several common named diets. Because they all avoid sweetened foods, processed meats, and ultra-processed grains while emphasizing vegetables and whole foods that look like themselves, these are all very compatible with Carb-craft.

TABLE 8. A Few of the Many Eating Plans Compatible with Carb-Craft

Name	Premise	Complication
Paleo	Let's eat like Paleolithic people. Paleo typically avoids dairy, grains, legumes, and root vegetables.	The diet of Paleolithic people was surprisingly diverse and in some places did include grains and root vegetables.
Keto	Very low-carb because it replaces carbs with healthful fats.	The strictest keto approaches want each meal—and sometimes each item on the plate—to meet a specific fat ratio.
Mediterranean	Let's eat like last-century Mediterranean people.	Specifics interpreted differently by different people
DASH	Eat to lower blood pressure, especially by reducing sodium and sugar.	Reducing sodium and sweeteners is great for most of us, but some versions of DASH recommend low-fat, which is outdated (chapter 17) and makes Carb-craft tough.
Anti-inflammatory	Eat foods that fight inflammation, especially omega-3 foods and foods with healthful phytochemicals.	Common lists of anti-inflammatory foods are playing the odds relative to allergies; nightshades and other foods are hard to place because of individual differences.
Plant-focused	Eat mainly, or only, plant-based foods.	Does this mean meat-free, meat-reduced, ovo-lacto, ovo-but-not-lacto, pescatarian, etc., etc. . . . ?
Vegan	Don't eat any animal product.	Some find it overly rigid compared with intent . . . others appreciate the clarity.
Climate Diet	Let's reduce our carbon footprint through food choices.	There is so much to know about how each item is grown, transported, and prepared. You'll have constant questions.

How does it mesh with low-carb?	Strength
Makes low-carb easy.	Highlights many healthful plant-based foods, along with healthful wild fish and meats.
Makes low-carb easy.	Helps us find and include healthful fats in our diet.
Makes low-carb easy.	Highlights healthful plant-based foods, wild healthful fish, and healthful fats.
Depends on specifics.	Highlights healthful plant-based foods.
Very compatible.	Highlights healthful plant-based foods and wild healthful fish.
Depends on specifics.	Highlights healthful plant-based foods.
Makes low-carb hard.	Highlights healthful plant-based foods.
Compatible.	Highlights locally sourced, healthful plant-based foods and wild healthful fish.

Keto was discussed in chapter 17, and anti-inflammatory on pages 201–203. Below are a few additional comments on particular diets.

Mediterranean

While there is some disagreement about exactly which foods and countries are Mediterranean, there is overall agreement that this diet should be high in olive oil or similar healthful oils, and in vegetables, whole grains, legumes, nuts, seeds, and fruits. Most versions of the Mediterranean diet include fish or seafood about twice a week and include modest amounts of meat and animal products. Many say we should speak of the Mediterranean *lifestyle*, emphasizing the importance of physical activity, and of minimizing stress and sharing meals with other people.

DASH (Dietary Approaches to Stop Hypertension)

Hypertension refers to high blood pressure. DASH advocates reducing sodium (salt) and added sugars, while encouraging whole plant foods that provide fiber and key nutrients, such as vegetables, fruits, grains, legumes, and nuts. Older versions of DASH limit saturated fat; this is an outdated approach (chapter 17). Today many modify DASH by adding healthy fats.

Plant-Focused

There is a whole continuum here from ovo-lacto-pescatarians to vegetarians to vegans. Plant-focused diets feature plants and avoid meat, but some allow eggs, dairy, or fish. One reason there are different approaches is that there are different motivations: from religious, to animal cruelty, to personal health, to environmentalism, to all of the above.

When I was a Carb-craft beginner, overwhelmed and feeling surrounded by hidden carb-sharks, my safety foods were animal-based foods because: zero carbs. But now that I've gained confidence and know how to play all the cards in my hand (activity, meds, insulin supplementation, and carb reduction), I'm back to eating the way I prefer, 90 percent plant-based.

During my learning journey, I was kind to myself—some days it was any port in a storm. Thank you, Parsley's turkey salad and Yodelin's chicken-rice-bowl-hold-the-rice, for letting me go out to eat with friends without panicking, obsessing, having a scary BG peak, or all three at once.

Just as with fat research, some past research on meat and health has been misinterpreted or poorly framed. I found studies out there claiming to show that a vegetarian or plant-based diet reduces odds of T2 diabetes. Whenever I looked closely at one of these studies, it did not show that eliminating meat improves health—but rather that diets rich in a variety of whole vegetables improves health. This will be true whether or not we get some of our protein from meat.

We do want to avoid *processed* meats (like hot dogs and lunch meat) because, as we saw in chapters 16 and 17, these have been shown to increase diabetes risk and other health risks.[41] Dr. Josefin Löfvenborg of Sweden's Karolinska Institutet writes: "Consumption of ***processed but not unprocessed*** red meat may increase the risk of LADA"[42] (my emphasis).

A 2021 review of vegetarian and vegan diets for T1 children concluded that vegetarian diets are often healthy, but vegan diets may be "too restrictive." According to Dr. Valeria Tromba, omega-3 fats, especially eicosapentaenoic acid (EPA) and docosahexaenoic acid (DHA), may be too low if we do not eat fish or fish oils; and "no food of vegetable origin contains enough [vitamin B_{12}]." Dairy, eggs, and fish are good sources of vitamin B_{12}. Dr. Tromba suggests that people restricting animal-based foods monitor or supplement vitamin B_{12}, calcium, iron, zinc, and O-3s (especially EPA and DHA). She adds that EPA and DHA are particularly important with LADA for "prolonging residual beta cells."[43]

As the Mediterranean approach shows, meat ***needn't be a yes-no dichotomy; it could be a rebalancing***.

Climate Diet

For those who wish to eat in an environmentally friendly way, there are good resources for learning the climate footprint of different types of foods.[44] The book *Climate Diet* explains why beef has a much higher climate impact than chicken; farmed salmon much higher than wild salmon; and lentils much lower than any of those. These resources will help you dig into the details of why food transportation (especially by airplane), food waste (a surprisingly significant impact), food packaging, deforestation, soil depletion by industrial agriculture versus soil-friendly methods available to small/traditional farmers, and other food impacts, are an astonishingly large part of *your* personal carbon footprint. "What you eat, where it's from, and what it's wrapped in account for a juicy 20 [to 30] percent of your carbon footprint," writes Natalie Fée.[45]

Analyses like these look at the *average* chicken or average lentil, so by moving even a little off average—more local, more seasonal, more sustainably raised—you can make a big difference.

Living in a planet-friendly way is a key motivation for many vegans. According to climate researchers, veganism is not the only way to eat in a climate-friendly manner. An occasional-meat-eater who de-emphasizes beef, buys food as locally as possible, avoids "flying food," and reduces food packaging and food waste could have a lower carbon footprint from food than her vegan neighbor, says climatologist Gidon Eshel.[46]

Depending on . . . a lot . . . about our personal situation, we might have more climate impact through creating a community garden in an old vacant lot than through buying a Prius. As Natalie Fée writes: "Despite being the problem, we're also the solution. Funny that."[47]

DIET CULTURE WARS?

Diet fanatics can be just so . . . fanatic. In the same way that I meander the farmers market, selecting what appeals from this or that stand, I now browse food philosophies, bringing home the best ideas without swallowing the lock, stock, and barrel.

While I eat keto-esque, I find ultra-rigid keto approaches unhelpful, such as those insisting every item on my plate should have some specific percentage of fat. While I love browsing paleo recipes, I'm not going to forgo a fabulous-looking roasted veggie dish just because it includes a few golden potatoes among the red peppers, broccoli, and asparagus. While I lean pro-plant-foods, I don't say no to Nancy's wild venison, Catha's pear-orchard sheep cheese, or Sarah's Seattle backyard honey.

Yes please to fun new food ideas and recipes, but no thank you to any more prohibitions, exclusions, or food guilt on top of what LADA has already dealt me.

One food author I enjoy jokes that he is "Pegan": a combination of paleo and vegan. Whaaaat? I wondered, how would that work? How could he combine a diet based on prohibiting legumes and grains and reliant on healthful meats—with a diet based on prohibiting meat and reliant on legumes and grains? Eventually I realized the only way it would work would be to stop focusing on what each diet *prohibits* and focus instead on what each *promotes*.

 ## KEY TAKEAWAYS

1. Carbs and grains are not inherently evil. When we have LADA, we pay for each carb with a card from our hand—for example, supplementing insulin or jogging farther. (If not, we'll pay by having unhealthy BG.)
2. Whether a food is whole or processed, how it is processed, and how it is raised can outweigh many other health considerations.
3. When you're able, choose organic produce; small wild fish; and meat, dairy, or eggs labeled *pastured, organic, arsenic-free, antibiotic-free, Certified Humane*, or *AGA*; or buy directly from a small farmer in your state.
4. Beverages and breakfasts were challenging for me in the beginning. This got better when I let go of old habits and allowed my food world to grow.
5. When it comes to named diets, I advocate stealing all the great ideas, but giving the prohibitions a bit of side-eye. Consider whether those "don'ts" work best *for you* as big-picture guidance, or rigid rules.

o o o

19 THE LADA HONEYMOON DILEMMA

Living with Change

Complete beta cell failure occurs in almost all [LADA] patients, but it may take up to 12 years.
  —Dr. Gunnar Stenström, Kungsbacka Hospital, Sweden[1]

TWO NEWLYWEDS WANDER UP A RIDGE, EACH FOOTSTEP WAFTING A sun-warmed pine bouquet into the air. At the top we gaze past a Realtor's sign to Sugarloaf Peak where we married. The grouse that charged our red Subaru when we drove up now prances on the hood, displaying his own bright red and drumming regally. A band of deer nibble past, so close we can watch their lashes blink, tugging pink-striped spring beauties out of the soft earth.

When sunset blushes the clouds, then fades, the lovesick grouse calls it a day. A few stars appear, then brighten . . . still we stay, turning to look this way, then that, too entranced to leave. We lie back in the soft spring grasses fragrant with wild onion, my head on Pierre's shoulder. The northern lights blossom, billowing electric green curtains across the sky.

The next morning we call the number on the Realtor's sign. We've found home.

"GET IT OUT OF HERE THIS WEEK AND IT'S YOURS FOR FIVE HUNDRED bucks," the owner said as we peered through the dusty doorway of a half-century-old Magnolia trailer. Seven and a half feet wide and twenty-three

feet long, built-in maple shelves and sliding maple doors, peeling lino-
leum, 1950s turquoise appliances: Pierre and I looked at each other and
grinned.

Only Judy, fisherwoman and boat-backer extraordinaire, could have
pulled it off: We sneaked the unlicensed Magnolia across the highway,
along twisty, rutted roads, then backward down a narrow track; hefted
a stump in front of the door, and popped open a bottle of champagne.
Home sweet aluminum home.

The next week Judy phoned: "You've got to watch *The Long, Long
Trailer*—that's your trailer!"

We rented the VHS (this was ancient times), carried the TV out to
its stump, popped popcorn, and snuggled up on the outdoors couch: the
ultimate drive-in theater.

The Long, Long Trailer is vintage Lucille Ball from the era of
"women-are-dingy-but-love-conquers-all." When loopy Lucy and manly
Ricky set off in their Magnolia, everything that can go wrong does: They
get stuck in mud, crumple a carport, and try to cook at sixty miles an
hour, juggling steaming pots that go ricocheting out of control.

Lucy charmingly fills the trailer with pretty rocks. Very, very large
pretty rocks, heaped unsteadily under foldout tables and falling out of
closets. Logical Ricky mansplains so often that even the audience gets it:
Lucy, this is too many rocks.

In the crisis moment, on a mountain grade straight out of an astronaut
simulation, the long, long trailer careens out of control, brakes smoking,
rocks flying, while Lucy and Ricky scream at each other all the way down
the mountain pass.

Awww, we said, holding hands.

As LADAs, OUR HONEYMOON—THE TIME BEFORE WE TOTALLY RUN
out of insulin—might last a few months . . . or a dozen years. Surprise!
They call it our honeymoon because *we expect it to end*: *not* because we've
somehow failed, but because that's the normal trajectory of this autoimmune condition.

Early research found that six years or less to the end of the honeymoon is common,[2] but a decade is possible;[3] and the length of our

honeymoon may be increasing as treatment of LADA improves thanks to earlier diagnosis, better beta cell pampering, and earlier insulin supplementation. In one small 2020 study, the majority of LADAs in the study still produced some insulin after eight years (although less than when they began); LADAs with higher levels of GAD antibodies lost insulin production more quickly.[4] Other research confirms that GAD levels, and also fasting or stimulated C-peptide, can give us a heads-up about whether our insulin decline is more likely to be fast or slow.[5]

Just like a long, long trailer, a long, long honeymoon is not necessarily easy to live in. There's a reason honeymoons are typically ten *days* long, not ten *years* long.

A T1's honeymoon is generally a few months long at most. "If only I had realized how much easier life was in the honeymoon," T1s write, adding "If you still have some working beta cells, take good care of them!"

Those whose honeymoon is gone for good remind us how precious our own honeymoon is, and how fortunate we are to have working beta cells to pamper. On the flip side, these folks weren't trying to live in that honeymoon for a decade. With Lucy and Ricky.

As our insulin shrinks, so does our carb ceiling. If we're trying to postpone supplementing insulin, our other choices are poor health (not really an option, right?) or learning to live well under a very low carb ceiling, a small and shrinking food space.

I've heard a wife describe her LADA husband as "eating now like he has an eating disorder—and his doctor just doesn't get it."*

It's true: Many LADAs are already fit, already eating healthfully when we're diagnosed. We can't simply cut out doughnuts and Wonder Bread because we weren't eating them. Now we're weighing cutting away healthful foods: yams, tamales, and granola bars.

If you were already eating healthfully when you were diagnosed, and "normal-healthful" meals now put big waves in your BG, Carb-craft sounds daunting. When I was managing my LADA only through diet and

---

* It turns out that eating disorders and disordered eating have a surprising connection with diabetes; more on this in part 4.

exercise, the food choices I faced pushed me right up against the line of unhealthy deprivation. *In my experience, few doctors or nutritionists grasp this.* Their heads may be full of *T2 food rules* that *are completely inadequate for LADA.* They may come back at us with, "Just limit rice to one-quarter of your plate," when we try to explain what a *quarter cup* of rice does to our BG.

"A quarter plate of rice!" I exclaimed. "I can't eat that much rice in three days!"

The nutritionist stared at me like we weren't speaking the same language.

And I guess we weren't. I was speaking LADA.

Take heart. We *can* balance our carbs and insulin and not become eating-disordered.

LIMITS? OR DEPRIVATION?

Maybe as a kid you wanted to be a dolphin trainer, a firefighter, a ballet dancer, an ice-cream-flavor inventor, a fighter pilot, and a bus driver. Now you probably have only one main career. The question is: Did you happily and consciously let go of being a bus driver in exchange for the rewards of being a firefighter—or did the option feel ripped away from you? Do you still, all these years later, feel bereft when a bus goes by?

Focus has often been my friend, but feelings of deprivation have train-wrecked me. Deprivation can be a tightrope between bitterness and loss. I have seen people eat *worse* after a diagnosis of diabetes. I've wondered if a sense of deprivation—along with our very human tendency to use food as a coping strategy—lay beneath their difficult struggle.

Whatever you enjoy eating right now, you're not eating *every single thing* on Safeway's shelves every day. Limits are intrinsic, built in to every moment. When limits are *your choice*, they bring you focus, success, and gratitude. But when I view limits as deprivation, I go into a rage at every stoplight. I have fought limits like a fish on a line, and all I did was wear myself into exhaustion.

When I began trying to Carb-craft, I wanted to find a magic number of allowable carbs per meal, and then stuff that many carbs into every single meal. I now see that this was a bit like trying to stuff too many shirts into a bulging, seam-split, overhead travel bag, when I would have been better off considering whether I really needed nine shirts for a four-day trip.

One part of joy is: Feel good and eat delicious food.

I've never heard anyone say joy is: Walk into Safeway this morning and, without pause, eat every single thing on every single shelf.

We all have to come to terms with limits, in every aspect of our life. The question is not whether your food choices will incorporate limits, but how you will view those limits, and whether you have room to be creative and joyous within them.

An act becomes art when natural limits shape and enhance beauty. An architect sculpts a mountain cabin to shed snow and hold heat, and a very different house to frame the view on a jutting ocean point, or to catch and pull in Louisiana breezes. In the same way, with Carb-craft we allow *our* specific limits (which we learn with the tools in part 2) to provide inspiration as we enjoy delicious meals. We focus on what we love.

Carb-craft can help anybody. **Its exact details will look different for everybody.**

GIVE IT TIME

My diabetes diagnosis went off like a mini bomb, disrupting all my daily habits. I needed to heal: cultivate the garden in my gut, repair chronic inflammation, reset body "thermostats," and retrain my sense of normal. I also had to make peace with the word *diabetes*, get comfortable saying it out loud, and figure out how to celebrate my heritage and family foods while protecting my health.

Profound change takes *time*.[6] I became a Carb-crafter in stages.

- **Step 1: Boot camp.** Absolute, unwavering rules. I set myself a strict boot camp to cleanse, reboot, and discover my safe space: foods that kept my BG healthy. In this first phase, set-in-stone rules and a temptation-free house helped me get clean and stay strong.
- **Step 2: Internship.** Questioning and experimenting. Having gotten solid, clear, and confident in boot camp, I now had the mental space and tools to see if I could *grow* my safe food space. I began asking questions, searching out new recipes, and experimenting. For me

there was a lot of learning-by-failing, and constant self-monitoring, in the internship. Some days we land it and some days we don't. I didn't beat myself up when something unexpected happened; that's part of the learning curve.

- **Step 3: Carb-craft.** Living happily in the moment. It struck me somewhat out of the blue one day that, *Hey, I've got this. I know how to take care of myself.* I realized I wasn't stressing about food, wasn't going high or low BG, had forgotten to use my food journal for a week, and had a full, happy life. *What can I eat?* was no longer an endless anxious soundtrack taking up too much brain space: it was muscle memory. It sneaked up on me—I'd been promoted—I wasn't an intern anymore, but a full-on Carb-crafter.

How long should *your* boot camp be? That depends on your personality. Many cleanses are ten days. Whole30 is a month. US Marine Corps boot camp is twelve weeks. My advice may sound counterintuitive, but: A *longer* stay in your personal food boot camp *makes everything that follows easier.* You are the expert on you, though, and what you can to commit to.

I set my boot camp at six weeks. The day I began, six weeks sounded like a frighteningly, insanely long time to survive without garlic naan. Looking back, it's the blink of an eye. Strict, simple rules, a maximum number of carbs per meal (established by my personal test-test-test) and a cleansed house holding only healthful low-carb options, helped me be successful in boot camp. Boot camp showed me that I always had a safe space, a successful place, I could return to anytime something beyond my control, like a death in the family, knocked me into a tough time.

There are things to love about boot camp: our body cleanses, our muscle builds, excess weight melts away. Boot camp built my endurance and my ability to withstand temptation. Cutting sugar can be like stopping smoking—your palate will become much more sensitive. Flavors explode, like colors in a tropical garden. As muscle builds, it gets steadily easier and more fun to participate in healthful activities: Zumba, yoga, walks with friends—whatever brings you happiness.

The body climbs to better health as if up a set of stairs, sometimes pausing awhile on a landing. A goal that seems utterly impossible in week two may earn you a gold star in week five. Stay the course. Trust time.

Boot camp is simple. But not easy. Boot camp demands commitment and faith. It's tough, it's worth it, and it's going to be over. All you have to do is survive, moment by moment. Mark off the days on the calendar, watching your goal get closer. Let time work its magic.

STOP STOPPING IT

In boot camp we build our safe space. But we don't want to live forever in a space so small and crammed with rocks—I mean rules—that we can barely turn around.

Stop eating dessert! society tells diabetics. The internship is the place to test for ourselves: Which desserts, and how much, can I still eat?

Stop eating fruit! a foodie told me. Evolutionarily, he said, we ate fruit only in a small season, but we gnawed on greens most of the year. Darn, my test-test-test says he's right that it spikes my BG to eat a whole apple at lunch now. Well, can I eat a quarter of an apple?

No hash browns, no challah, no tamales, no pancakes, and definitely no potato chips, chided the internet. In my internship, I read the label on the potato chip bag and did the math. Interesting: For this brand at least, one potato chip is about one gram of carb. Huh. The math says I can safely eat a few chips (if I'm sure I can stop after those few).

Dark chocolate: same. Again, the math surprised me. Many family-size artisan dark chocolate bars are thirty to forty grams of *non-fiber* carb; so if you can eat fifteen grams of carb in a meal you can eat several squares of dark chocolate tonight, assuming you didn't spend those carbs on other things.

I found enormous relief in knowing that I wouldn't have to give up completely and forever on *any* food I love. Chocolate, pancakes, potato chips, cheesecake, garlic naan, nachos, and beer—we can eat anything, just not everything-at-once. Today I **spend carbs like gold**.

IT DIDN'T HAPPEN FOR ME OVERNIGHT

When I was a boot camp beginner, I came upon a recipe: "Here's a substitute for mashed potatoes—made from cauliflower—natural and low-carb!"

So I steamed cauliflower, tossed it in my blender, whipped in the recipe's additions, set it on my table in a beautiful bowl, breathed, smiled, and took that first bite. Disgusting! Get this baby-food mashed-yuk out of here! I rarely throw out food, but that dish went straight to the compost bucket.

At the time, the memory of "real" mashed potatoes and how much I loved them outshone cauliflower mush. Same with a recipe for low-carb nachos. Calling squishy veggies "nachos" made me miss the real thing like crazy, and despise what was in front of me.

With hindsight I see that it was *me*, not the food. I had to *get through boot camp first*. I couldn't just rocket straight to the internship. Ironically, a year later, I "invented" similar recipes "all by myself" and thought: *Wow, tasty!* Today I'm all about substituting this for that, finding ways to keep the flavors I love while eliminating many of the carbs. But it took time before I could get there.

I couldn't step off a train going sixty miles an hour onto the station platform. I had to transition. I had to change my body—and even more, my mind—to get off the train hurtling me to an early grave, and onto the stage where the lovely party of life was going on.

A LADA CAN GO FROM THE HONEYMOON TO . . . THE *SECOND* HONEYMOON?

If we have the support, good fortune, and access to begin supplementing insulin while we are still making some insulin of our own, we'll preserve beta cells while also having more leeway in what we eat. If our food space was becoming just too small without supplemental insulin, beginning insulin can raise our carb ceiling back to a more livable level, and give us a *second* honeymoon.

In this second honeymoon, supplemental insulin pampers our beta cells, lowers BG spikes, and adds more freedom to our food world. Meanwhile the insulin we still make ourselves lets us inject smaller amounts, makes dosing decisions easier, may allow us to use only one type of insulin (chapter 13), and reduces our risk of dangerous BG lows.

I was very med-avoidant when I began my LADA journey. I thought: *If the top of the diabetic class is managing without meds, I want an A+, too!* Now I understand that with diabetes we each begin in a different place, with our own challenges. My insulin tank had nearly run dry by the time I was diagnosed, and my cells that could refill it were steadily dying, not because I'd done wrong but because of the mystery that is autoimmunity.

I'd been living in a deficient state for so long, I wasn't fully aware of the extent to which low insulin was impacting everything from my energy level and joy to whether my liver repeatedly dumped too much sugar into my blood. Today it feels like a no-brainer to add metformin, vitamin D, and insulin to my toolbox. Thanks, meds, for making my food world larger.

KEY TAKEAWAYS

1. The LADA dilemma: How long is a good honeymoon, and how good is a long honeymoon?

2. LADAs expect to run out of insulin, but we don't know when! Two to six years is common, but be ready for anything from six months to twelve years. In fact, with early diagnosis and good beta cell pampering, no one knows how long we might go. You might make medical history!

3. A LADA *can eat anything*. We just can't eat everything. The better questions are: How much? How often?

4. Cutting sugar can make eating more fun! Flavors explode.

5. Profound change takes *time*. At first I needed strict rules and a temptation-free house to get strong and clean (boot camp). After I felt solid, clear, and safe around food, I could experiment, ask questions, and try to grow that safe space (internship). Today—Carb-craft: I enjoy a full, happy life, where *What can I eat?* is muscle memory, not an endless anxious soundtrack.

6. When our first honeymoon begins to feel too limited, uncomfortable, or like disordered eating, we can begin supplementing insulin. This will raise our carb ceiling, prolong the lives of our beta cells, and begin our second honeymoon.

o o o

To live happily in a small space for a long time—or in a long, long trailer—you have to make it beautiful, and you have to make it yours. You plant mint and hops. You take the old couch left behind by the droll, Kundera-quoting roommate, put it out on the porch, and watch the sun set and the white-headed woodpeckers build their nest.

There was so much room in our tiny Magnolia. Pierre's mother, June, lived there with us for months after her heart attack. Unused to the bright sun of eastern Washington after living in Juneau for decades, June carried a sassy parasol, twirling it as we wheeled her around town. She planted flowers, tended to the hummingbirds, and wrote impassioned letters to the editor in exquisite calligraphy.

Our son Raven was born just months after we lost June. As a threesome, we fell in love all over again, in a new way. I will always remember Pierre on the weather-warbled porch, rocking Raven, heart against heart, Pierre humming a deep, quiet song, when a mother coyote and two pups trotted across the meadow blazing with wild sunflowers. I also remember my first squirt-in-the-eye of diaper-changing baby-pee: that happened on the porch of the Magnolia, too.

Now teenage Raven and his friends laugh and joke on the porch steps of the Magnolia. And every spring, a wild rose, a rhubarb plant, and a patch of mint that June planted burst up into the sunshine.

BIG PICTURE

BIG PICTURE 3 AND PART III SUMMARY: TWENTY-TWO STEPS TO CARB-CRAFT SUCCESS

- Carb-craft—balancing carbs and insulin—is the foundation for diabetes health.
- Carb-craft honors each person's unique limits and location along the diabetes spectrum.
- Carb-craft lets us revel in healthy delights, whatever our food preferences.
- Carb-craft is built on twenty-two rules we can each carry out in our unique way, expressing our identity and culture.

THE TWENTY-TWO STEPS

1. **Eat foods Great-Grandma would recognize.**
2. Enjoy **whole foods** that look like themselves. Eat a **rainbow.** Colorful, and heavy toward the many shades of green.
3. **Veggie-centered meals.** Veggies at the heart. Veggies as the centerpiece. Light on the root veggies. Build each meal around veggies.
4. **Cut the carbs, keep the joy.** No deprivation, no self-punishment. Reinvent favorite traditional foods in lower-carb versions. Don't abandon flavors and foods you love—just learn how much and how often they work best for you.
5. **Spend carbs like gold.** When insulin is limited, carbs are precious. Let them make life rich, whether you spend them on wine and chocolate, fresh mango, or one butter-melting piece of just-baked bread.
6. **Let the pancreas rest between meals.** A LADA's pancreas has to run hard to digest a meal. LADAs do better when we minimize grazing, and separate our meals by at least four hours. Some will find even longer rests helpful (intermittent fasting).

7. **Light on beans and grains.** LADAs don't need to abandon the many health benefits of beans and grains. We do need to think carefully about portion size. For most of us, these are no longer the centerpiece of our meal.

8. **Fiber is friendly. Eat pro-garden and anti-inflammatory.** Fiber is friendly, "free," and filling. One of the best things a LADA (and most of us) can do to promote our health is cultivate a healthy microbiome.

    Most LADA-love foods (appendix B)—especially berries, nuts, greens, and wild salmon—are anti-inflammatory for most people; but never be afraid to test-test-test for yourself.

9. **Fermented foods** help the health of our garden. Pickles are a great starter fermented food. Enjoy yogurt, kefir, tempeh, kombucha, kimchi, or sauerkraut. The label should say KEEP REFRIGERATED (chapter 11).

10. **Enjoy healthful fats.** A splash of healthful fat is a perfect way to add calories without carbs, keeps BG calm, and can lower cardiovascular risks and quench hunger. While omega-3s are the champions, many types of fats are both heart-healthy and improve diabetes health (chapter 17).

11. **Both animal and plant foods can be healthy.** Carb-craft is compatible with carnivorous, omnivorous, vegan, vegetarian, and many other approaches. Processed meats (like hot dogs) raise health risks, but other meats do not (chapter 17), and eggs and dairy can improve our health with LADA.

12. **Eat the yolk.** Eggs don't harm our heart or raise cholesterol—and they are a great source of protein and vitamins. While egg white has good protein, only the yolk contains the vitamins (A, D, E, K, and B), minerals (calcium, zinc, phosphorus), and antioxidants.

13. **Toxin-free food and small fish.** Solid research shows that when we eat "standard" produce, meat, eggs, or dairy; standard farmed fish; and fish at the top of the food chain, chemicals in and on these foods increase our risk of diabetes (chapter 18).

14. **Named diets: Harvest the best ideas.** Like the author who jokes that he is *Pegan* (paleo plus vegan), we can choose the best ideas and recipes from among many named diets.

15. **Superfoods.** Enjoy foods rich in vitamins and antioxidants, like avocado, blueberries, leafy greens, crucifers (broccoli, cauliflower, arugula), coconut, green tea, nuts, and seeds. (You don't have to call them superfoods if you don't want. But it is kind of a cute word.)

16. **Breakfast: Go global.** Try omelets, fry-ups, tofu scrambles, idli, avocado bakes, huevos montañeros, Scandinavian cold cuts, poached fish, feijoada, and other international delights.

17. **Keep a safe space in your back pocket** . . . I began by figuring out my safe space: foods that keep BG happily out of the danger zone.

    - **Zero-carb.** Healthful fats and animal protein (meat, eggs, hard cheeses).
    - **Freebies.** Foods like a slice of lemon, a sprinkle of onion, spices, or a scoop of salsa we can consider "freebies," in part because of low carbs, and in part because of low quantity.
    - **So low, you can feel free.** There are few carbs in lettuce, spinach, broccoli, bok choy, collards, cauliflower, and similar LADA-love veggies (appendix B). So few, I don't bother to count—minimize math! Two thumbs-up as well to mushrooms, which are a healthful mix of carb, protein, and fiber. It can be helpful to pair these low-carb/low-cal foods with low-carb/higher-cal foods like avocado, coconut, dressings, nuts, seeds, nut butters, olives, olive tapenade, healthful oils such as fish oil, or meat/fish/dairy/soy.
    - **In moderation.** Foods I eat often but do track carb amounts include carrots, tomatoes, cucumber, zucchini, yellow squash; berries, cherries, apricots, plums, and citrus fruits; unsweetened yogurt and nut milks.

18. **. . . and know when and how to let yourself off the leash.** I don't let my safe space become a prison cell. I add fun foods, **spending carbs like gold:**

    - Fruits are healthful and delicious, but with LADA I eat them less often and in smaller portions: the cherry on top!
    - I'm moderate with beans and grains.
    - When spending carbs like gold, I budget for occasional treats: croissant, rice, waffle, chocolate, cheesecake . . . Yes, guy in

my diabetes class: Once in a while we absolutely are meant to savor an ice cream with the woman we love.

19. **Exercise like kids play.** Can you up your activity level 15 percent? Keep it playful, switch it up, keep it moving, keep changing the rules—on a whim, because there are no rules. If you feel safe to do so, add a sprint, a full-speed burst, mixed in with your slower steady pace. Try something new. Remember fun?

20. **Play with getting out of the supermarket.** I'm not dissing lovely little community grocers, and I'm not trying to make your life harder. But sometimes the easiest way to shop smart is to leave the store where much of what you see is bad for you and go where everything you see is good for you: like your local farmers market. Speaking of easy: Sign up for a CSA (community-supported agriculture) and receive a weekly bag of locally grown veggies. Today these options are not equally accessible to all, but—is there a small independent farmer in your state who needs you as much as you need her?

    Consider your power to transform your own backyard; or if you have no yard, your local community garden; or if there is no nearby community garden—how do you think they get started?

21. **Let food love you back.** It's science, peoples: When we eat from small, pretty dishes, eat fragrant foods, and have a pleasing acoustic environment while eating, we eat less and are happier. Equally important and—for me—even harder: Do your best to notice your food, to eat only because you're hungry, and to avoid multi-tasking while eating. Do your best to treat yourself like a person you love, and to serve yourself well.

22. **Spark joy.** As with riding a bike, skiing, or life's greatest pleasure, there can be a learning curve. Trust time. Don't give up too soon.

    The principles of Carb-craft are the same for everyone, but we each sculpt the fine details depending on our identity, heritage, tastes, and preferences.

    LADA has put enough on our plates; we don't need to add self-punishment. If you hope to sustain healthful eating *long-term*, craft your personal version to bring you joy.

PART IV

CRUISING WITH CARB-CRAFT: GO THE DISTANCE

Learning about my microbiome, pricking my fingers, and memorizing the carbs in my favorite foods seemed hard. But here's what was harder for me: my late-night self, standing in the blue light of the fridge, spooning ice cream straight from the carton into my mouth—that self who came out of the shadows and in fifteen minutes undid all the bullet-sweating twenty-three and three-quarter hours of effort by my cheery, rational daytime self.

Food is deeply tangled with our hearts, our heritage, our coping mechanisms, our romances, our despair, and our celebrations. The psychology of food is enormous. And partly biochemical. There is nothing remotely simple about "just" changing what we eat. While I can't do full justice to the psychology of food here, I think the gazillions of books telling diabetics what to eat, while never once acknowledging the psychological and cultural aspects of eating, are disingenuous.

I'd changed what was on my pantry shelves, changed my recipes, gotten more comfortable with my identity and more clear about my needs. But could I prevent moods and emotions from undermining my rational self? Could I heal my lifetime of challenges and dysfunctions around food? Honestly, I wouldn't have bet on myself.

The next few chapters explain why **the same body chemistry that predisposes us to diabetes** may also make it harder for us to have an emotionally healthy relationship with food.

20 HUNGER

I know that hunger is in the mind and the body and the heart and the soul.
    —Roxane Gay[1]

As a kid I delighted in climbing trees, somersaulting across lawns, and leaping off the roof of the toolshed. But somewhere between the alphabet and long division, it became less likely to find me in the crab apple's branches, and more likely to find me in front of the mirror, sucking in my stomach. If I could log all my hours in dressing rooms searching for the mythic pair of jeans that would make me look skinniest, and all the hours I've wasted trying to "fix" my body, would they reach to the moon, or just spin the Earth's equator?

When I hit fifty I thought: *Never again!* Gather all the women I love and admire, and the collective mental energy we've put over the years into dieting, not-dieting, researching, wondering, obsessing, taking a bite of this, jiggling a pound, pinching an inch—there'd be a cure for cancer and a colony on Mars if we'd put all that focus into something worthwhile. I will diet no more forever. This is my freedom song.

A month later, I was diagnosed with diabetes. Ironic. Since *when we have diabetes, managing weight is the first critical step* to caring for our health.

HOW WE BALANCE

Have you seen a balance scale? It's a perfectly balanced bar with a plate or basket on each end. We could put a stack of gold coins on one side, and a gold nugget on the other, to see if they weigh the same. (Or, like Monty Python, a witch on one side and a duck on the other.)

We can picture our brain using a balance scale to decide if we're hungry, piling the no votes on one side and the yes on the other.

Ghrelin is the star *I'm hungry* hormone. It stimulates appetite, increases food intake, and sharpens both the senses and imagination, making scents sweeter and sharper and making colors—whether of fruit or Twinkie packages—gleam brighter. Ghrelin levels increase as we age, contributing to the spare tire many wake up to in late middle age. *I'm hungry* ghrelin, produced mainly by our empty stomach, reveals our short-term needs.

Leptin. As Layla's story illustrates (chapter 10), we need leptin to weigh in on the other side of the balance. *I'm full* leptin, a hormone produced by our body fat, reflects our long-term status.

The brain wants to balance our short-term situation—what we've eaten in recent hours—with our long-term energy reserves. The brain monitors demand from muscles, how much food is in our tummy, how well we're supplied with vitamins, minerals, and other building blocks, what our microbiome wants, how the immune system is feeling, whether we're running a fever, how much total body fat we have, the level of energy sources in our bloodstream, and more. It learns all this by reading hormone levels; checking out what other organs are posting on Instagram. Then the brain integrates all this information into one conscious thought, such as: *For some reason, I'm craving an orange right now.* Or the thought: *I couldn't eat another bite.* Or: *We still have three miles to hike to reach our car, and all I can think about is pizza and beer.*

 The brain piles *I'm hungry* hormones on one side of the scale, and *I'm full* hormones on the other, to balance our short-term and long-term food needs.

o o o

WHEN THE BALANCE BREAKS

Just as we can develop resistance to the hormone insulin, we can develop resistance to leptin. Leptin-resistant people often have very high levels of leptin, yet leptin can't do its work. Many obese people struggle with leptin resistance.[2]

Losing significant weight may drop our leptin levels below normal, making us hungrier at the same time that our body has become more efficient, running on fewer calories.[3]

And while leptin makes a "normal" person more sensitive to insulin, it makes prediabetics less sensitive to insulin, according to the research team of Dr. Simona Bungau. Dr. Bungau also found that high insulin levels "impair the . . . response to leptin . . . [and] generate weight accumulation leading to a vicious cycle."[4]

Ghrelin signaling can also get disrupted. For some people who struggle to control their weight, ghrelin does not drop after a meal; they are nearly as hungry after the meal as before.[5] For some, after we successfully reduce to a more healthful weight, ghrelin may rise, and stay elevated for years, or perhaps permanently. And in bad news for us insulin-limited folk, ghrelin reduces release of insulin from our beta cells.[6]

Not only do men and women store fat differently (chapter 10), but we also differ in the effect of weight loss on our ghrelin/leptin balance; and we differ in whether our likelihood of weight regain is more influenced by ghrelin or by leptin.[7]

GET OTHER HORMONES ON YOUR SIDE

1. **Defuse the cortisol bomb.**

     It's hard to change food habits without experiencing stress, and stress can fill our scale with hormones that urge us to eat. Studies have shown that simply counting calories (not reducing them, just counting them) can raise stress and increase levels of the hormone cortisol.[8] High cortisol levels are strongly linked to overeating and weight gain, turn more of a given meal to fat, and put that fat in the least healthy places (abdominal fat). *Reducing cortisol by managing stress* in healthful ways is one of the best things a diabetic can do for her health.[9]

2. **Enlist the satiety hormones.**

Meet the friends I call Glip, Pip, and Chik.* Like three singing chipmunks, they can sometimes make enough noise (they might say: "music") to drown out growling, gotta-eat ghrelin. Cueing off the *quality* of the food we eat, Glip, Pip, and Chik pile into the *I'm full* side of the scale and tell the brain: We're good.

Research found that people who took Glip at breakfast reported feeling more satisfied and ate fewer calories at lunch.[10] Glip not only helps us feel well fed and happy, it also heals the garden in our gut, reduces inflammation, protects beta cells, increases insulin production, and tells the liver not to dump sugar.[11] Glip is so awesome that medications to mimic or increase Glip have been created; but these medications are new enough that some have questions about their safety (chapter 12). Luckily eating high-quality, high-nutrient food can promote our three amigos.

- **Glip** makes us feel full and stabilizes our blood sugars. Glip increases when we eat *leafy greens, fiber, and protein*. It's reduced by chronic inflammation.
- **Pip** reduces food intake and obesity. It thrives on *fiber and protein*. High blood sugars impair Pip.
- **Chik** flourishes on *healthy fats, fiber, and protein*. Like the first two friends, Chik is produced in the intestines and reduces food consumption.

3. **Shut down the craving hormone.**

   NPY (neuropeptide Y) stimulates appetite, particularly for carbohydrates. It's produced by our brain when we're food-deprived or in times of other stress. To fight this carb-craving hormone, eat plenty of fiber and protein. Whaaat, eating my spinach could obliterate my doughnut craving? Who knew?

4. **Get your rest.**

   When we lack sleep, we produce more ghrelin, more cortisol, and less leptin. Which is a fancy way of saying: lack of sleep makes us grumpy and hungry. (What a stunner.)

---

* GLP-1 or glucagon-like peptide-1, PYY or peptide YY, and CCK or cholecystokinin.

Diabetics may have sleep apnea and be unaware of it; addressing this can help us feel enormously better. Sleep apnea can cause weight gain, diabetes, heart arrhythmia, cardiac arrest, and more. If this may be an issue for you, ask about the simple screening test where, sleeping at home as normal, you wear a small device on your finger measuring oxygen levels.

5. **Stay active or get more active.**

Exercise and activity, even mellow activity like gardening or strolling by a river, increase *adiponectin, testosterone, adrenaline,* and *growth hormone*: hormones that burn fat and give us energy, drive, and alertness (chapter 10).

STAY A STEP AHEAD OF HUNGER

Ten different people may have ten different experiences of hunger. Food cravings can vary with genetics, microbiome, age, sex, stress levels, hormone levels, and more. Just as there are many kinds of hunger, there are many kinds of fullness, and we can use all of them to battle hunger:

1. **Volume.** Bulk; a pleasantly full tummy. Thank you fiber, salads, and green veggies. Thank you broccoli, cauliflower, collard greens, and green beans.
2. **Calories.** Did you get *enough* of them in this meal to make it for four hours (or through the night) without crashing?
3. **Fat.** Appropriate amounts of healthful fat. A splurge of velvety dressing on the salad, unsweetened peanut sauce on the broccoli, or cream in Thai tea blankets our hunger, soothing away pangs.
4. **Nutrients.** Nutrient-dense foods stimulate satiety hormones.
5. **Hydrate.** It's healthful and can help you feel full.
6. **Visual cues.** Studies show that when we eat from attractive dishes right-sized for the meal portion, eat in pleasant surroundings, eat slowly, and notice what we're eating, we feel more satisfied and eat less. "The eye eats first," my chef-friend says.

21 CARBS AND OUR BRAIN, HEART, AND HERITAGE

*There are moments in this life that I recall not as visual
snapshots but as tastes and fragrances. They make sense to
me, to who I am, in ways that . . . are profoundly rooted . . .
those moments seem as deeply etched into the matter of my
body as anything can be.*
　　　—Gary Paul Nabhan, *Coming Home to Eat*[1]

IN A STUDY, RANDOM PEOPLE WERE ASKED TO SOLVE COMPLICATED puzzles (and, oh, don't touch this food please, it's for the next user of the room), then left alone in a room. On the table nearby lay either a plate of fresh-baked chocolate chip cookies or a bowl of radishes. All test subjects faithfully followed instructions; no one sneaked a cookie or a radish.

The puzzle solvers in the radish room wildly outperformed the cookie room. People in the cookie room couldn't make as much progress on the puzzles, quit sooner, and reported feeling exhausted and depleted.

Other studies confirm these findings: Resisting food steals our mental sharpness and exhausts us mentally, physically, and emotionally.[2]

Having diabetes or losing significant weight—either or both—can throw off the body's natural feedback systems. While most people can listen to the body and trust its messages about when, what, and how much to eat, this will not always be true when we have diabetes.

If I can't trust my body's signals, and must rely on food rules to stay healthy, does this lock me in the cookie room for the rest of my life?

As the book Devoured explains, right in the subtitle, "what we eat defines who we are."[3]

It's hard to eat a traditional or celebratory meal from any heritage and not eat a significant amount of carbohydrates. Challah. Injera. Tortillas. Lefse. Garlic naan. Fresh-baked biscuits. Moo shu. Pizza. Biryani. Thai curry *goes on* rice. Hand-rolled pasta. Danish breakfast sandwiches. Christmas tamales and hallacas. Grits. Pad Thai. Blintzes. Paella. Picnic potato salad. Pho. Flan. Corn on the cob at the county fair. Posole. Pick a culture, almost any culture: The glory is in the carbs.

What are our celebration foods? What are our "treats"? Carbs, nine times out of ten. The carb-treat connection in our brains gets wired so early: in pre-memory days for most of us. Celebrate birthdays with cake. Celebrate Christmas with gingerbread houses, Mexican wedding cookies, krumkaker, eggnog, ponche crema. Celebrate Easter with chocolate bunnies and marshmallow peeps. Would it really be Thanksgiving without the stuffing and mashed potatoes, the pumpkin, apple, and pecan pies? Would camping be the same without s'mores?

From the day we are born, food is commingled with our deepest psychological needs: love, safety, and human connection. When we are diagnosed with diabetes, food stays tangled with love. But now food is also a thing to fear: a thing that might literally kill us, with each and every bite.

On top of this, access to healthful foods is much more difficult for some, which can layer anger, frustration, guilt, and other complex emotions on top of the rest.

That's . . . complicated.

For any one of us, food may not be everything listed below, but for many:

Food is love.

Food is identity.

Food is family.

Food is heritage.

Food is reward.

Food is a numbing strategy for anxiety.

Food is energy.

Food is adventure.

Food is play.

Food is art.

Food is addiction, for many.

Food is creativity.

Food is companionship.

Food is sensual, and sometimes sexual.

Food is (was) the perfect gift, as close to universally appreciated as a gift can come.

Food is shelter and safety.

Food is a barrier against pain.

Food is self-harm, and self-loathing, for some.

Food is the tangible heart of celebrations.

Food is community.

For me, food is (was) all of these. I wonder if anyone in the world has a simple relationship with food.

FOOD FEAR

Food was already complicated for me . . . then when I was diagnosed with diabetes, I plunged into true food fear. Unexpected traps were everywhere. A bowl of vegetable soup and a salad zoomed my BG into the red? Farm-fresh strawberries? Cottage cheese? These random food bombs made me twitchy.

More fears: Now I'll be the chronic dieter, the tattered Dickens character staring through the window at "food glorious food" after my daily inadequate morsel—I'll be on the outside looking in . . . *forever.*

Now I'll just gnaw down calories without carbs, grinding through broccoli stems like a beaver. I'll be like my friend who puts a chunk of butter, along with heavy cream, in her coffee every morning: calories without carbs! Breakfast today, tomorrow, and every day: butter-choked-coffee and a bowl of raw cabbage. Yum.

For many of us, it was already hard to be normal about food. **Diabetes can triple our risk** of self-harming eating patterns.

DISORDERED EATING

One in twenty Americans have an *eating disorder* (such as anorexia, bulimia, and others). Many of the rest of us have *disordered eating*—an obsessive relationship with weight, food, body size, or exercise.

Both eating disorders and disordered eating affect all ages, races, and genders. On any given day 45 percent of American women, and many men, are on a diet. Eighty percent of thirteen-year-old girls have dieted. Among women over fifty, about one in eight have disordered eating.[4] A survey found that about 80 percent of women are dissatisfied with their appearance, and 40 percent said they would trade three to five years of their lives to achieve weight loss goals.[5]

Psychologists view eating disorders as a form of mental illness, and disordered eating as a type of OCD (obsessive-compulsive disorder). What is OCD? Many of us experience unwanted, distressing thoughts or feelings we casually refer to as obsession or compulsion. But when these thoughts or behaviors *feel out of our control, destroy our goals, relationships, or health, run counter to our values, or interfere with our daily life*, they cross the line into OCD.

Disordered eaters include:

- **Social switchers.** Eating only salads when with friends, then anything and everything when kicked back on the couch.
- **Food restrictors.** Counting every last calorie, sometimes to the point of developing nutrient deficiencies or triggering the body's starvation response.
- **Orthorexics.** Combatively judgmental about what others eat, and avoiding social situations where food will not be within our control.
- **Compulsive dieters.** Following faddish or dangerous diet plans.
- **Compulsive exercisers.** Exercising obsessively and only for weight loss, sometimes even when injured or exhausted.

Disordered eating may become more extreme over time, progressing to a full-blown eating disorder. Conversely, disordered eaters may be "recovered" anorexics.

Both eating disorders and disordered eating steal joy and energy, and measurably harm working intelligence. Eating disorders have the highest mortality rate of any mental illness; are often linked to substance abuse and suicide; and arise from a combination of genetics and environment.[6]

HARD AS IT ALREADY WAS TO BE NORMAL ABOUT FOOD, *DIABETICS, statistically, have it even harder.*[7] According to the National Association of Anorexia Nervosa and Associated Disorders:[8]

- Female diabetics have almost *four times the prevalence of eating disorders* as the average American female.
- *Over a third* of diabetic women have disordered eating behaviors.
- Diabetic disorders include *diabulimia*, systematically underusing insulin, risking blindness and brain damage in the hope of losing weight. *Diabulimia triples our risk of death.*

WHEN DISCUSSING DISORDERED EATING, THE MEDICAL COMMUNITY often adds, down in the small print: but if you're restricting or obsessing about food *due to a legitimate health concern* then never mind, what you're doing is healthy.

Gosh, thanks.

I mean: Wait, whaaat?

Does this mean all the stresses of disordered eating don't affect a diabetic? Or don't matter? Or they do matter, but not as much as a heart attack? Or . . . what, exactly?

CAN FOOD BE ADDICTIVE?

Ahh, sugar, sugar, you got me wanting you, sang the Archies. Our bodies and brains are built to love sugar. Carbohydrates trigger the release of dopamine, lighting up pleasure centers in our brains in much the same way that opiates do. Dopamine is the neurotransmitter of euphoria, bliss, motivation, and concentration.

Lab rats chose sugar over cocaine in one study, prompting headlines like: "Is Sugar More Addictive than Cocaine?" Nope, is the current scientific consensus: Sugar is roughly as addictive as nicotine. Addiction research finds many similarities between addiction to food and addiction to cigarettes.[9]

"Palatable foods can promote an addictive process akin to drugs of abuse," writes Dr. Revi Bonder of New York University.[10] Separate studies from Finland, China, and Canada found that diabetics have triple to six times greater risk of food addiction.[11]

In addiction, a substance hijacks our brain reward pathway. First a trigger says, *This is marvelous.* Second our brain adds: *Let's make this happen again.*

First the brain releases a rush of dopamine, making us giddy with pleasure. Then the amygdala and hippocampus sear associated visuals, smells, and colors into our memory to help us find this experience again. (That's the simplified overview; the brain's a complicated place, and other neurotransmitters and hormones get involved.)

But it's never as good as the first time. Each subsequent time we "use," our brain releases less dopamine, and also *prunes away* some of our dopamine receptors. This means that between times of using, we become dopamine-*deprived*: needy, cranky, angry, or anxious.

This is the tolerance effect. Actual use gives us less of a rush (less dopamine) each time. Meanwhile those visual and scent cues that make us *anticipate* use produce *ever-stronger* chemical rushes in the brain, impelling us to crave, foretaste, and seek. As neuroscientist and addict in recovery Dr. Judith Grisel explains, for her at this point, "It wasn't enhancing my life any more . . . I was just using it to cope with the effects of not using it."[12]

THE AMERICAN PSYCHIATRIC ASSOCIATION DEFINES ADDICTION AS "a brain disease that is manifested by compulsive substance use despite harmful consequence." Food addiction, like other addictions, physically alters our brain.[13] And as is typical of addiction, those with a food addiction have greater risk of other addictions.[14]

Scientists estimate that in the US and other countries, about one in six have an addiction to food; similar to the percentage with an alcohol or tobacco addiction.[15] Within particular groups, the percent food-addicted can range from 10 to 55 percent, or even up to 96 percent in those with a full-blown eating disorder.[16] A person with a food addiction may be at, above, or below their healthy weight.[17]

Genetics loads the gun and environment pulls the trigger. Our susceptibility to food addiction is linked to our genetics and shaped by our earliest experience: Beginning in the womb, very high *or* very low levels of sugar increase our risk of food addiction.[18]

Food addiction is a one-two punch. First, boom, dopamine. Second, your memory is etched with associated sights, smells, and sensations. That's why smelling cookies baking, watching someone else eat ice cream, seeing the bright color of a favorite food label—or just reading this sentence—can release chemicals in your brain that trigger intense craving. While the pleasure rush keeps decreasing over time, the memory-trigger pathway gets more intense each time, until you get more jacked up from smelling and craving the chocolate chip cookie than you're going to get pleasure from eating it.

Never Enough, the title of Dr. Grisel's book on addiction, captures the heartbreaking essence of this hunger. Some of us are more vulnerable to addiction, explains Dr. Grisel, particularly those whose baseline endorphins are lower than usual, because when an addictive substance floods these people with endorphins, that's a rare feeling they are deeply driven to repeat. When Grisel encountered her first addictive substance, "Suddenly I was full and okay in a way I had never been," she explained in an NPR interview with Terry Gross.

RESEARCH SHOWS THAT OUR MOST ADDICTIVE FOODS ARE:[19] (1) ultra-processed and highly sweetened foods with very fast carbs; (2) fat-infused carbs such as potato chips and doughnuts; and (3) salty foods.

As in other addictions, food addicts:

- Suffer intense cravings, particularly for ultra-processed foods that are high-carb or high-carb-high-fat.

- Use compulsively; may binge.
- Frequently fail in attempts to not use; are often unable to resist temptation.
- Build a tolerance, requiring ever more of the substance, until eventually we use not for a high, but to pull ourselves out of a low.
- Suffer withdrawal symptoms.
- Continue using though we know we are harming ourselves.
- May sacrifice relationships and other important aspects of life for our addiction.

FIGHTING BACK AGAINST ADDICTION

The brain loves "normal," and is always trying to rebalance. The tolerance effect happens because our brain is trying to bring us back to normal. That's why it prunes away dopamine receptors. It says, *I'll get out ahead of you; now when you use it will have less effect—voilà!*

The brain begins this prebalancing before we even put the substance into our mouths (or veins or lungs). The brain starts smiting dopamine the moment it believes a "hit" is probably on the way.

So when an alcoholic in recovery pulls up to the tavern, planning to see pals and just sip a Coke, at the sight of that neon sign, her brain begins to destroy her dopamine. As she's pushing open the tavern door, her dopamine and happiness are plummeting. The longer she's in that tavern, the more drained she'll be, and the more desperately her body/mind will crave a hit.

Learning this hit home: I closed my eyes, re-seeing my breakfast with friends at O'Grady's. So that's why I felt like a drooly dog who had a steak waved under her nose. Not because I'm weird or weak, but because my brain was doing to me what all brains do.

For this reason, many deal with addiction in stages. When we're starting out, vulnerable and shaky, we stay away from the tavern. But later, perhaps we don't avoid a memory-steeped place: We might decide to deliberately desensitize to it, on a day we're confident we have lots of support and the tools to do so successfully. The first few times may be very difficult, but *we can retrain the brain.* Oh, says the brain—eventually—the tavern doesn't always equal alcohol . . . my favorite coffee shop doesn't always equal a flaky chocolate croissant . . . guess I won't zap away all dopamine as the hand opens the door.

HUNGER HAS THREE LAYERS

Three hungers stack inside us like a pyramid. We all have the base: hormonal (body) hunger. Some have the middle layer, emotional (heart) hunger, and some also the cap: addictive (neural-loop) hunger.

If we have more than one type of hunger, all our layers, connected and codependent, confront us simultaneously. Yet they may be best dealt with the way cool kids deal with Oreo cookies: one layer at a time.

Body Hunger

Body hunger keeps us directed toward survival yet doesn't interfere with the tasks of survival. Body hunger sharpens our senses, brightening colors and scents, while allowing us to focus and work hard. For some lucky humans, this is the only kind of hunger they know. This does not mean that physical hunger is a lightweight. *Chronic* physical hunger and food insecurity can etch deeply into our body and mind, and even pass down through generations.

Emotional Hunger

Emotional hunger, heart hunger, is where compulsions, rituals, self-soothing, and bingeing reside. This is the realm of "what fires together wires together." This is why I "need" to soothe and reward myself with "a treat," ideally a salted-caramel-dark-chocolate one, after a discouraging day. "I was haunted by a wild hunger for something I couldn't name, and while food didn't fill it, having more of what I didn't want was better than having nothing at all," writes Geneen Roth in *Messy Magnificent Life*.[20]

Addictive Hunger

Addictive hunger is a hostile takeover of the pleasure centers of the brain, similar to what a nicotine addict experiences. "Highly palatable foods, such as processed foods with added sugars and fat, could be as addictive as drugs, acting via the same neurocognitive . . . processes," writes Dr. Aymery Constant of University Rennes.[21]

DO CARBS MAKE US HAPPY?

There's some silly misinformation on the internet riffing off the fact that serotonin (a natural antidepressant in your brain) is synthesized from carbohydrates. Some will hyperbolize this to frighten us that we'll become depressed if we don't eat enough carbs.

Small amounts of carbs are needed to make our brain run, that's true. But we can get that small amount of carbs just from veggies like bok choy and broccoli. There are a few carbs in avocados and in kale, in cabbage and unsweetened almond milk—and these few are plenty to keep your happiness chemistry sparkling.

It's almost as simple as Mom used to say. Just eat your veggies (the non-starchy ones: Mom was pointing to the spinach on your plate, not the potatoes) and you'll be fine.

IT'S NOT A LEVEL PLAYING FIELD—BUT WE CAN STILL WIN THIS GAME

Either running low on insulin *or* insulin resistance may make us more vulnerable to food addiction,[22] so all types of diabetes are vulnerable to food addiction—and us lucky LADAs get it from both sides.

A diabetic may have been self-medicating with food before diagnosis. In doing so she may have strongly reinforced a neural pathway of craving food when tired, depressed, or anxious. A long history of self-medicating can make it hard for us to tell the difference between our stress response and our hunger response.

When we can't trust our body's signals, we become more at risk for disordered eating. Diabetics are much more likely than non-diabetics to have disordered eating or an eating disorder.

"When you are addicted to drugs you put the tiger in the cage . . . when you are addicted to food you . . . take [the tiger] out three times a day for a walk," notes Dr. Kerri-Lynn Murphy Kriz.[23]

Some of us have to work harder to get to the same place as others; yet *we can* triumph.

> ### KEY TAKEAWAYS
>
> 1. Food is deeply entwined with identity. To be forced to drastically change what we eat can be a deep loss.
> 2. Resisting food measurably steals working intelligence and exhausts us.
> 3. Food can be literally addictive, and ultra-processed highly sweetened foods are most addictive.
> 4. We have three types of hunger—of body, heart, and neural pathway—and they can be hard to disentangle. One strategy is to take them one at a time: deal with addiction, then emotional eating, and then learn to interpret your body's sometimes misleading signals with some grains of salt.
> 5. With LADA, or with a long history of disordered eating, or both, it becomes hard to trust our body's signals. The next chapter offers strategies for reinterpreting and recalibrating signals we suspect.

o o o

I PARK AT THE SNOQUALMIE RIVER TRAIL AS THE SKY GRAYS WITH dawn. My footsteps crunch grass blades spiky with frost. Gauzy fog wafts like ghosts along moss-draped alder branches. A mallard rustles her wings; one drop of water glints down her back. *Exercise* seems a silly word for being present for this whispered symphony. Small flitterers flutter in a blackberry tangle. Sunrise backlights the fog with gold but cannot break through.

After my walk, chilled, smiling, and hungry, I push open the heavy door of the Grateful Bread coffee shop. I step up to the counter and tentatively ask whether it is possible to get the breakfast sandwich without the sandwich. Everything but bread, please, Ms. Grateful Bread.

The flour-dusted server pauses, thinking, then nods: Of course.

It's not unlike a ham and cheese omelet, or so I tell myself, as I attack with plastic fork the thick slab of salty ham, the melting Swiss cheese and fluffy egg, trying to focus on what they *are*, instead of what they aren't.

To one side of my table, there's a family: a two-year-old in pink rubber boots stands on a chair clapping powdered sugar into the air. To the other side, two men in camo. I open my computer and begin to write.

I wasn't eavesdropping. Really. Especially given the body language of the men in camo, the way they lean over coffees, the way they speak in low tones, like men talking in code about a secret fishing hole. But try not to smell a cinnamon roll. Try not to hear what someone next to you is saying.

The man closest to me, a beard covering his acne-scarred face, keeps his back to the room and hunches over his coffee, staring down into his cup. The steely-haired man beside him sits tall and with an air of balance; like someone waiting in a deer blind, like someone good at waiting. I hear "meeting," "sober," "power," "faith," and "struggle."

The younger man is asking, vulnerable. The older man doesn't seem to be offering an automatic yes.

Up at the counter, a curly-haired dude in Tevas, his bakery box over-flowing with muffins and scones, hesitates as if wondering: maybe just one more. By the window a couple bookended by matching ponytails flirts, backlit by shifting fog, while a muscled man whose tattoo patterns take up where his biking jersey leaves off, intently journals.

The men in camo stand. Their wooden chair legs scrape sighs from the painted floor. "Tuesday, then," the younger man says.

There's a long pause. They are looking into each other's eyes. The girl in pink boots is pulled down to sitting in her chair and gently shushed.

"The decision you make now is for your life," the older man finally says. "But you can reverse it . . . and not hurt nobody but yourself."

Driving home, I keep thinking about the gray-haired man's words. About how they apply to me. Perhaps to many of us reading this book.

The door swings both ways. Every minute of every day. That's what makes us crazy, and that's what gives us hope.

22 BUILDING A BETTER RELATIONSHIP WITH FOOD

The body is not an apology.
—Sonya Renee Taylor

BUILDING A HEALTHY RELATIONSHIP WITH FOOD CAN BE A CHALLENGE for anyone, and becomes more difficult with diabetes (chapter 21). Many of us can no longer simply "listen to our body" to stay in our healthy zone.

The diet industry rakes in billions of dollars by targeting our deepest fears, needs, and vulnerabilities and tying them psychologically to food and to how others rate our bodies. For too many, yo-yo dieting makes us sick, destroys our self-confidence, and breaks our hearts. The diet industry thrives when we believe that getting healthy is too complicated, with all these molecules, hormones, mitochondria—when we fear we can't do this by ourselves. But we can do this. We absolutely can.

Regaining our health will blossom from profound changes in how we live, and in how we relate to food.

Just as a marriage counselor won't say all your marital problems can be solved by wearing higher heels and glossier lipstick, nor by going to two of your daughter's soccer games instead of none, don't expect a quick fix for a profound, intricately rooted issue. Improving a valued and complex relationship requires honest self-assessment, meaningful change, and a lifetime commitment.

Some with diabetes wish to gain weight, and struggle to do so. Many with diabetes have a goal to lose weight, in order to improve the effectiveness of insulin, lessen chronic inflammation, and improve immune response. For some with diabetes, body fat is at a healthy level, and we may wish to improve our relationship with food in a different way, such as choosing more nutritious foods, choosing foods that align with moral values, or breaking free from disordered eating.

And we can.

WEIGHT MANAGEMENT CAN PUT INSULIN RESISTANCE INTO REMISSION

For many with diabetes, losing even ten to twenty pounds, or 5 percent of body weight, can radically cut insulin resistance. A recent study in the UK of T2s of a range of ages and BMIs (body mass indices) asked a random half of the group to stop all meds and instead rely on a structured, supported diet. The average person in this supported-diet group lost twenty pounds and *put their diabetes into remission*; the odds of remission were highest (86 percent) for those who lost the most weight. Even two years later, many had put their insulin resistance solidly into remission and did not need any antidiabetic drugs.

"Remission of type 2 diabetes is a practical target for primary care," wrote the lead researcher.[1]

DO DIETS WORK?

That depends: What do we *mean* when we say "diet"?

- What most people mean doesn't work in the long term. Ninety-five percent of people who attempt a diet, fail (do not achieve and sustain their goal).
- Individually, *diets can work*: Hundreds of thousands of us have gone from unhealthy weights to healthy and stayed there.

As the UK study above shows, a diet can work if it's our "relationship counselor," helping us build a permanent new relationship with ourselves. This is so different from what many mean by the word *diet*, we might need to use a different word. *Diaita*, the original Greek word, simply means "a way of life."

Superficial fixes give short-term results. In the short term, counting calories can work; but over the long term, food quality becomes more important.

DO DIETS WORK?

If *diet* means learning about food and our body, making foundational changes in our approach to food, and joyfully crafting a new food identity: Yes, diets work.

If *diet* means a deprivation crash-course to "fix" our weight without addressing deeper issues and then a return to old habits: Nope, unlikely.

○ ○ ○

EXERCISE IS KEY

Research shows that of ***those who successfully lose weight, 95 percent incorporate exercise***.

Exercise doesn't just burn up yesterday's bag of chips. It alters our metabolism, energy levels, and hormones. It also builds muscle; and muscle burns fat. Having more lean muscle mass raises our metabolism. Turn a pound of fat into a pound of muscle, and after that, just sitting around breathing, you'll burn more calories than you did before.

"Diet and exercise are both vitally important to good health in diabetes . . . the adoption and maintenance of physical activity [is] critical," writes Dr. Andrea Bolla of the IRCCS Diabetes Research Institute.[2]

LET GO OF DICHOTOMOUS THINKING

Research shows that the biggest impediment to weight loss is dichotomous thinking, which is when our view of ourselves flips from "good" to "utter failure" with one slip.

Nutrition coach Sherry Winslow finds that women are particularly vulnerable to dichotomous thinking. "If women make one mistake and go off their diet . . . they seem more likely to give up and just go off the diet all together," says Winslow. "My male clients . . . say, 'So what, I had a beer' and get back on the program."[3]

As women, we may have been conditioned against valuing ourselves equally with others. We may do much of the cooking and shopping for our family; may be around food all day; and may prioritize children's or partner's preferences instead of the eating patterns and foods that would be healthiest for us. To be present and healthy for our loved ones long-term—there is no substitute for self-love, self-care, and for prioritizing ourselves.

REALISTIC GOALS

Setting a clear, realistic goal is crucial.[4] For those who desire to reduce body fat, a slow steady pace of losing a pound or two a week is optimum. Faster weight losses may crash us into starvation mode and make long-term weight loss ultimately harder. A goal to have a healthy amount of fat is realistic; a goal of looking like an airbrushed supermodel is not.

Your goal(s) can set you up for success or failure. Choose goals:
  > That are measurable.
  > That are personal, kind, realistic, and healthy.
  > That build progressively toward health.
  > You can reward yourself for meeting.

You might set goals for:
  > Movement and fitness (aka exercise).
  > Meal spacing.
  > Lowering BG peaks.
  > Minimizing low BG depths.
  > Time in range—reducing the frequency of highs and lows.
  > A1c.
  > Weight.
  > Nutrition goals (for fiber, veggies, omega-3s, superfoods, et cetera).
  > Stress management.
  > Reversal of complications such as nerve pain, or improved results at dental and eye exams.

o o o

RETRAIN THE BRAIN

Many people are triggered by particular foods, environments, stresses, or other triggers; we have the power to unlearn these triggers. "Food craving . . . [is] a conditioned response that . . . can also be unlearned," writes Dr. Adrian Meule of University Hospital in Munich.[5]

Frame it for success. After a successful boot camp (chapter 19), in a safe space, with support, you may choose to gently desensitize yourself to triggers, so that you won't be at their mercy down the road.

RE-STORY

To live well with LADA, we have to understand food on all the levels it matters. Cell level to society level. Mind, body, and culture. Physical, emotional, and even spiritual. To build a healthier relationship with food, we triumph like a gardener, not like Superman. Weeds poke their little heads up every day. It's all about incessantly starting over. It's about our inner narrative and self-talk. Ultimately, the story we choose to tell ourselves about food will determine who we are.

RECOVERING FROM EMOTIONAL EATING

When we silence our authentic voice, the body itself tells our story.

"Your silence will not protect you," wrote Audre Lorde. "You will merely die without ever having had a voice."

We heal emotional hunger by changing habitual unhelpful behaviors. We recognize the futility of our Band-Aid behavior, identify our triggering situations, turn away from self-harm, and reach out to a support system. We begin again, as often as we need to, with perseverance and self-love.

Allowing ourselves to start again, without judgment, is the most important, and often the hardest, task we face when we take on a significant change.

My meditation teacher Ginger says that when something bad happens to us, it strikes us like an arrow. Our dog dies. We lose our job. We get diabetes.

Many of us respond by immediately shooting ourselves with additional arrows. *I should have called the vet an hour earlier. I should have told my*

*boss yada yada yada. Diabetes happens to people who eat wrong, I brought
this on myself, I really am a worthless person.*

There's no avoiding the first arrow. Pain is not optional.

The second, third, fourth, and fifth arrows—the blame, story, and
judgment—we do that to ourselves. We become cartoon cowboys, with
dozens of arrows sticking out of our hat. We begin to move through life
covered with arrows instead of learning how to be with our pain and focus
on it, so the pain can move through and past us.

When a storyteller (and we're all storytellers) asks herself: "What else is
also true?"—she is beginning the journey toward true healing. *

1. Name it. This is sorrow. This is pain. This is loneliness.
2. Question self-doubt and negative self-talk. Ask: Is that
    really true? Is that *always* true, or have there been moments
    of my better self?
3. Look directly at the first arrow. Feel it. Breathe it. Be with it.
4. Release it.

o o o

The physiological life span of an emotion is ninety seconds, says neuroscientist Jill Bolte Taylor.[6] When we stay stuck, it is because we are
choosing to retrigger a difficult emotion over and over, perhaps to avoid
dealing with the first arrow.

"Choosing to keep struggling with food," writes Geneen Roth, "is a
choice to stay in the burning building of suffering while telling ourselves
we can't help it."[7]

RECOVERING FROM ADDICTIVE EATING

Addiction is strange and ordinary, disturbing and vanilla, pathologically
absurd and eerily normal. Somewhere between one in six and one in eight
Americans struggle with addiction.[8]

---

* Thank you, Elizabeth Austen.

We can get through the physical withdrawal phase of food addiction in *just three days*. For three days, eliminate all carbs, sweets, and your addictive foods (you know which foods boss you around). It won't be the easiest three days of your life but it's Just. Three. Days. Ask for support, if possible. (Support groups include Overeaters Anonymous and Food Addicts in Recovery Anonymous.)

After physical withdrawal, we next reset our habits. Resetting a habit takes about forty days, so for many it works well to make boot camp (chapter 19) at least forty days long. Addiction research shows it then takes an additional two to three months to regrow healthy neural pathways.

Finally, desensitizing yourself to food triggers—sights, smells, and settings that make it hard for you to resist—may take the best part of a year or more. While Dr. Grisel writes that it took her *nine years* to fully disconnect from her triggers,[9] triggers can lose their sharpest intensity after three months, a milestone to celebrate.

Even now, when I'm exhausted from a tough day, or heading into something unfamiliar that makes me anxious, I crave the "reward" of chocolate. Or ice cream. Or anything. I'm dreaming of chocolate, but I'm also ready to scour the pantry, dig crystallized honey out of a dust-caked jar, and smear it on a freezer-burned onion bagel. What's in this old box? Is there really a board-like chunk of graham cracker left from the teens' s'more party two years ago? Sweet!

When I feel this way, I ask myself: What if I were craving a cigarette right now? What would I say to myself?

BUILDING A HEALTHY FOOD RELATIONSHIP WHEN WE HAVE LADA

With LADA it can be a challenge to eat in a way that keeps us physically healthy, yet does not become emotionally unhealthy. We want to be committed, but not obsessive. We want to recognize when our place along the spectrum has shifted to the point where it's time for a major change, such as supplementing insulin.

The frustratingly pervasive misconception that T2 food rules apply to LADA makes eating well with LADA so much harder. Many times, friends and loved ones never really get it: When we have little insulin left, "eating healthy" is very, very different.

Honeymoon LADAs who are trying to postpone using insulin, and trying to manage BG just through lifestyle and food, are often described by loved ones as "eating like someone with an eating disorder." I have to admit this would have been a fair description of me in my first year after diagnosis, when I achieved a very healthy BG just through exercise, metformin, and an extreme focus on foods.

"Is what you're doing *sustainable?*" doctors would ask, when I explained how few carbs I ate each day.

"Yep, sure." I nodded, prepared to obsess indefinitely.

Sustainable, I didn't then realize, was code for: emotionally healthy.

Even with my early success and strict carb control, my food ceiling kept shrinking and shrinking, while my BG control worsened. That's the way of LADA: We hope to slow beta cell death, but most of us can't halt it. For most, our beta cells will keep dying, our insulin production keep falling—and we don't know whether we've got months or decades of our own insulin. For me, beginning to supplement insulin raised that sinking ceiling, and opened a window, letting fresh air and sunshine back into my life.

How could I possibly be grateful to diabetes? And yet . . . it wasn't until I was diagnosed with diabetes, and began to regulate it through diet, that I realized I had been having a completely different experience of hunger than many people around me. And that the hunger I'd been struggling with for so long was: *optional*. Silly Dorothy, the universe and Oz said to me, you've been wearing the ruby slippers all along.

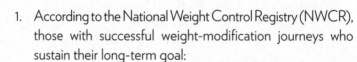

1. According to the National Weight Control Registry (NWCR), those with successful weight-modification journeys who sustain their long-term goal:
    - Often have a wake-up call; a major life event.
    - Quickly get back on track when we slip; don't give up after a slip.
    - Use self-monitoring tools such as journals.
    - Exercise regularly.

2. Those who **successfully reach the *two-year mark*** of maintaining a weight goal are likely to maintain it permanently.
3. When a doctor asks if your eating plan is sustainable, she likely means: Is it emotionally healthy?—and may not even herself fully understand the difference.
4. A successful journey begins in your mind:
   - Set realistic goals.
   - Retrain the brain.
   - Re-story.
   - Build your support network.
   - Let go of dichotomous thinking.
5. Tools for achieving/maintaining desired weight:
   - Exercise.
   - Hydrate.
   - Process stress with practical, healthful, daily techniques (chapter 14).
   - Eat high-nutrient, fiber-filled foods, especially stem/leaf veggies.
   - Eat enough calories to avoid starvation mode but a bit fewer than you're burning.
   - Let the pounds drop slowly and steadily. You've got your whole life ahead of you.
   - Restful sleep calms hunger hormones and promotes satiety hormones.
   - Choose an approach to food you can embrace as a permanent, joyful, healthy life.

o o o

23 COMPLETING THE JOURNEY

Finding Support from Structure, Not Ruled by Rules

*With an adventurous heart and the right maps, we can travel
anywhere and never fear losing ourselves.*
    —Brené Brown[1]

WHEN I WAS A KID, MY DAD WOULD TAKE OVER THE KITCHEN ON SUNday mornings. Some mornings, we'd see the waffle iron emerge, watch as he separated whites from yolks, and start salivating for melting butter and real maple syrup. Other mornings we watched the metal mixing bowl go into the freezer, and then we'd get excited for his famous Norwegian pancakes mounded with freshly whipped cream and the fragrant strawberries I washed and my sister sliced as the pans heated. Yet other mornings, we'd hear pots banging, the timer ticking, and slight swearing under his breath. Then we'd know we'd have to come instantly to the table when summoned because: Eagle's Nests!

Eagle's Nests was just a silly term for poached eggs on spinach on toast, but it totally worked on us kids.

In the first six months of my diagnosis, if you'd tried to offer me a toast-free version of Eagle's Nests—of Eagle's Nests!—I'd have scowled and rolled my eyes. *You **can't** have Eagle's Nests without toast. End of story. Leave me alone. I'm going to sit here chewing down eggs and lettuce and feeling sorry for myself.*

Funny . . . one peaceful Sunday morning two years after my diagnosis, alone in my kitchen where morning sun lights up the snowy peaks of Sleeping Lady with rose and cinnamon, I sliver leek greens, sauté them lightly with crisp cabbage, add spinach to wilt, and top these every-color-of-spring greens with two poached eggs. As the rich yolk blends with the fragrant spinach, out of nowhere comes a memory I haven't thought of in a long time: Eagle's Nests. The flavors carry me away, and for a moment I'm a kid at the table of a still-whole family, all of us young and healthy, with delicious food at the center.

I guess I'm just saying: Wait for it. Then revel in it.

If We Let Go of Rigid Rules, What Will Support Us?

I began this journey asking *What can I eat?* and expecting the answer to be like third-grade flash cards. I wanted lists, strategies, and techniques. *Whaaat? Look inward and build a peaceful relationship with my body? I don't think so!* Fortunately karma has a delightful sense of humor.

In the beginning, to get to physical health, I needed rules, rules, rules. Now, for the sake of my mental health, I needed to *move away from rules* toward something easier, freer, that *I could still trust* to keep me safe.

I now think of a LADA meal as a table with four legs:

1. Your powerhouse: Stem/leaf/flower veggies, and other low-carb veggies (the LADA-love foods in appendix B). Your happy place. No limits!
2. Super-charged carbs: Nutrient-dense and fiber-rich root veggies, berries, and other superfoods add vitamins and zest, and zap cravings. Keep these under your personal carb limit.
3. Protein: Be Goldilocks.
4. Healthful fats: "Round up" to meet minimal quantity (calories), feel good, and quash cravings.

To make the four legs work, we need to know our carb limit and our quantity (or approximate calorie) goal.

o o o

Carb Limit

Testing your BG after numerous meals has shown you how many carbs you can eat without sending your BG too high. This is your personal carb limit. Your carb limit is situational: different when you're marathoning than when you're telecommuting in your p.j.'s. A carb limit changes over time—increasing as we gain muscle or become more active, or decreasing as our ability to make insulin dwindles —so it's good to keep an eye on it through continued periodic testing (or a continuous glucose monitor).

When we begin supplementing insulin, this becomes less a limit and more a dosing decision. Lower-carb meals make insulin dosing easier: Finessing our insulin dose so it's both *successful* and minimal can minimize insulin's fat-building bias.

Quantity Goal

Like our BG, food quantity is something we keep in a Goldilocks range, neither too high nor too low, because if the body believes we are starving, it slams in place metabolic changes that can torpedo weight management. I find that an approximate calorie goal—not scrutinizing to the precise calorie but rounding meals to the nearest hundred or so calories—helps me track my meal quantity. Calories can be problematic (chapter 16), and you may find a different way to keep an eye on quantity that works best for you.

Our quantity goal is situational and individual. Online calculators can suggest an approximate calorie goal based on height, weight, age, sex, and activity level. And your doctor can connect you with a nutritionist for a personal session (often free for a diagnosed LADA).

Protein: Also Goldilocks

Too little *or* too much protein is bad for us. The guidelines for a healthful upper limit have recently been revised upward (chapter 16); and remember that it's preferable to have protein in each meal, rather than a big wad at dinner.[2] So when building your LADA "table," all meals can have a similar protein leg.

LESS MATH, MORE ART

I began with head scratching and back-of-the-napkin math, multiplying grams of protein by four calories per gram, grams of fat by nine, dividing by Santa's reindeer and carrying three. Then it dawned on me than I was making this all much harder than necessary. (Who, me?)

Now I just:

1. Put a healthy portion of protein into my meal (like two eggs for breakfast; or tofu and cashews in my stir-fry).
2. Ignore all the freebies and low-carb veggies not worth counting (broccoli, salsa, lemon slice).
3. Ballpark and add up the carbs in other foods—either to double-check they're under my carb ceiling or to calculate my insulin dose.
4. Ball-park-check that calories aren't too low—if they are, I toss on a favorite calories-with-few-carbs food (avocado, salad dressing), often a food high in healthful fat.

That's it!

THINK OF A MEAL AS A STRUCTURE. (SAY, THE "LEANING TOWER OF pizza.")

Before I was diagnosed, I built my meal's foundation from carbs (rice, potatoes, pasta, bread, pizza dough, pancakes). Onto this structure, I added toppings. If my structure was pizza, my foundation was the dough; then I added sauces, cheeses, veggies, and more. If my structure was pasta, I might add pesto, a side of green beans, and a salad.

Today I do the same, except that *my foundation is low-carb vegetables.* I start with this structure and layer on protein, calories, and superfoods—the toppings, the spicing-up of my LADA life.

For example, I put my broiled cauliflower steak (tasty, filling, fiber-rich structure) on a bed of wilted greens (nutrient-dense superfoods) that I've drizzled with lime and olive oil, and top it all with pasture-raised cheddar, toasted walnuts, and olive tapenade (protein and calories).

GETTING STARTED

It can be hard to get started as a LADA. I say, "Test to learn what works"— but where does a beginner begin? With appendix B: LADA-Love and LADA-Limit Foods.

LADA-love foods are my tried-and-true go-to foods. Enjoy the no-limit veggies to feel full and add healthful fiber and nutrients. Other foods in the LADA-love table help us wisely target our quantity goals.

LADA-limit foods, I may need to limit. If I'm eating two LADA-limit foods in a meal, I eat half as much of each; if three, a third as much; and so on. Find the quantities that work well for you using the techniques explained in chapters 8 and 9.

STAYING SAFE

At the beginning of this journey, I accumulated safe meals. I loved having a mental list of safe meals I could whip up in a hurry without having to google or do math.

Safe breakfasts—for me. Unsweetened yogurt with berries and toasted nuts. Cauliflower grits. Scrambled eggs with a side of steamed green beans and avocado slices. Shakshuka. Tofu-feta-broccoli scramble (caloried-up with sunflower seeds or toasted coconut or olive tapanade). Breakfast raita. Veggie custards: veggies baked with eggs and cheese—bake them in muffin cups for a quick breakfast-on-the-go. Huevos rancheros over stir-fried greens (light on the black beans) topped with fresh salsa and melted cheese.

Safe lunches—for me. Chef's salad with carrots, tomatoes, cubed chicken, cubed cheese, and no stinting on healthful-fat dressing. Salmon, tuna, or sardine salad with garlic sauce on a bed of spinach. Caprese salad—so simple! Peanut butter cucumber roll-ups in kale or lettuce leaves. Quiche (for some reason, with Good Mood Food quiche, I can even *eat the crust*, woo-hoo!) My personal limit of a tasty off-the-shelf soup (often about one measuring cup) supplemented with bone broth and handfuls of chopped veggies; if I'm taking it to work, it travels well in a canning jar. Frittatas (in their nearly endless variations). "Naked" ratatouille tartines (this gorgeous medley doesn't need bread—try it on lettuce, kale, or straight on the plate). A stir-fry of any favorite vegetables, caloried-up with nuts or peanut sauce or coconut milk or meat or eggs or tofu.

Safe dinners—for me. Pesto on zucchini zoodles. Pesto on any favorite veggie melange. Coconut-chicken curry (no rice). Rosemary turkey with steamed veggies and one exquisite bright dab of fruit-sweetened cranberry sauce. Soups and stews (low-carb versions). Burger on a salad, not a bun (the burger can be beef, fish, chicken, a moderate-carb brand of veggie burger, or grilled eggplant). Roasted veggies, heavy on cauliflower, light on root veggies. Black beans and salsa over sautéed summer squash, red peppers, and chard. Brussels sprouts with caramelized onions, walnuts, and sheep feta. Pho made with cabbage instead of noodles. Dishes at a favorite Thai restaurant where the sauces aren't too sugary. At Wenatchee's new Japanese restaurant: seafood soup with tofu-avocado salad. Grilled portobellos, asparagus, and peppers. Parsley's Pantry's "everything" salad. Sautéed zucchini and tomatoes from Kari's garden, topped with a tasty sample of the lasagna my son and his girlfriend brought to share. Wild Alaskan salmon on a bed of greens. Unbreaded eggplant parmesan. Spinach-mushroom-basil soufflé. Tempeh and green bean lemon tagine.

> It's simple: Let nutrient-dense low-carb vegetables be your foundation. Add a tasty accompaniment of protein and fat to keep you full, happy, sharp-minded, and energetic.
>
> That's it!

o o o

TO THE INTERNSHIP—AND BEYOND!

Six months along, I'd learned the rules, I'd accumulated safe meals, but I was still food-focused, still intense and mathy about food, always reading books like this one, and generally behaving in a way some silly people might call obsessive.

But there did come a day I wasn't pulling food lists out of my wallet, or googling the carbs in sweet potato versus daikon. There did come a day I no longer felt like a person defined by their food limits, defined by dozens of don'ts, and ruled by rules. Instead I felt supported by a vision of a meal as a structure—something I could throw together out of whatever was in the fridge with as little drama as I throw together an outfit to wear around the house on a weekday evening.

What a relief. I was done being Buzz Lightyear: "To Carb-craft and beyond!" To my surprise: I'd arrived. I could relax . . . *and* be healthy. With LADA! *And* eat food I loved. I could have my cake and eat it, too, because I knew how to Carb-craft.

In the beginning, time may feel like the enemy, like molasses we have to wade through. Over time, time becomes our friend. Each small success makes the next success easier. Every healthy day makes the next healthy day easier. Eventually food rules become muscle memory, and we can gently transform rigid rules into lightly held guides.

Carb-craft is the path. It's okay to fall off. Just get back up again. You are not a failure. Unless or until the day you cease to try.

24 FOOD FOR THOUGHT

Access and Equity

Despite the fact that insulin has been used for nearly 100 years, an estimated 1 in 2 people who need it cannot afford and/or access this much-needed medicine.

—Dr. Margaret Ewen, senior projects manager for
Health Action International and former adviser to the
World Health Organization[1]

New Year's Day, I wave goodbye to my son at the airport, blinking back tears. He'll be gone for a year—but how can I not be thankful for the term in Iceland and other adventures taking him off into the world?

Our meditation feels especially compelling that Sunday. We ponder this story: When asked, "Roshi, what's the most important thing?" Roshi answered: "To find out what's the most important thing."

The most important thing is finding our most important thing. If we could set our most important thing like a light at the bow of our ship (or, in my case, paint-chipped rowboat), it would be easier to know which way to go.

In the meditation circle, Ginger passes around strands of silky red bamboo yarn, and we each tie three knots. As we tie the middle knot, we think of our most important thing. Then we tie a knot on each side: one for something we aspire to in the coming year, and one for something we hope to let go. A neighbor helps tie our thread around wrist or ankle like a friendship bracelet.

When I tie my middle knot, I think of seven generations: my grand-parents, my parents, sister, children, grandchildren (theoretical at this point—I hope!). Not just my Christmas card list, but the whole genera-tion; not just the friends my son camped with last month, but the ones he may meet in Iceland.

The Iroquois concept of seven generations has been explained to me as beginning with our children and stretching six more generations into the future. But my middle knot travels in all directions, past and future, uniting those I love, those my parents remember, and those I have yet to meet . . . and the world they will someday walk through. "May you walk in beauty," the Diné (Navajo) say.

As I sit by my fire that evening, my puppy in my lap, my fingers wander to the red thread. I stare into the flames, asking myself: What is the bigger picture of diabetes, bigger than myself?

DIABETES AND OUR MEDICAL SYSTEM

Time magazine points out that while the US spends the most per capita of any nation on health care, Americans' life expectancy ranks forty-third in the world, and poor diet has been identified as Americans' main cause of death.[2]

"Today's health care system simply isn't equipped to manage diabetes properly," writes diabetic educator Gary Scheiner. "Health care providers consistently come up short when it comes to time, expertise, and access. This is not from a lack of desire; most physicians are talented, motivated, caring people who wish they had the time and resources to do more for their patients."[3]

By 2050, the CDC estimates, one in three Americans will have diabe-tes. Worldwide, 422 million have diabetes, and an additional 350 million have prediabetes.

These statistics are posted on the walls of my local clinic's exam rooms:

- Two out of five US adults will develop diabetes in their lifetime.
- One of four people who have diabetes *do not know* they have it.
- One in three US adults have prediabetes (stage one diabetes).
- Of those with prediabetes, three out of four *do not know* they have it.

- One-third of prediabetics will progress to full diabetes within five years.
- The risk of death for adults with diabetes is double the risk for non-diabetics. (This statistic is helpfully illustrated with a twice-as-large tombstone.)

I've tried to imagine what it's like to be a doctor treating diabetes. I picture the endless, heartbreaking stories a doctor encounters: a talented youngster brain-injured by a graduation-night car wreck; a pregnant mother diagnosed with cancer weighing risks to her own life against risks to her child. Then the doctor walks in to see a T2. This person, thinks the doctor, may only need to lose weight and be physically active to be completely healthy.

As we've explored in this book, weight issues are complicated, beset by raging hormones and broken body thermostats. But the typical American, and many doctors, don't know just *how much harder* achieving a healthy weight is for some of us than others.

On top of this, there's a one-in-ten chance that this patient is actually LADA, not T2, and is **running out of insulin**, needs different treatments, and must prepare for different outcomes. But today the doctor is extremely unlikely to do the simple test to find out.

So as the doctor opens the door to walk into the room, the situation may already be fraught.

Focused on trying to save us from horrific complications, the doctor has little time to discuss *living well* with diabetes. She has fifteen minutes to explain everything in this book. Some doctors, particularly those serving less-wealthy populations, receive enormous patient loads. A doctor's frustration at the situation may unintentionally come across as frustration at the patient.

Meanwhile, the diabetic may be feeling enormously confused—overwhelmed by a tsunami of conflicting "expert" advice. He may feel surrounded by sharks—or possibly life rafts?—but unable to tell which are which. His friends and family probably misunderstand diabetes and may act in unhelpful ways. His doctor doesn't have enough time for him. The free nutritionist session that should be offered with a diabetes diagnosis may not be offered—or may not hit the right level: "This is called whole wheat bread. See, it looks brown." His diabetes class may be designed for T2, and may imply that T2 advice, although completely inadequate for LADA, should be all he needs.

Finding excellent medical care as a LADA is possible; but most of us will have to advocate for ourselves. Some of us (the undocumented, un-housed, incarcerated, institutionalized, and others) will have to fight much harder for good care.

We can *support our doctors* and other medical professionals as they cre-ate better resources and do their best in a difficult situation. Understanding that diabetes is tough for doctors too can help patients put ourselves *on the same side* as caring medical staff.

WHAT'S AGRIBUSINESS GOT TO DO WITH IT?

The modern world was built on carbs. A grain- or potato-based agricultural revolution gave birth to all of the large civilizations around the globe, from Egypt, Rome, Greece, and China to the Americas.[4]

Homo sapiens used to die mainly from diseases of famine and poor sanitation. But today we are most likely to die from chronic diseases of the industrial lifestyle. This profound transformation is on a scale with the birth of agriculture ten thousand years ago.[5]

Industrialization of the food supply—mass production first of flour and sugar, and then of ultra-processed foods that are inexpensive, highly ca-loric, and packed with sugar, salt, and fat—has transformed the way many today eat and created a global health crisis.[6] Most experts agree that, as with other addictive substances, "societal level, supply-side interventions on food will be more effective than individual acts."[7]

Current commodity programs in the US transfer your tax money into the pockets of the largest producers of factory-farmed corn, soy, dairy, and sugar.[8] The giants at the top of this food pyramid invest this profit into advertising and political donations. At the same time, many smaller farmers—for example, many whose land, lives, and hands put cheap chicken on our tables—have lost their independence and must follow oppressive requirements.[9]

Our food industry is only doing what we incentivize it to do. As with doctors, this is about putting ourselves *on the same side* as farmers. We have a right to have a voice in how our tax dollars are spent, and an imperative to protect the health of ourselves, our children, and our grandchildren.

YOUR MONEY OR YOUR LIFE

I've frequently seen this cartoon shared on diabetes forums: The customer at the pharmacy counter asks, "What is the main side effect of this drug?"

"Bankruptcy," the pharmacist replies.

THE RESEARCHERS WHO WON THE NOBEL PRIZE FOR DEVELOPING insulin sold the patent to University of Toronto for $1 each, so that this life-saving medicine could be available to all. Instead, explains BBC reporter Rita Prasad, "Retail prices in the US are around the $300 range . . . Even accounting for inflation, that's a price increase of over 1000%."[10]

Today three companies—Eli Lilly, Novo Nordisk, and Sanofi—control 90 percent of the insulin market and earn billions annually. These drug-makers have been accused of repeatedly raising insulin prices in lockstep to "maintain monopoly pricing,"[11] and this seeming price-fixing (*tripling in price over ten years **synchronously** by all three international companies*) has spurred lawsuits.[12]

Insulin's price explosion has also been fueled by pharmacy benefit manager (PBM) profits;[13] by "pay for delay"—paying competitors not to enter the market[14]—and by "patent evergreening"—building thickets of patents around drugs.[15] Sanofi, for example, has filed seventy-four patent applications on Lantus, creating the potential for thirty-seven more competition-free years on this one drug.[16] To renew a patent, which extends your monopoly, you have to *change* the formulation; but you don't have to show you've *improved* it.[17]

INTERNATIONALLY, THE PRICE OF A VIAL OF INSULIN CAN RANGE FROM $1.50 to $75.00.[18] In the US we pay seven times more for insulin than consumers in peer countries such as Canada.[19] Due to deductibles or other situations, many Americans say insulin costs them more per month *than their rent.* Of those in the US who rely on insulin, its cost throws one in

seven into what researchers term *catastrophic spending*—after the minimum for housing and food, insulin consumes more than 40 percent of
their remaining income.[20]

We pay higher prices for insulin in the US than in almost any other
country, and are more likely to ration insulin due to cost than any other
high-income country.[21]

"Cost-related insulin underuse [is] associated with adverse clinical outcomes. Healthcare providers fac[e] patients . . . who struggle to afford insulin," writes Dr. Luo of the University of Pittsburgh's School of Medicine.[22]

Separate surveys by Yale Diabetes Center, Georgetown University,
and others have found that a quarter or more of US insulin users have
"stretched" insulin—used less insulin than desired because of cost—and
these patients were likely to have poor glycemic control and worse health.[23]
In an Atlanta hospital, a survey of patients admitted with life-threatening
ketoacidosis found that for two-thirds the cause was not having sufficient
insulin; asked why, most said they were trying to "stretch insulin" due to
lack of money or access.[24]

Americans die every year from lack of insulin. The nonprofit T1Inter-
national shares story after heartbreaking story of young Americans: "Our
Jesy, gone too soon," "Josh died because his insulin cost too much," "Losing Andy," "Rationing while waiting on a refill took Kayla's life," "Honoring Antavia as I fight for affordable insulin," "My sister Jada should never
have died," "My son Jeremy couldn't afford his insulin and now he's gone,"
"I lost Allen because he was forced to ration insulin," "Losing Rachel, our
only daughter," "Fighting in Micah's memory" . . . and on and on.

"The fact that type 1 diabetes has gone from a death sentence to a
survival condition [and] back to a death sentence in the United States is
shameful," writes James Elliott, a T1International trustee.[25]

IN AUGUST 2022, A PROPOSAL TO CAP INSULIN COSTS AT $35 PER
month for every American with health insurance came within a few votes
of passing Congress. Due to the lack of those few votes, and a last-minute
political tactic, the insulin cap was ultimately granted only to Medicare
recipients.

Some states are moving to limit insulin costs,[26] and legislation to make insulin more affordable nationwide is reintroduced in Congress nearly every year. As we go to press, the bipartisan *INSULIN Act*—endorsed by thirteen diabetes organizations—is before Congress: It would extend the $35 per month insulin cap to everyone with health insurance (sadly, this still excludes many of us) and would tackle PBM profit-siphoning.

In a joint letter of support for the *INSULIN Act*, the thirteen health organizations write: "Without this legislation . . . there is a continued risk that one in four insulin-dependent patients will have to keep rationing their supply, skipping doses and risking their lives because they cannot afford the medication needed to keep them alive . . . The COVID-19 pandemic made this legislation even more urgent. We know that unmanaged and under-treated diabetes has made our community deeply vulnerable to the worst of the pandemic's outcomes. Tragically, 40 percent of those who have died from COVID-19 have been Americans with diabetes, making the diabetes community 12 times more likely to die of COVID-19 than others. We know that affordable, accessible insulin saves lives."[27]

"ON A GLOBAL LEVEL THE MAIN CAUSE OF MORTALITY FOR A CHILD with type 1 diabetes is a lack of access to insulin, and in sub-Saharan Africa the life expectancy of a child with type 1 diabetes can be as low as 1 year," writes Dr. Beran of the University of Geneva.[28] Globally 50 percent of people who require insulin to survive cannot reliably obtain it, due either to complete unavailability or to cost, according to a 2015 report by Health Action International.

Sixty-three percent of households in low-income countries cannot afford insulin.[29] The cost of insulin relative to average income can be staggering: Insulin can cost up to 56 percent of average income in Kenya, 77 percent in Syria, 82 percent in Brazil, and 80 percent in Fiji. In rural Mozambique, the life expectancy of a child diagnosed with T1 is less than eight months.[30] "A lack of insulin is the number one cause of death for children living with type 1 diabetes," writes Dr. Margaret Ewen, former adviser to the World Health Organization.[31]

ONE PARTIAL FUTURE ASSIST: GENERIC INSULINS

A *generic* is a medicine with the same chemical composition and the same effect as the brand-named version. Because modern insulins mimic a complex biological molecule, *biosimilars* is the technically correct term for insulin, and the process for regulating biosimilars is different than regulation of generics. In 2020 the FDA finally loosened regulation of insulin biosimilars, opening the door for what are commonly (if slightly incorrectly) termed *generic insulins.*

So far only a trickle of biosimilar insulin has reached the market, and at high prices. However, several new manufacturers, including nonprofits, hope to reach full production of insulin biosimilars by 2024, and are promising to offer vials for $30 apiece, and a set of five pen cartridges for $55.[32]

WHO HAS ACCESS TO SAFE EXERCISE AND HEALTHFUL FOOD?

The US is riddled with neighborhoods lacking food sovereignty, where fresh produce and other healthy items are hard to find. Typically, these neighborhoods also lack good public transportation to the adjacent world of well-stocked grocery stores. Neighborhood features such as lack of safe greenspaces and parks can discourage physical activity, and this may be equally important to residents' health.[33]

Diabetes reveals how our systemic disparities in health insurance, income, built environment, food access, and more play out in shockingly different health outcomes for different subpopulations the US.[34]

In the US today, whether for T1, T2, or LADA, both a person's risk of diabetes and her health with diabetes are most dependent on two things: *her income, and whether she has health insurance.*[35]

WHO HAS HEALTH INSURANCE IN THE US TODAY?

Although about 80 percent of Americans between the ages of 25 and 54 are employed,[36] a significant number of the employed have no health insurance.

Virtually all Americans 65 or older (over 99 percent) have health insurance: either Medicare, private, or a combination.[37]

For Americans *under* 65, just over half (57 percent) are insured through an employer. The rest of us either privately purchase, purchase through an exchange, receive public assistance such as Medicaid, or are uninsured.[38]

More than one in ten Americans younger than 65 (about 32 million of us) have no health insurance.[39] In 84 percent of uninsured households, at least one person is employed.[40] Most of the uninsured are US citizens in an employed household, and most say they want but cannot afford health insurance.[41]

Commonly the uninsured go to extreme lengths to minimize medical costs; one in three go without needed medical care. When they are forced to seek care, they pay much more for it than the rest of us and are vulnerable to crippling medical debt they may never be able to clear.[42]

With diabetes, having health insurance is the single strongest predictor of quality of care and of health outcomes.[43]

o o o

"Perhaps we have focused too much on the medical/biological aspects of the disease and we have not fully addressed educational, social, financial, psychological and cultural determinants of health and disease," writes Dr. Enrique Caballero of Harvard Medical School.[44]

One in three chronically ill adults report that they are sometimes unable to afford food, medication, or both; they are food insecure and sometimes "noncompliant" with medications and treatments. Most of these struggling patients who are noncompliant out of economic desperation never discuss this aspect with their physician, and many physicians are unaware of which of their patients struggle to comply for purely economic reasons.[45]

"The association of [diabetes] risk with low income," writes Dr. Wylie Burke, chair of Bioethics and Humanities at the University of Washington, "speaks to . . . root causes . . . such as access to adequate housing, food security, education, jobs, [and] safe neighborhoods."[46]

Systemic inequities contribute: Latinos, African Americans, indigenous Americans, and others who have been historically economically disadvantaged through systemic racism, are disproportionately affected by diabetes.[47] In the US, African American children with diabetes are twice as likely to die as white or Latinx children with diabetes.[48] Our disparities in diabetes outcomes are not *caused* by race/ethnicity, research shows, but by differences in income and in access to medical care, healthy food, and a healthy environment.[49]

Diabetes is quadruply troubled by historically rooted ongoing inequities: first in access to and quality of health care; second in access to and quality of healthful food; third in access to and quality of built environments that promote activity and community; fourth in escape from environmental toxins.[50]

o o o

Raj Patel, British author of *Stuffed and Starved*, explains that today's food system is unsustainable. "Not everyone will eat tomorrow because of how we eat today . . . a complex web of social and ecological subsidies . . . produces food that appears as a bargain but is increasingly likely to contribute to chronic disease and ecological destruction," he writes.[51] When an unsustainable system is created, someone, someday, somewhere will bear the brunt, and pay all the past-due costs. Diabetics are among the canaries in the mine of our broken food system.

Internationally, we see heartbreaking situations, such as the many children in Mexico today who drink Coke more often than water; for many of them, clean water is not available.[52] We also see inspiring stories, such as the country of Bhutan, which chose as an entire nation to go 100 percent organic.[53]

People without housing and people in institutions are particularly vulnerable to having only low-nutrient, high-carb, chemically contaminated food options.[54] From schools in low-income neighborhoods, to nursing homes, to those who cognitively can't live independently, to those swept up by questionable incarceration policies: Access to fresh vegetables, which seems it could be such a simple thing, is all too often out of reach.

Yet ironically concern for healthy food is sometimes painted as elitist— something only rich, white snowflakes can afford to care about . . . while at the same time the economically disadvantaged may be chided, patronized, or pathologized for not "eating healthy." To me this sounds like divide and conquer: an old, old, old, tired strategy. We don't have to fall for this. All food consumers *are on the same side.* We all want and deserve sovereignty, access, and healthy options.

BE THE CHANGE

All across the US people are transforming their communities, a rising groundswell empowering and benefiting us all. Like Reverend Heber Brown III, pastor at Pleasant Hope Baptist Church in Baltimore, who decided: "I wanted to do more for people than just pray."

In Baltimore, 34 percent of Black residents live in neighborhoods lacking access to healthful foods, compared with 8 percent of white residents; and Black communities here have much higher levels of obesity and diabetes.

Brown began with a garden: a fifteen-hundred-square-foot plot of land in front of the church, which was soon producing a thousand pounds of produce a year. Next he reached out to local Black farmers, helping create pop-up markets. Then he launched a grassroots initiative: The Black Church Food Security Network.

"We have people contacting us from all over—different religions, different parts of the city . . . The phone is always ringing, the emails are always coming in from churches saying, 'Hey, we want in,'" says Brown.[55]

AGROECOLOGY OFFERS HOPE NOT ONLY FOR OUR URBAN NEIGHBOR-hoods, but also for rural revitalization: rebuilding soils and farming communities, supporting cleaner drinking water, and returning farming toward a chemically safer, "greener" job that adequately compensates the people on the ground.

A groundswell of revitalizing initiatives is springing up both in the US and internationally, including: Farm to School programs, Edible School-yard programs, doubling SNAP (food stamp) value at farmers markets, Meatless Mondays, Minnesota Thursdays, Health Care Without Harm, food networks like Detroit's Black Community Food Security Network, regional coalitions of small farmers, subsidizing or easing creation of community gardens, taxes on junk food and sugary beverages in Mexico and Chile and, in more than a dozen countries, limiting the targeted marketing of junk food to children. Often-cited success stories include India's Zero Budget Natural Farming Program, Denmark's program to reduce agricultural antibiotics, and France's agroecology initiative.[56]

In the US we are beginning to take a few small, experimental steps toward increasing food sovereignty in low-income neighborhoods, increasing diabetes-appropriate food at food banks, and improving the safety and walkability of neighborhoods.[57] Initiatives to improve neighborhood safety and greenspaces are already making people healthier. Safe access to recreation, public transit, walking, biking, parks, and recreation facilities, says Professor James Sallis of San Diego State University, "have widespread and sustainable effects."[58]

Dr. Hill-Briggs of John Hopkins University writes, "The most effective interventions will be at the population level, through policy and regulation, with a particular focus on protecting marginalized and underserved populations . . . Structural . . . interventions are needed to address . . . root causes of diabetes inequities, rather than compensatory interventions assisting the individual to adapt to inequities."[59]

As economist Heather McGhee has shown, addressing inequities doesn't carve up the "pie" into smaller pieces: It grows a bigger pie. When our neighbors have the tools to be healthy, the cost of our whole system drops, and *we all save money*.[60] Working together, we can put the costs where the profits are, and create more inclusive solutions.

"If we as a health care system make insulin out of reach for people, not only is that ethically wrong, but it's also going to cost us more in the long term," says Dr. Kasia Lipska of Yale School of Medicine, noting that complications, emergency room visits, and poor outcomes not only make individuals suffer, but raise costs system-wide, "so it's really shortsighted."[61]

"Companies must be held accountable," writes Elizabeth Pfiester Rowley. "Several patient-led groups and organizations focused on insulin access do exist. People living with diabetes all over the world are petitioning . . . and marching . . . patients will be at the frontline of change."[62]

In America today, we don't all have equal access to needed medicines, clean water, healthy vegetables, or a safe place to walk. Democracy means we can choose to create that America, and that world, for our children and their children.

"BASED ON ITS IMPACT ON HEALTH, THE ENVIRONMENT, AND THE economy, nutrition is the leading issue of our time," writes Dr. Mozaffarian of Tufts University. I can't do full justice here to the social issues around insulin, healthy food, and clean water. But here are a few resources:

- *Food, Inc.* An Oscar-nominated documentary featuring interviews with farmers and consumers, with commentary by Michael Pollan. Called "smart," "gripping," "comprehensive," and "compelling" by newspaper reviewers.
- The Small Planet Institute. Its mission is to foster democratic solutions in hunger, agriculture, and the environment. It was founded by Frances Moore Lappé, author of *Diet for a Small Planet* (selected as one of 75 Books by Women Whose Words Have Changed the World). Lappé's recent books include *World Hunger: 10 Myths* and *EcoMind*.
- Native American Food Sovereignty Alliance.
- Black Dirt Farm Collective.
- US Food Sovereignty Alliance (and its many member organizations).
- Food Chain Workers Alliance (and its member organizations).
- Rural Coalition / Coalición Rural.

    SOURCE: More resources and health equity organizations can be found at https://guides .lib.berkeley.edu/publichealth/healthequity/orgs

Asked in a 2020 interview whether she was an optimist, Frances Moore Lappé replied: "We are all connected and . . . change is the only constant.

If those two things are true . . . then it is simply not possible to know what is possible . . . I'm not an optimist. I am a possible-ist."[63]

ALL WE HAVE TO DO

I heard this quote on the radio: "Thomas Edison remarked over a hundred years ago that we live in this planetary home like a squatter, burning the front porch for heat, and not like an owner. Or at least the average person does, the dominant cultures. But *the average person is a numbers game*. All we have to do to change is change."

Whether we begin with insulin affordability; our local farmers market; city-wide composting; suggesting to a local parent group that fundraising for healthy school lunches might be as reasonable as fundraising for the basketball team; fighting racism; advocating that if we have agricultural subsidies, they should support family farms, soil sustainability, and human health; planting basil on a windowsill; fighting for the rights of people without housing and fighting against the criminalization of poverty; helping plan a new bike trail; signing up for a CSA; supporting the Disparities Solutions Center or a similar local organization; a soda tax; the American consumer's role in tropical deforestation; a community garden; affordable housing; more greenspace and safer parks; volunteering at a local food bank; advocating for better availability of medical translators; planting a garden at a school, church, or mosque . . . on and on, fill in the blank . . . they're all connected, and they all fight diabetes and create a better world for our children and grandchildren.

In the end it's less important where we start than that we *do* start and take just a step or two on the path every day.

25   GO BIG *AND* GO HOME

Sometimes the truth is like a second chance.
   —Dar Williams

What we play is life.
   —Louis Armstrong

AT NEW YEAR'S MEDITATION, WE EACH WRITE DOWN AN INTENTION for the coming year.

"I will fearlessly express my creativity," I write, uncreatively, copying from the woman sitting next to me.

Now can I live up to that? I ask my puppy, as I pack two bags—clothes, journals, and computer for me; squeaky snake and bouncy ball for her. Off we head to another writers' gathering on Whidbey Island.

Between classes, wind whipping our hair, we writers walk on a curve of fist-round stones where a Salish longhouse once stood. Goldeneye and bufflehead ducks dive into foam-flecked waves, and a harbor seal studies us through curious eyes. Perhaps her ancestors studied the people in the longhouse.

In classes, we ponder how to go deeper in our writing. What else is also true?

"What do we want; what do we get; what do we realize?" asks our teacher.

The perfect question.

For writing, also.

After two days of hard thinking and difficult honesty, I sink seal-like into the water in a tiled soaking tub. I pop my head out, take a big bite of the chocolate bar I'm hiding from these supportive friends, sigh, and submerge.

All day I've acted the role of the courageous person. I *have* been courageous. Ish. Just not enough to eat chocolate in front of my friends after reading them passages all day about how I have this food thing figured out.

I guess courage is a destination. I guess courage is like diabetes, or like changing our relationship with food: They all require learning to begin again, again.

On the last day of class, snow falls thick and fast—Whidbeyites are calling it snowmaggedon. The mountain pass I need to cross to get back home is closed as trees and power lines topple across the highway. Sixty-six inches on the pass over the next six days. Highway crews send a low-flying helicopter to try to wind-shake snow off the trees.

It's almost a week before the pass opens and I can make the sketchy, white-knuckle drive over the pass on icy roads threading aggressive semis. Hours later, tense and exhausted, I'm at the foot of my snowy three-mile driveway, not plowed in winter. Now comes the adventure.

When I dig out my snowmobile, nothing's broken—hooray!—but the cargo sled I pull behind is frozen to the ground. I free the sled, load it up, and off we—ergh. The snowmobile won't pull the cargo sled up the hill. I unpack everything, tip the sled on its side, and carefully scrape every trace of ice off the runners. I dry the runners with my sleeve. Boot step by boot step, I pack a spot in the snow, set the sled there, load up everything again, tie it all down, and try again. Fail. I jump off the snowmobile, pack the snow, reposition the sled, and try again. Fail. Once, twice, three times. It's no use. It won't budge.

I shut off the snowmobile. Arms crossed, I study the sleeping bag, just-purchased groceries, books, suitcase, puppy, and puppy toys I'm trying to take home. Which are the most important things? I stuff my day pack as full as it will go with computer, papers, and a few of the groceries. I unhook and tarp the cargo sled and drag it to the edge of the road, out of the way of other travelers.

But even without the sled attached, the snowmobile refuses when I try to drive up the steep hill. Beneath the fresh snow is slick ice. The snowmobile digs straight down to the ice, the track spins, the engine revs and whines, and I go nowhere.

Each time the snowmobile spins down to ice, I get off, carefully pack the snow beside it with my feet, then struggle the heavy machine sideways, lifting first the back, then the front, then the back again, until the track is resting on packed snow instead of ice. Holding my breath, I start the engine, delicately accelerate and: Whoosh! My packed snow flies out sideways and the snowmobile burrows straight down to ice. By the fourth try I'm sweating, jacket off.

Finally, I grab the skis on the front of the snowmobile and drag it 180 degrees so it's facing downhill. I put on my ridiculously heavy daypack, coax my puppy onto my lap, and drive downhill praying I'll be able to maintain enough speed through a tight U-turn to keep enough power to send my snowmobile uphill. All while with one hand holding an excitedly flopping thirty-five-pound puppy in my lap—which doesn't make steering a tight turn in deep powder any easier!

Some days, all we ask is to just get home.

I somehow make the precarious turn, missing the drop-off by inches; accelerate, accelerate, then don't slow down and don't look back. I'm dodging snow clumps as a wild foam of snow fountains into my face. The mantra for deep powder is: Keep moving no matter what. "If you go fast enough, you can go over anything," a mountain-biking friend once told me—not a philosophy I usually test, but today, yes!

Two hours after I arrived at the snowmobile, I'm at my own front door.

What a relief to turn off the noisy stinky engine and allow the deep silence to settle around me. So quiet. The world is a fluffy garden of whimsical sculptures, sparkling in the last rays of the sun. A few snowflakes whisper down my jacket sleeve. Amen, Dorothy of Oz: there's no place like home.

That night, still aching from snowmobile wrestling, I treat my tired muscles to a luxurious hot bath. I gaze at the red thread around my ankle and ponder the months and years of my journey from diagnosis to here.

BEFORE LADA, I BELIEVED WE COULD DRAW A LINE, WRITE HEALTHY on one side, UNHEALTHY on the other, and confidently place any food squarely on one side or the other. But then . . . brick wall therapy.

Whaaat, rice and beans from Los Camperos sends my BG high? Hummus dip? A salad with cottage cheese?

I only believed these startling discoveries because my personal super-power repeatedly and patiently showed me: Now that I have LADA, foods affect me differently than they did in the past, and differently than they affect people with abundant insulin. To be healthy now with LADA I would need to make significant changes in my food choices, timing of eating, patterns of exercise and activity, sleep health, stress management, and more.

To make an important change, we need clear rules.[1] And we need time. We need boot camp (chapter 19). Boot camp is a place to learn and get strong, but it's not a destination resort. We pass through boot camp because we're determinedly heading somewhere else.

For me, *the twenty-two rules of Carb-craft* were crucial. But equally crucial was to eventually loosen my death grip on these rules, let them transition into muscle memory, and turn my life toward joy. Today I'm expanding my food-world and re-creating childhood recipes in new formats. It might sound trite, but it's true: I needed to heal emotionally as well as physically.

Not that long ago, I didn't even know there was such a thing as LADA—and like so many of us, I didn't learn about LADA from my doctor, skilled and experienced though he was. LADA was a wake-up call to advocate for myself: for starters, to demand the very simple test that diagnoses LADA. And I had to keep advocating, searching for support, information, resources, and a doctor on my wavelength. It slowly sank in that having LADA wasn't going to be like getting over the mumps: I'd have to embrace new *lifelong* ways of living. Ultimately, advocating for myself entered a larger framework: advocating for all diabetics, and for others who eat—advocating for all of our children.

TODAY'S GOOD NEWS

Today a quarter of diabetics are healthy and in the 5 percent club (chapter 6). Whatever our A1c is today, we can maintain, or radically improve, our health. Good health is easiest when we have support and information, advocate for ourselves, are diagnosed early, and have access to healthy food and water and good medical care.

To be our healthiest, we begin keeping records and counting carbs, noticing our personal patterns, not with a self-punishing attitude, but the way we'd count our change at the grocery store—we need to know our budget. We build our understanding of fat-the-organ, not in a shaming way, but in the same way we learn how our pancreas rolls out insulin.

LADAs are very diverse. That's why one of the most important things we can do is learn where *we* are on the spectrum and have a self-reliant attitude. Through test-test-test, we learn what's *best for us* **now** and, aware that our situation will change over time, continue to test-test-test often to track how we're changing.

"Taking care of yourself when you have diabetes takes serious work," says Gary Scheiner, "and at times it may seem quite thankless . . . Taking care of diabetes is really just an ongoing series of small sacrifices, costs, mental efforts, and time commitments."[2]

As we take control of our LADA, we'll notice immediate and long-term benefits:

- Increased energy and stamina.
- More restful sleep.
- Clearer thinking / improved memory.
- Better moods / mental health.
- Healthy eyes.
- Healthy kidneys.
- Strong heart.
- Successful pregnancy.
- Good nerve function.
- Healthy feet.
- Flexible joints.
- Healthier skin and gums.

Metformin and vitamin D are gold-star medicines for most LADAs (chapter 12). Watch out for T2 medications like sulfonylureas, which burn up a LADA pancreas more quickly. Bumping up our activity level a notch becomes a best friend, our most effective "pill."

The medical community is moving toward *earlier* supplementation of insulin for LADAs: This pampers the beta cells and can offer a second honeymoon. And an international panel has recommended that *everyone diagnosed as T2 be screened for LADA.*[3]

LADAs have a lot of cards in our hand, and we do best when we are able to play them all.

I used to think of LADA as a double whammy, because most of us have insulin resistance *on top of* autoimmunity. But now I wonder: double whammy . . . or gift? Having both meant my blood sugars ran into trouble sooner, while I had more beta cells left. Having more of these crucial cells makes it easier for me to pamper them—and they return the favor, improving my blood sugars . . . which makes it easier to pamper them—it's a positive feedback loop. Pampering my beta cells makes my life easier every day, helps me enjoy occasional splurges, and keeps my "sleeping beauties" alive (chapter 4), which could have a big payoff down the line.

THE LADA GOLDEN RULE: PAMPER THE BETA CELLS

To pamper the beta cells:
1. **Carb-craft.**
   - Spend carbs like gold.
   - Embrace **fiber**: Eat a rainbow, heavy toward green, of foods that look like themselves.
   - Right-size **carbs**, within your unique *limit*, and tip them toward nutrient-dense veggies.
   - Enjoy healthful **fats**.
   - Be Goldilocks with **protein**.
2. **Reduce stress**, or convert it to energized readiness.
   - Channel stress into action, engaging adrenaline's *let's go-go-go* rather than cortisol's *I'm trapped* (chapter 10).
   - Tactical breathing, box breathing, meditation, prayer, going to our happy place . . . whatever you call it, science shows it makes us physically healthier and lowers blood sugars (chapter 14).
   - Enjoy ample restful sleep.
3. Keep the **garden in the gut** healthy (chapter 11). May your minions be friendly!
4. **Love and right-size fat-the-organ**, so it doesn't helicopter out of control and interfere with remaining precious insulin (chapter 10).

5. Frequent joyous **physical activity** keeps our "locks" sparkling, so that each precious insulin "key" can have its maximum effect (chapter 3).
6. Get **feedback loops** spinning in a positive direction.
   - Inflammation — microbiome — fat-the-organ is a trifecta: Each of these constantly impacts the others. At the time we are diagnosed, this loop may be spiraling down toward disaster. We can start it spinning in a positive direction, toward health.
7. Ideally we **begin insulin**, in consultation with our doctor, while we still have working beta cells left (chapter 13).

TOMORROW'S POSSIBILITIES

T1

The future looks bright for T1s as researchers learn more about genetics, antibodies, and drugs to slow autoimmune attack such as Tzield (teplizumab-mzwv), approved by the FDA just as we go to press.[4] Antibodies may be detected years before symptoms appear, helping T1s get diagnosed earlier, with more of their pancreas and insulin intact. T1 technology improves every year: New insulins better match our natural insulin, CGMs are becoming increasingly reliable, and we are on the cusp of integrating pumps and CGMs. Making these advances available to all would lower costs system-wide.

T2

The future looks hopeful for T2s as new research on diet, inflammation, and healthful fats corrects the mistaken advice of past decades. Although many T2s have to work harder than the average person to have a healthy weight, they now have better tools and information and can work *with*, instead of against, the hormones that control hunger. Genetics are powerful, but lifestyle is more powerful.

LADA

The things that help T1 and T2 also help LADA. Advances in antibody testing help LADA diagnosis, and *early diagnosis* is the best gift we can give ourselves, since the scariest health effects of diabetes happen cumulatively over time. LADA offers us a honeymoon . . . and then a second honeymoon. The art of prolonging these two honeymoons is a door that medicine is just beginning to open.

Research is on the cusp of exciting advances: interventions for our microbiome; immunotherapies like Tzield to slow the attack on the pancreas; and regrowing, reinserting, or extending the life of beta cells.[5]

As we saw in chapter 4, to hide from our immune system, a last few beta cells *dedifferentiate*. Can these sleeping beauties be woken? Not yet . . . but researchers are working hard on this, which "hold[s] promise for efforts to restore beta cell function well after diagnosis."[6] Recent findings, says the University of Exeter's Dr. Oram, "have raised a number of questions regarding how the remaining beta cells have escaped immune destruction, whether pools of 'sleeping' or dysfunctional beta cells could be rejuvenated and whether there is potential for new growth of beta cells."[7] LADAs are more likely than most diabetics to have significant reservoir areas of our pancreas undamaged, so LADAs may be particularly well placed to benefit from coming next-level discoveries in beta cell pampering.[8]

Protect the beta cells you still have, as much as you can, because who knows what's just around the corner.

SPARK JOY

I'm not sure how Marie Kondo did it, but she made "clean your room!" sound joyous and empowering. Similarly, fun activities, meditative breathing, connection, community—these aren't a list of chores. They are a recipe for happiness. They are play, presence, and vacation.

Let the little indulgences make life sweet; whether a curl of cinnamon bark in your morning coffee; pausing, on your way to fold the laundry, to tip your forehead against a loved one's; or stopping mid-stride to watch the sunlight dance on a fountain.

We spark joy when we go out into the fresh October sunshine and kick our feet through red maple leaves, or when we walk our dog as the moon lights up a field of freshly fallen snow. But for some reason I need a little push, at times, to get off the couch and go do that.

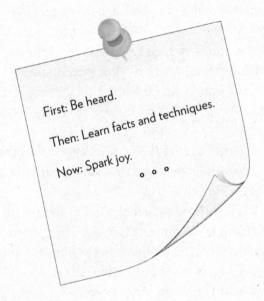

First: Be heard.

Then: Learn facts and techniques.

Now: Spark joy. ○ ○ ○

HOW'S THE DIABETES GOING?

Just diagnosed, I stared into a bakery case, afraid I would never again taste these fabulous foods I loved. I literally ran away—well, tried to—from the question stuck in my head: *What can I eat?*

Over time, I learned that while my body, and my place on the diabetes spectrum, are slightly unique (so I have to think for myself), they also follow the path of many who have gone before (so I can learn from my diabetes community). Thanks to community, test-test-test, and daily record keeping—and most of all thanks to Carb-craft—I feel confident and comfortable around food again.

My question has changed. It's no longer *What can I eat?* It's *How can I eat what I want? How can I eat the things I love while protecting my health?*

I've learned: I can eat anything; just not everything.

I've learned: With diabetes we can feel good, be healthy, and eat delicious food.

FRIENDS STILL ASK ME: "HOW'S THE DIABETES GOING?"

I smile, remembering how frustrated this question made me right after I was diagnosed. Back then, trying to answer this question felt like staring at a sled-dog harness that the dogs had hopelessly tangled—where would I even start?

Today LADA is still a dog-sled harness—complicated!—everything connects to everything! But now I can view this complex web with understanding, respect, and optimism. One thing about these interconnections: They mean that any place I start is a good place to start. Each is one part of the solution.

Life is built of small moments. Each success makes the next success easier. Build in little indulgences and find your heart's way to revel in the pleasures of eating.

No matter what happened yesterday, start in this moment. Stride forward from here. Caring for ourselves, and coming home to ourselves, allows us to support and care for others. Let your own footprints, making slow but steady progress, be your inspiration.

It's a beautiful world out there, and it's yours.

PART IV | SUMMARY

1. Food is tangled with our hearts, heritage, and coping mechanisms. There is nothing simple about "just" changing what we eat.
2. Diabetics and prediabetics have increased risk of food addiction and disordered eating.
3. Ultra-processed sweetened carbs are the most addictive. Food addiction is about as common and as difficult to kick as a nicotine addiction.
4. I once feared hunger: a beast that could hurt and control me. Now I realize: This experience of hunger, while common, is *optional*.
5. With the correct attitude, system, and support, those with a goal to change their weight can reach a healthier weight and maintain it. The successful have strong motivation, keep written records, incorporate exercise, value persistence, and are willing to begin again as often as it takes. We frame it for success.
6. By thinking of a meal as a structure, we can simplify our approach to food: Have we included all four legs of the table?
   - Low-carb veggies: the foundation.
   - Protein (be Goldilocks).
   - Healthful fats (round up to needed calories).
   - Carbier foods, especially superfoods (enjoy within your personal limits).
7. Getting healthy is not about deprivation and sacrifice: It's about empowered choices within a guiding framework.
8. Staying healthy means letting go of obsession and overly rigid rules. If our body's signals about food can no longer be trusted, we steer by lightly held guides.

9. Insulin, the lifesaving medicine all LADAs expect to one day depend upon, is not equally available to all in the US or around the globe.
10. At the beginning of my LADA journey, I learned I'd have to advocate for myself. By the end, I'd realized: To advocate for myself, I must advocate for all.

ACKNOWLEDGMENTS

I WOULDN'T BE HEALTHY TODAY, OR SANE, OR CORRECTLY DIAGNOSED were it not for my fabulous friends. Thank you for being there for me even after I abandoned you in coffee shops; thank you for the long walks where you listened to my rants and voiced important questions. And the deepest thanks to sharp-eyed, clear-speaking Shannon, who taught me the magic word LADA, and also kept saying: whaaat? . . . that doesn't make sense . . . have you thought about getting another opinion?

I don't know of words big enough to thank someone who has literally saved my life. Thank you, Shannon, forever and from the bottom of the Mariana Trench to the top of the sky. The gift you have given me—I hope this book can be that gift for someone else.

To my beloved Mom, Dad, Sis, and Son: your love holds me up, always.

To Maury, for being a stickler, and patient and clear, while I struggled to get it right.

To guide, mentor and friend Laura Pritchett—together with my Fish-trapping partners Adam, Beth, Janet, Maggie, and Victoria—you brought this book to life.

To the "Doctor Right" in my life, Dr. Lorena Wright, for supporting me and this book, and for her advocacy and care of the wider community.

Special thanks to my discerning agent Regina Ryan: You transformed this dream into reality. Special thanks to my inspiring editor Renee Sedliar for expanding my thinking and continually making the room larger, while gently and patiently nudging her foot across rabbit holes. Thank you to many other unsung sheroes and heroes at Hachette who turned this pile of words into a thing of beauty.

To A Book For All Seasons, the phenomenal family bookstore who adopted me—thank you Pat, Stephen, Donica, and the whole gang.

To Ana Maria Spagna and the warm, wise generous NILA community, with thanks to Elizabeth George for the scholarship that set my feet on the writer's path. To writing mentors Aaron Abeyta, Kathleen Alcalá, Elizabeth Austen, Bonny Becker, Carmen Bernier-Grand, John Calderazzo, Larry Cheek, CMarie Fuhrman, Tess Gallagher, Claudia Castro Luna, Kathleen Dean Moore, Beth Piatote, Bruce Holland Rogers, Derek Sheffield, Kim Stafford, David Wagoner, and many, many others—thank you for your wisdom, your generosity, and for showing me what is possible— as did fellow writers Ann, Bren, Chanelle, Chris, Claire, Deborah, Erika, Evonne, Frances, Heather, Ian, Iris, Jane, Jim, Lailani, Leonie, Lois, Mare, Marina, Marlene, Mattie, Nadine, Nancy, Rachel, Sandy, Sarah, Stephanie, and many more than I can name.

Deep gratitude to Elk River Writer's Workshop, Fishtrap, and Tin House Writer's Workshop for the glorious work you do, and for gracing and shaping this book.

To Barb, who has walked far beyond me, and shines with stunning grace. Thank you for grand adventures.

My forever gratitude to Amy, Ann, Anna, Barbara, Bekah, Catha, Dean, Debbie, Diane, Fred, Ginger, Holly, Jenny, Judy, Karen, Kari, Karl, Karla, Kathy, Larry, Leona, Lisa, Marileta, Nancy, Pierre, Susan, Tammy, and so many more: you make the world beautiful, and you made this book possible.

Heather, thank you for believing that no space is too small to share, and creating a comfy bed on your floor so I could meet Fabulous Doctor Five. Thank you to rivers, trails, and not-trails of the Cascades. Thank you to coffee shops, bakeries, cafes, hogans, farms, and campgrounds where many of these words met the page. With humble appreciation, and a pledge to stand against whitewashing, lemlmtš and pidamayape to the P'squosa, the Wahpekute, and other nations upon whose unceded lands

I have written and lived. To my ancestors and the wise ones over generations. To Cascadia. Mni Wiconi. And to the future, the only reason any of it matters.

"Our children cannot dream unless they live," wrote Audre Lorde, "they cannot live unless they are nourished, and who else will feed them the real food without which their dreams will be no different than ours?"

APPENDIX A

Food-by-Food Summary

Carb-craft is compatible with virtually any inclusion or exclusion and many named diets: with kosher, halal, plant-based, keto, paleo, meat lovers, and more. There are no required foods in Carb-craft—only healthy balance. This table assumes you are not allergic to the food being discussed, and that you have chosen a version of the food that is not highly processed, sweetened, or chemically contaminated.

Table A: Food-by-Food Summary

Food	Positives	Cautions
Eggs	Zero-carb. A safe space. Great source of vitamin B_{12} for those who do not eat meat. The yolk is packed with vitamins and minerals.	An allergen for some.
Dairy	Full-fat dairy, especially cheese and yogurt, can improve diabetes health.	An allergen for some.
Fish	Zero-carb, omega-3, anti-inflammatory.	Can be toxin-laden, so choosing the right fish is very important. An allergen for some.
Unprocessed meat (meat that looks like itself)	Zero-carb.	Be Goldilocks with any protein. Watch for carbs in toppings and sauces.
Processed meat (lunch meat, hot dogs, et cetera)	—	Raises risk of diabetes, heart disease, and other scary diseases.
Legumes and grains	Can be great sources of fiber, iron, vitamins, minerals, essential fatty acids, and antioxidants.	Often high-carb. Choose whole or less processed forms.
Tree nuts and seeds	Excellent sources of protein, fiber, healthful fats, vitamins, minerals, and antioxidants. Walnuts and flax are the O-3 stars among nuts.	Because they are energy-dense (high-calorie), keep serving size moderate. An allergen for some.

More to consider	Verdict
A vitamin-packed protein food that is comparatively easy to raise healthfully and locally in a wide range of communities.	Excellent staple for LADA.
See "What Our Food Ate" and "Climate Diet."	Excellent staple for LADA.
See "Choosing Healthful Fish."	Specific healthful varieties are an excellent staple for LADA and an excellent source of O-3s.
See "What Our Food Ate" and "Climate Diet."	Can provide a safe space for beginners and in tricky situations like eating at the homes of others or dining out.
—	Enjoy your uncle's homemade elk sausage, but hot dogs aren't as innocent—or as cheap (big picture)—as they seem.
See "Lectins." For grains: See "Gluten."	Healthful, but at the serving size that protects BG, won't offer much protein or calories.
See "Kidney Stones And Nuts."	Excellent staple for LADA.

TABLE A CONTINUES

TABLE A CONTINUED

Food	Positives	Cautions
Peanuts	Good source of protein, fiber, healthful fats, and many vitamins and minerals.	An allergen for some.
Soy	It's complicated. Read "Soy."	It's complicated. Read "Soy."
Mushrooms	Great source of protein and other nutrients, with relatively few carbs.	Typically healthier when cooked.
Avocado, olives, coconut (unsweetened), healthful oils	Good sources of calories with few carbs. Great add-ons to a veggie-centered meal.	Oils can be extracted in a healthful or unhealthful manner.
Stem/leaf/flower veggies	The stars of the LADA show. Filling, nutritious, packed with vitamins, minerals, antioxidants, and more, yet low-carb.	–
Root veggies	Many are great sources of vitamins. Most are high-carb.	Count carbs and adjust serving size.
Fermented foods	Improve diabetes health and our microbiome.	Remember to choose those labeled KEEP REFRIGERATED.
Fruits	Nutritious: packed with vitamins, minerals, and antioxidants.	Count carbs and adjust serving size.
Berries	Among fruits, berries are often lower-carb while high in vitamins and antioxidants.	"Standardly" grown berries may have a high toxin load and large carbon footprint (flying food).

More to consider	Verdict
See "Aflatoxins" and "Lectins."	Good protein source for LADA.
See "Lectins" and "Organic Produce."	Good protein source for LADA.
–	Good protein source for LADA.
–	Healthful fats, healthful calories.
–	The centerpiece of a typical LADA meal.
–	Often healthful, but at the serving size that protects BG, these won't be major players in most LADA meals.
See chapter 11.	Excellent for LADA.
–	For most LADAs, portion sizes will be small. A slice or two makes a delicious, healthful treat: the cherry on top.
Look for local options in season; easy to freeze yourself.	Berries are the new candy! Delicious.

APPENDIX B

LADA-Love and LADA-Limit Foods

Table B1 gives a visual impression using example foods. Tables B2 and B3 offer more complete food lists.

TABLE B1: VISUAL OVERVIEW: ENJOY FREELY, LIMIT, OR SPEND LIKE GOLD

	ENGINEERED FOODS	GRAINS	ROOT VEGGIES AND SQUASHES
Spend Like Gold	ultraprocessed sweet or salty (Ding-Dongs, doughnuts, chips)		
		homemade desserts, breakfast cereals	
		waffles, pancakes, granola	
		couscous, healthful white bread, grits	cassava, potatoes
Craft Your Personal Limit		rice, pasta, oats, whole-wheat bread	yams, sweet potatoes
		quinoa, corn, millet, hominy	most winter squashes and pumpkin
		teff injera, sprouted bread, barley	rutabagas
			spaghetti squashes
			beets, parsnips
Enjoy and Note Carbs			carrots, daikon, jicama, summer squashes, turnips
Enjoy Freely		All the LADA-Love Foods in chart B2 including fish, nuts, seeds, meats, mushrooms, avocados, olives, oils, stem and leaf veggies, and more	

LEGUMES	FRUITS	DAIRY AND OTHERS
	raisins, figs, dates	
baked beans	bananas, pineapple, grapes, mangoes, kiwis	sweetened yogurt, milk chocolate
chickpeas (garbanzos), kidney, pinto, navy beans	apples, pears, cantaloupe, watermelon	cottage cheese and other soft cheeses
black beans, black-eyed peas	oranges, cherries, papayas	dark chocolate
lentils, split peas, soybeans	grapefruit, strawberries, blueberries, blackberries	cow milk, oat milk, kefir
tofu, tempeh, green peas, edamame	bell peppers, eggplant, okra, tomatoes	unsweetened yogurt, lightly sweetened nut/soy milks
	cucumbers	unsweetened nut/soy milks, hard cheeses

increasing carb speed and density →

TABLE B2: LADA-LOVE FOODS

Great Foundation	
	Minimize math [a] asparagus, artichoke, bamboo shoots, bok choy, broccoli, brussels sprouts, cabbage, cauliflower, celery, chard, collard greens, cucumber, dandelion greens, green beans, jicama, kale, lettuce, nettle greens, radish, spinach, sprouts
Little Luxuries	
	Minimize math [b] fresh lemon, fresh lime, garlic, ginger, onion, turmeric, other spices, pure unsweetened cocoa/cacao, salsa
Add Protein [c]	
	Minimize math [a] mushrooms (common culinary types)
	Respect calories beef, chicken, pork, venison, other meats, fish (healthful types) eggs, hard cheeses, tree nuts (almonds, Brazil nuts, cashews, hazelnuts/filberts, pecans, pistachios, walnuts, others), peanuts, seeds (chia, flax, hemp, pumpkin, sesame, sunflower, others), nut butters
Add Energy [d]	
	Respect calories avocado, nuts, seeds, fish oil, olives, olive oil, other healthful oils, cream, unsweetened coconut (fresh, dried, and other forms)
	Track carbs and respect calories bone broth, garlic sauce, peanut sauce, curry sauce, tomato sauce, and other culinary sauces half and half, yogurt, milks (dairy, nut, and grain-derived)
Pamper Your Garden [e]	
	Minimize math [a] kimchi, pickles, pickled vegetables, sauerkraut
	Track carbs and respect calories tempeh, tofu, kefir, kombucha, unsweetened yogurt

[a] So low-carb that I don't count carbs.

[b] So low-quantity (at normal serving sizes) that I don't count carbs.

[c] Aim for protein in most meals. Aim for foods raised and produced without diabetes-triggering chemicals.

[d] Easy to keep on hand to add to a finished dish when you wish to round up calories/energy so a meal will carry you 4+ hours. Aim for healthfully extracted oils. Foods in "add protein" section also add energy.

[e] Fermented foods that say *KEEP REFRIGERATED* and/or *LIVE CULTURES*.

TABLE B3: LADA-LIMIT FOODS

ENJOY AT YOUR PLEASURE, BUT NOTE CARBS
Within Soy:
edamame, tempeh, tofu
Within Fruits and Veggies:
blackberries, blueberries, grapefruit
bell peppers, carrots, daikon, eggplant, green peas, jicama, okra, snow peas, sugar peas, summer squashes, tomatoes, turnips, zucchini
Within Dairy and Other:
unsweetened yogurt, lightly sweetened nut/soy milks
CRAFT YOUR PERSONAL LIMIT
Within Beans and Grains:
Baba ghanoush, black beans, black-eyed peas, chickpeas (garbanzos), fava beans, hummus, lentils, pinto beans, navy beans, soybeans, split peas
barley, chapati (whole wheat), corn, hominy, injera (teff), millet, oats, pasta, pita (whole wheat), quinoa, rice, tortilla, sprouted breads, wheat berries, whole-grain breads
Within Fruits and Veggies:
apples, bananas, cantaloupes, cherries, figs, grapes, guavas, kiwis, mangos, oranges, other melons, papayas, pears, pineapple, plums, pomegranate, raisins, strawberries, watermelon
acorn squashes, beets, Hubbard squashes, Jerusalem artichokes (sunchokes), other winter squashes, parsnips, potatoes, pumpkins, rutabaga, spaghetti squashes, sweet potatoes, turnips, yams
Within Dairy and Other:
chocolate, cottage cheese and other soft cheeses, cow milk, sweetened yogurt including Greek yogurt, moderately sweetened alternative milks including soy, almond, coconut, oat, rice
SPEND LIKE GOLD
Within Grains:
couscous, crackers, grits, sorghum, bagels, breakfast cereals, granola, healthful white breads (including chapati, naan, pita, sourdough), homemade desserts, pancakes, waffles
chips, ultra-processed sweets (including fast-food desserts and most store-bought desserts)
Within Fruits and Veggies:
fruit juices, jam, preserves
cassava, potatoes
Within Dairy and Other:
ice cream, sodas

SOURCE CITATIONS

Aaboe K, Knop FK, Vilsbøll T, et al. Twelve Weeks Treatment with the DPP-4 Inhibitor, Sitagliptin, Prevents Degradation of Peptide YY and Improves Glucose and Non-Glucose Induced Insulin Secretion in Patients with Type 2 Diabetes Mellitus. Diab Obes Metab. 2010 Apr;12(4):323–33. doi: 10.1111/j.1463-1326.2009.01167.x. PMID: 20380653.

Abbasnezhad A, Falahi E, Gonzalez MJ, et al. Effect of Different Dietary Approaches in Comparison with High/Low-Carbohydrate Diets on Systolic and Diastolic Blood Pressure in Type 2 Diabetic Patients: A Systematic Review and Meta-Analysis. Prev Nutr Food Sci. 2020 Sep 30;25(3):233–45. doi: 10.3746/pnf.2020.25.3.233. PMID: 33083372; PMCID: PMC7541922.

Abboud M, Rizk R, AlAnouti F, et al. The Health Effects of Vitamin D and Probiotic Co-Supplementation: A Systematic Review of Randomized Controlled Trials. Nutrients. 2020 Dec 30;13(1):111. doi: 10.3390/nu13010111. PMID: 33396898; PMCID: PMC7824176.

ACCORD (Action to Control Cardiovascular Risk in Diabetes) Study Group, Gerstein HC, Miller ME, Byington RP, et al. Effects of Intensive Glucose Lowering in Type 2 Diabetes. N Engl J Med. 2008 Jun 12;358(24):2545–59. doi: 10.1056/NEJMoa0802743. Epub 2008 Jun 6. PMID: 18539917; PMCID: PMC4551392.

ADA (American Diabetes Association) website. 2020. https://www.diabetes.org/diabetes/complications/stroke.

Afshin A, Micha R, Khatibzadeh S, Mozaffarian D. Consumption of Nuts and Legumes and Risk of Incident Ischemic Heart Disease, Stroke, and Diabetes: A Systematic Review and Meta-Analysis. Am J Clin Nutr. 2014;100(1):278–88. PMID: 24898241.

Aguirre M, Venema K. The Art of Targeting Gut Microbiota for Tackling Human Obesity. Genes Nutr. 2015;10(20). doi: 10.1007/s12263-015-0472-4.

Akimbekov NS, Digel I, Sherelkhan DK, et al. Vitamin D and the Host-Gut Microbiome: A Brief Overview. Acta Histochemica et Cytochemica. 2020;53(3), 33–42. doi: 10.1267/ahc.20011.

Al-Goblan AS, Al-Alfi MA, Khan MZ. Mechanism Linking Diabetes Mellitus and Obesity. Diab Metab Syndr Obes. 2014 Dec 4;7:587–91. doi: 10.2147/DMSO.S67400.

Al-Shoumer KA, Al-Essa TM. Is There a Relationship Between Vitamin D with Insulin Resistance and Diabetes Mellitus? World J Diab. 2015;6(8):1057–064. doi: 10 .4239/wjd.v6.i8.1057.

Al Theyab A, Almutairi T, Al-Suwaidi AM, et al. Epigenetic Effects of Gut Metabolites: Exploring the Path of Dietary Prevention of Type 1 Diabetes. Front Nutr. 2020 Sep 24;7:563605. doi: 10.3389/fnut.2020.563605. PMID: 33072796; PMCID: PMC7541812.

Alarim RA et al. Effects of the Ketogenic Diet on Glycemic Control in Diabetic Patients: Meta-Analysis of Clinical Trials. Cureus. 2020 5 Oct;12(10):e10796. doi: 10. 7759/cureus.10796.

Alkayali T, Ricardo J, Busari K, Saad I. Sitagliptin-Induced Pancreatitis: Chronic Use Would Not Spare You the Complication. Cureus. 2020;12(3):e7389. 2020 Mar 24. doi: 10.7759/cureus.7389.

Allard C, Desgagné V, Patenaude J, et al. Mendelian Randomization Supports Causality Between Maternal Hyperglycemia and Epigenetic Regulation of Leptin Gene in Newborns. Epigenetics. 2015;10:342–51.

Allison MB, Myers MG Jr. 20 Years of Leptin: Connecting Leptin Signaling to Biological Function. J Endocrinol. 2014 Oct;223(1):T25–T35. doi: 10.1530/JOE-14-0404. PMID: 25232147; PMCID: PMC4170570.

Alvarez-Bueno C, Cavero-Redondo I, Martinez-Vizcaino V, et al. Effects of Milk and Dairy Product Consumption on Type 2 Diabetes: Overview of Systematic Reviews and Meta-Analyses. Adv Nutr. 2019 May 1;10(Suppl 2):S154–S163. doi: 10.1093 /advances/nmy107. PMID: 31089734; PMCID: PMC6518137.

American Diabetes Association. Standards of Medical Care in Diabetes — 2014. Diabetes Care. 2014 Jan;37(Suppl 1):S14–S80. doi: 10.2337/dc14-S014.

ANAD (National Association of Anorexia Nervosa and Associated Disorders) website. https://anad.org.

Andersen MK. New Insights into the Genetics of Latent Autoimmune Diabetes in Adults. Curr Diab Rep. 2020 Jul 28;20(9):43. doi: 10.1007/s11892-020-01330-y. PMID: 32725517.

Andersen MK, Hansen T. Genetic Aspects of Latent Autoimmune Diabetes in Adults: A Mini-Review. Curr Diab Rev. 2019;15(3):194–98. doi: 10.2174/1573399814666 180730123226.

Aneklaphakij C, Saigo T, Watanabe M, et al. Diversity of Chemical Structures and Biosynthesis of Polyphenols in Nut-Bearing Species. Front Plant Sci. 2021 Apr 6;12:642581. doi: 10.3389/fpls.2021.642581. PMID: 33889165; PMCID: PMC8056029.

Anthony K, et al. Attenuation of Insulin-Evoked Responses in Brain Networks Controlling Appetite and Reward in Insulin Resistance: The Cerebral Basis for Impaired Control of Food Intake in Metabolic Syndrome? Diabetes. 2006;55:2986–92.

Anton SD, Lee SA, Donahoo WT, et al. The Effects of Time Restricted Feeding on Overweight, Older Adults: A Pilot Study. Nutrients. 2019;11(7):1500. Published 2019 Jun 30. doi: 10.3390/nu11071500.

Anton SD, Moehl K, Donahoo WT, et al. Flipping the Metabolic Switch: Understanding and Applying the Health Benefits of Fasting. Obesity (Silver Spring). 2018;26(2):254–68. doi: 10.1002/oby.22065.

Arenas DJ, Thomas A, Wang J, DeLisser HM. A Systematic Review and Meta-Analysis of Depression, Anxiety, and Sleep Disorders in US Adults with Food Insecurity. J Gen Intern Med. 2019;34:2874–82.

Astrup A, Magkos F, Bier DM, et al. Saturated Fats and Health: A Reassessment and Proposal for Food-Based Recommendations: JACC State-of-the-Art Review. J Am Coll Cardiol. 2020 Aug 18;76(7):844–57. doi: 10.1016/j.jacc.2020.05.077. Epub 2020 Jun 17. PMID: 32562735.

Athinarayanan SJ, Adams RN, Hallberg SJ, et al. Long-Term Effects of a Novel Continuous Remote Care Intervention Including Nutritional Ketosis for the Management of Type 2 Diabetes: A 2-Year Non-Randomized Clinical Trial. Front Endocrinol (Lausanne). 2019;10:348.

Atkinson MA, Roep BO, Posgai A, et al. The Challenge of Modulating β-Cell Autoimmunity in Type 1 Diabetes. Lancet Diab Endocrinol. 2019 Jan;7(1):52–64. doi: 10.1016/S2213-8587(18)30112-8. Epub 2018 Oct 24. PMID: 30528099; PMCID: PMC7322790.

Attia P. Is the Obesity Crisis Hiding a Bigger Problem? TED Talk. 2013 Jun 25.

Avena NM, Bocarsly ME, Hoebel BG. Animal Models of Sugar and Fat Bingeing: Relationship to Food Addiction and Increased Body Weight. Methods Mol Biol. 2012; 829:351–65. doi: 10.1007/978-1-61779-458-2_23. PMID: 22231826.

Avena NM, Gold MS. Food and Addiction—Sugars, Fats and Hedonic Overeating. Addiction. 2011 Jul;106(7):1214–15; discussion 1219–20. doi: 10.1111/j.1360-0443 .2011.03373.x. PMID: 21635590.

Avena NM, Rada P, Hoebel BG. Evidence for Sugar Addiction: Behavioral and Neurochemical Effects of Intermittent, Excessive Sugar Intake. Neurosci Biobehav Rev. 2008;32(1):20–39. doi: 10.1016/j.neubiorev.2007.04.019. Epub 2007 May 18. PMID: 17617461; PMCID: PMC2235907.

Avena NM, Rada P, Moise N, Hoebel BG. Sucrose Sham Feeding on a Binge Schedule Releases Accumbens Dopamine Repeatedly and Eliminates the Acetylcholine Satiety Response. Neuroscience. 2006;139:813–20.

Azad MB, Abou-Setta AM, Chauhan BF, et al. Nonnutritive Sweeteners and Cardiometabolic Health: A Systematic Review and Meta-Analysis of Randomized Controlled Trials and Prospective Cohort Studies. CMAJ. 2017 Jul 17;189(28):E929–E939. doi: 10.1503/cmaj.161390. PMID: 28716847; PMCID: PMC5515645.

Babar ZU, Ramzan S, El-Dahiyat F, et al. The Availability, Pricing, and Affordability of Essential Diabetes Medicines in 17 Low-, Middle-, and High-Income Countries. Front Pharmacol. 2019;10:1375. Published 2019 Nov 19. doi: 10.3389 /fphar.2019.01375.

Babcock, BA. Iowa Ag Review. Fall 2001;7(4):1–3. Center for Agricultural and Rural Development.

Bailey A, Gilmer E. Jul 9, 2019. Colorado's Insulin Price Cap: A Foundation to Build Upon. T1International.com. https://www.t1international.com/blog/2019/07/09 /colorados-insulin-price-cap-foundation-build-upon.

Bailey TS, Zisser HC, Garg SK. Reduction in Hemoglobin A1C with Real-Time Continuous Glucose Monitoring: Results from a 12-Week Observational Study. Diab Technol Ther. 2007;9(3):203–10. doi: 10.1089/dia.2007.0205.

Bakkila BF, Basu S, Lipska KJ. Catastrophic Spending on Insulin in the United States, 2017–18. Health Affairs. 2022 Jul;41(7). https://doi.org/10.1377/hlthaff.2021.01788.

Balaji S, Napolitano T, Silvano S, Friano ME, Garrido-Utrilla A, Atlija J, Collombat P. Epigenetic Control of Pancreatic Regeneration in Diabetes. Genes (Basel). 2018 Sep 7;9(9):448. doi: 10.3390/genes9090448. PMID: 30205460; PMCID: PMC6162679.

Bamberger C, Rossmeier A, Lechner K, et al. A Walnut-Enriched Diet Reduces Lipids in Healthy Caucasian Subjects, Independent of Recommended Macronutrient Replacement and Time Point of Consumption: A Prospective, Randomized, Controlled Trial. Nutrients. 2017;9(10):1097. Published 2017 Oct 6. doi: 10.3390/nu9101097.

Banel DK, Hu FB. Effects of Walnut Consumption on Blood Lipids and Other Cardiovascular Risk Factors: A Meta-Analysis and Systematic Review. Am J Clin Nutr. 2009 Jul;90(1):56–63. doi: 10.3945/ajcn.2009.27457. Epub 2009 May 20. PMID: 19458020; PMCID: PMC2696995.

Baraz J, Alexander S. *Awakening Joy: 10 Steps to Happiness* (Ballantine Books, 2012).

Barclay E. Fruit Juice vs. Soda? Both Beverages Pack in Sugar, Health Risks. The Salt. NPR. 2014 Jun 9. https://www.npr.org/sections/thesalt/2014/06/09/319230765/fruit-juice-vs-soda-both-beverages-pack-in-sugar-and-health-risk.

Barkan AL, Dimaraki EV, Jessup SK, et al. Ghrelin Secretion in Humans Is Sexually Dimorphic, Suppressed by Somatostatin, and Not Affected by the Ambient Growth Hormone Levels. J Clin Endocr Metab. 2003 May 1;88(5):2180–84. doi: 10.1210/jc.2002-021169.

Barnard N. *Dr. Neal Barnard's Program for Reversing Diabetes: The Scientifically Proven System for Reversing Diabetes Without Drugs* (Rodale, 2007).

Battistini C, Ballan R, Herkenhoff ME, et al. Vitamin D Modulates Intestinal Microbiota in Inflammatory Bowel Diseases. Int J Mol Sci. 2020 Dec 31;22(1):362. doi: 10.3390/ijms22010362. PMID: 33396382; PMCID: PMC7795229.

Baynes HW, Mideksa S, Ambachew S. The Role of Polyunsaturated Fatty Acids (n-3 PUFAs) on the Pancreatic β-Cells and Insulin Action. Adipocyte. 2018;7(2):81–87. doi: 10.1080/21623945.2018.1443662. Epub 2018 Mar 14. PMID: 29537934; PMCID: PMC6152539.

Bear TLK, Dalziel JE, Coad J, et al. The Role of the Gut Microbiota in Dietary Interventions for Depression and Anxiety. Adv Nutr. 2020 Jul 1;11(4):890–907. doi: 10.1093/advances/nmaa016. PMID: 32149335; PMCID: PMC7360462.

Beckles GL, Chou CF. Disparities in the Prevalence of Diagnosed Diabetes—United States, 1999–2002 and 2011–2014. MMWR Morb Mortal Wkly Rep. 2016;65(45):1265–69. Published 2016 Nov 18. doi: 10.15585/mmwr.mm6545a4.

Bellan M, Andreoli L, Mele C, et al. Pathophysiological Role and Therapeutic Implications of Vitamin D in Autoimmunity: Focus on Chronic Autoimmune Diseases. Nutrients. 2020;12(3):789. doi: 10.3390/nu12030789.

Bellerba F, Muzio V, Gnagnarella P, et al. The Association Between Vitamin D and Gut Microbiota: A Systematic Review of Human Studies. Nutrients. 2021

Sep 26;13(10):3378. doi: 10.3390/nu13103378. PMID: 34684379; PMCID: PMC8540279.

Beran D, Ewen M, Laing R. Constraints and Challenges in Access to Insulin: A Global Perspective. Lancet Diab Endocrinol. 2016;4(3):275–85. doi: 10.1016/ S2213-8587(15)00521-5.

Beran D, Ewen M, Lipska K, et al. 2018a. Availability and Affordability of Essential Medicines: Implications for Global Diabetes Treatment. Curr Diab Rep. 2018;18(8):48. Published 2018 Jun 16. doi: 10.1007/s11892-018-1019-z.

Beran D, Hirsch IB, Yudkin JS. 2018b. Why Are We Failing to Address the Issue of Access to Insulin? A National and Global Perspective. Diabetes Care. 2018 Jun;41(6):1125–31. doi: 10.2337/dc17-2123. Published correction in Diabetes Care. 2018 Sep;41(9):2048. Epub 2018 Jun 15. doi: 10.2337/dc18-er09a.

Beran D, Yudkin JS, de Courten M. Access to Care for Patients with Insulin-Requiring Diabetes in Developing Countries: Case Studies of Mozambique and Zambia. Diabetes Care. 2005;28(9):2136–40. doi: 10.2337/diacare.28.9.2136.

Berger S, Raman G, Vishwanathan R, et al. Dietary Cholesterol and Cardiovascular Disease: A Systematic Review and Meta-Analysis. Am J Clin Nutr. 2015 Aug;102(2):276–94. doi: 10.3945/ajcn.114.100305. Epub 2015 Jun 24. PMID: 26109578.

Bergman Å, Heindel JJ, Jobling S, et al. State of the Science of Endocrine Disrupting Chemicals 2012 (World Health Organization, 2013).

Bernstein RK. Dr. Bernstein's Diabetes Solution: The Complete Guide to Achieving Normal Blood Sugars. 4th ed. (Little, Brown, 2011).

Berridge M. Vitamin D Deficiency and Diabetes. Biochem J. 2017 Mar 24;474(8):1321–32. doi: 10.1042/BCJ20170042.

Berry SE, Bruce JH, Steenson S, et al. Interesterified Fats: What Are They and Why Are They Used? A Briefing Report from the Roundtable on Interesterified Fats in Foods. Nutr Bull. 2019;44:363–80. doi: 10.1111/nbu.12397.

Bettelheim A. Proposed Insulin Price Cap Poses Test for Dems. Axios. June 23, 2022. https://www.axios.com/2022/06/23/proposed-insulin-cost-cap-poses-test-for-democrats.

Beydoun MA, Fanelli Kuczmarski MT, Beydoun HA, et al. Associations of the Ratios of n-3 to n-6 Dietary Fatty Acids with Longitudinal Changes in Depressive Symptoms Among US Women. Am J Epidemiol. 2015 May 1;181(9):691–705. doi: 10.1093 /aje/kwu334. Epub 2015 Apr 7. PMID: 25855645; PMCID: PMC4408948.

Beysel S, Unsal IO, Kizilgul M, et al. The Effects of Metformin in Type 1 Diabetes Mellitus. BMC Endocr Disord. 2018;18(1):1. doi: 10.1186/s12902-017-0228-9.

Bibbò S, Dore MP, Pes GM, et al. Is There a Role for Gut Microbiota in Type 1 Diabetes Pathogenesis? Ann Med. 2017;49(1):11–22. doi: 10.1080/07853890.2016 .1222449.

Bielka W, Przezak A, Pawlik A. The Role of the Gut Microbiota in the Pathogenesis of Diabetes. Int J Mol Sci. 2022 Jan 1;23(1):480. doi: 10.3390/ ijms23010480.

Biswas A, Oh PI, Faulkner GE, et al. Sedentary Time and Its Association with Risk for Disease Incidence, Mortality, and Hospitalization in Adults: A Systematic Review and Meta-Analysis. Ann Intern Med. 2015 Jan 20;162(2):123–32. doi: 10.7326 /M14-1651. Published correction in Ann Intern Med. 2015 Sep 1;163(5):400. PMID: 25599350.

Bittman M. *Animal, Vegetable, Junk: A History of Food, From Sustainable to Suicidal* (Houghton Mifflin Harcourt, 2021).

Black JL, Macinko J. Neighborhoods and Obesity. Nutr Rev. 2008 Jan;66(1):2–20. doi: 10.1111/j.1753-4887.2007.00001.x. PMID: 18254880.

Black PH. The Inflammatory Consequences of Psychologic Stress: Relationship to Insulin Resistance, Obesity, Atherosclerosis and Diabetes Mellitus, Type II. Med Hypotheses. 2006;67(4):879–91. doi: 10.1016/j.mehy.2006.04.008. Epub 2006 Jun 15. PMID: 16781084.

Black PH, Garbutt LD. Stress, Inflammation and Cardiovascular Disease. J Psychosom Res. 2002 Jan;52(1):1–23. doi: 10.1016/s0022-3999(01)00302-6. PMID: 11801260.

Blaser MJ. The Theory of Disappearing Microbiota and the Epidemics of Chronic Diseases. Nat Rev Immunol. 2017 Jul 27;17(8):461–63. doi: 10.1038/nri.2017.77. PMID: 28749457.

Bliss ES, Whiteside E. The Gut-Brain Axis, the Human Gut Microbiota and Their Integration in the Development of Obesity. Front Physiol. 2018 Jul 12;9:900. doi: 10.3389/fphys.2018.00900. PMID: 30050464; PMCID: PMC6052131.

Blitstein JL, Lazar D, Gregory K, et al. Foods for Health: An Integrated Social Medical Approach to Food Insecurity Among Patients with Diabetes. Am J Health Promot. 2021;35(3):369–76. doi: 10.1177/0890117120964144.

Bolla AM, Caretto A, Laurenzi A, et al. Low-Carb and Ketogenic Diets in Type 1 and Type 2 Diabetes. Nutrients. 2019;11(5):962. Published 2019 Apr 26. doi: 10.3390/nu11050962.

Bolte Taylor, Jill. *My Stroke of Insight: A Brain Scientist's Personal Journey* (Penguin, 2009).

Bonaccio M, Di Castelnuovo A, Pounis G, et al. A Score of Low-Grade Inflammation and Risk of Mortality: Prospective Findings from the Moli-Sani Study. Haematologica. 2016;101:1434–41. doi: 10.3324/haematol.2016.144055.

Bonder R, Davis C, Kuk JL, Loxton NJ. Compulsive "Grazing" and Addictive Tendencies Towards Food. Eur Eat Disord Rev. 2018 Nov;26(6):569–73. doi: 10.1002/erv.2642. Epub 2018 Sep 26. PMID: 30259593.

Boyle JP, Thompson TJ, Gregg EW, et al. Projection of the Year 2050 Burden of Diabetes in the US Adult Population: Dynamic Modeling of Incidence, Mortality, and Prediabetes Prevalence. Popul Health Metr. 2010;8:29. Published 2010 Oct 22. doi: 10.1186/1478-7954-8-29.

Bradford A. Gluten-Free Diet: Benefits and Risks. Livescience. 2015 Dec 11.

Brady H. Red Skittles Spilling onto Wisconsin Highway Were Headed for Cattle. National Geographic. 2017 Jan 23.

Brandhorst S, Choi IY, Wei M, et al. A Periodic Diet that Mimics Fasting Promotes Multi-System Regeneration, Enhanced Cognitive Performance, and Healthspan. Cell Metab. 2015 Jul 7;22(1):86–99. doi: 10.1016/j.cmet.2015.05.012. Epub 2015 Jun 18. PMID: 26094889; PMCID: PMC4509734.

Brawerman G, Thompson PJ. Beta Cell Therapies for Preventing Type 1 Diabetes: From Bench to Bedside. Biomolecules. 2020;10(12):1681. Published 2020 Dec 16. doi: 10.3390/biom10121681.

Breit S, Kupferberg A, Rogler G, Hasler G. Vagus Nerve as Modulator of the Brain-Gut Axis in Psychiatric and Inflammatory Disorders. Front Psychiatry. 2018;9:44. Published 2018 Mar 13. doi: 10.3389/fpsyt.2018.00044.

Bremner JD, Moazzami K, Wittbrodt MT, et al. Diet, Stress and Mental Health. Nutrients. 2020 Aug 13;12(8):2428. doi: 10.3390/nu12082428. PMID: 32823562; PMCID: PMC7468813.

Brophy S, et al. Interventions for Latent Autoimmune Diabetes (LADA) in Adults (Review). Cochrane Database Syst Rev. 2011 Sep 11;9. doi: 10.1002/14651858 .CD006165.pub3.

Brophy S, Yderstraede K, Mauricio D, et al. Time to Insulin Initiation Cannot Be Used in Defining Latent Autoimmune Diabetes in Adults. Diabetes Care. 2008 Oct;31(10):2077. doi: 10.2337/dc07-1308.

Brown B. *Daring Greatly: How the Courage to Be Vulnerable Transforms the Way We Live, Love, Parent, and Lead* (Penguin Random House, 2012).

Brunkwall L, Orho-Melander M. The Gut Microbiome as a Target for Prevention and Treatment of Hyperglycaemia in Type 2 Diabetes: From Current Human Evidence to Future Possibilities. Diabetologia. 2017 Jun;60(6):943–51. doi: 10.1007/s00125 -017-4278-3. PMID: 28434033; PMCID: PMC5423958.

Bueno NB, de Melo IS, de Oliveira SL, da Rocha Ataide T. Very-Low-Carbohydrate Ketogenic Diet v. Low-Fat Diet for Long-Term Weight Loss: A Meta-Analysis of Randomised Controlled Trials. Br J Nutr. 2013;110(7):1178–87.

Bungau S, Behl T, Tit DM, et al. Interactions Between Leptin and Insulin Resistance in Patients with Prediabetes, With and Without NAFLD. Exp Ther Med. 2020 Dec;20(6):197. doi: 10.3892/etm.2020.9327. Epub 2020 Oct 14. PMID: 33123227; PMCID: PMC7588790.

Burke W, Trinidad SB, Schenck D. Can Precision Medicine Reduce the Burden of Diabetes? Ethn Dis. 2019;29(Suppl 3):669–74. Published 2019 Dec 12. doi: 10.18865 /ed.29.S3.669.

Burrows T, Kay-Lambkin F, Pursey K, Skinner J, Dayas C. Food Addiction and Associations with Mental Health Symptoms: A Systematic Review with Meta-Analysis. J Hum Nutr Diet. 2018 Aug;31(4):544–72. doi: 10.1111/jhn.12532. Epub 2018 Jan 25. PMID: 29368800.

Buse JB, Bethel MA, Green JB, et al. Pancreatic Safety of Sitagliptin in the TECOS Study. Diabetes Care 2017 Feb;40(2):164–70. doi: 10.2337/dc15-2780.

Buzzetti R, Di Pietro S, Giaccari A, et al. Non Insulin Requiring Autoimmune Diabetes Study Group. High Titer of Autoantibodies to GAD Identifies a Specific Phenotype of Adult-Onset Autoimmune Diabetes. Diabetes Care. 2007 Apr;30(4):932–38. doi: 10.2337/dc06-1696. PMID: 17392553.

Buzzetti R, Tuomi T, Mauricio D, et al. Management of Latent Autoimmune Diabetes in Adults: A Consensus Statement from an International Expert Panel. Diabetes. 2020 Oct;69(10):2037–47. doi: 10.2337/dbi20-0017. Epub 2020 Aug 26. PMID: 32847960; PMCID: PMC7809717.

Buzzetti R, Zampetti S, Maddaloni E. Adult-Onset Autoimmune Diabetes: Current Knowledge and Implications for Management. Nat Rev Endocrinol. 2017;13(11):674–86. doi: 10.1038/nrendo.2017.99.

Caballero AE. The "A to Z" of Managing Type 2 Diabetes in Culturally Diverse Populations. Front Endocrinol (Lausanne). 2018;9:479. Published 2018 Aug 28. doi: 10.3389/fendo.2018.00479.

Caesar R. Pharmacologic and Nonpharmacologic Therapies for the Gut Microbiota in Type 2 Diabetes. Can J Diab. 2019 Apr;43(3):224–31. doi: 10.1016/j.jcjd.2019.01.007. Epub 2019 Jan 31. PMID: 30929665.

Calder PC. Omega-3 Fatty Acids and Inflammatory Processes: From Molecules to Man. Biochem Soc Trans. 2017 Oct 15;45(5):1105–15. doi: 10.1042/BST20160474.Epub 2017 Sep 12. PMID: 28900017.

Calsolari MR, Rosário PW, Reis JS, et al. Diabetes auto-imune latente do adulto ou diabetes melito tipo 2 magro? [Latent Autoimmune Diabetes of Adult or Slim Type 2 Diabetes Mellitus?]. Arq Bras Endocrinol Metabol. 2008;52(2):315–21. doi: 10.1590/s0004-27302008000200019.

Camacho S, Ruppel A. Is the Calorie Concept a Real Solution to the Obesity Epidemic? Glob Health Action. 2017;10(1):1289650. doi: 10.1080/16549716.2017.1289650.

Carabotti M, Scirocco A, Maselli MA, Severi C. The Gut-Brain Axis: Interactions Between Enteric Microbiota, Central and Enteric Nervous Systems. Ann Gastroenterol. 2015;28(2):203–09.

Cardoso CRL, Leite NC, Moram CBM, et al. Long-Term Visit-to-Visit Glycemic Variability as Predictor of Micro- and Macrovascular Complications in Patients with Type 2 Diabetes: The Rio de Janeiro Type 2 Diabetes Cohort Study. Cardiovasc Diabetol. 2018;17:33.

Carlsson S. Etiology and Pathogenesis of Latent Autoimmune Diabetes in Adults (LADA) Compared to Type 2 Diabetes. Front Physiol. 2019a;10:320. Published 2019 Mar 26. doi: 10.3389/fphys.2019.00320.

Carlsson S. Environmental (Lifestyle) Risk Factors for LADA. Curr Diab Rev. 2019b;15(3):178–87. doi: 10.2174/1573399814666180716150253. PMID: 30009710.

Carré A, Richardson SJ, Larger E, Mallone R. Presumption of Guilt for T Cells in Type 1 Diabetes: Lead Culprits or Partners in Crime Depending on Age of Onset? Diabetologia. 2021 Jan;64(1):15–25. doi: 10.1007/s00125-020-05298-y. Epub 2020 Oct 21. PMID: 33084970; PMCID: PMC7717061.

Carter A, Hardman CA, Burrows T. Food Addiction and Eating Addiction: Scientific Advances and Their Clinical, Social and Policy Implications. Nutrients. 2020 May 20;12(5):1485. doi: 10.3390/nu12051485. PMID: 32443731; PMCID: PMC7284368.

Cassin SE, Buchman DZ, Leung SE, et al. Ethical, Stigma, and Policy Implications of Food Addiction: A Scoping Review. Nutrients. 2019 Mar 27;11(4):710. doi: 10.3390/nu11040710. PMID: 30934743; PMCID: PMC6521112.

Castelblanco E, Hernández M, Castelblanco A, et al. Low-Grade Inflammatory Marker Profile May Help to Differentiate Patients with LADA, Classic Adult-Onset Type 1 Diabetes, and Type 2 Diabetes. Diabetes Care. 2018 Apr 1;41(4):862–68. doi: 10.2337/dc17-1662.

Celiac Disease Foundation website. https://celiac.org. Accessed 2022 Mar 3.

Centers for Disease Control and Prevention. *Diabetes Report Card 2017* (Centers for Disease Control and Prevention, US Department of Health and Human Services, 2018).

Centers for Disease Control and Prevention. *National Diabetes Statistics Report, 2020* (Centers for Disease Control and Prevention, US Department of Health and Human Services, 2020).

Cha, AE, Cohen RA. Demographic Variation in Health Insurance Coverage. CDC National Health Statistics Report Number 169, 2022 Feb 11.

Charlotte Observer. The "A" List. 2008 Oct 8.

Chauhan S, Kodali H, Noor J, et al. Role of Omega-3 Fatty Acids on Lipid Profile in Diabetic Dyslipidaemia: Single Blind, Randomised Clinical Trial. J Clin Diagn Res. 2017;11(3):OC13–OC16. doi: 10.7860/JCDR/2017/20628.9449.

Chaurasia B, Talbot CL, Summers SA. Adipocyte Ceramides—The Nexus of Inflammation and Metabolic Disease. Front Immunol. 2020 Sep 23;11:576347. doi: 10.3389/fimmu.2020.576347.

Chen B, Sun L, Zhang X. Integration of Microbiome and Epigenome to Decipher the Pathogenesis of Autoimmune Diseases. J Autoimmun. 2017 Sep;83:31–42. doi: 10.1016/j.jaut.2017.03.009. Epub 2017 Mar 23. PMID: 28342734.

Chen C, Yu X, Shao S. Effects of Omega-3 Fatty Acid Supplementation on Glucose Control and Lipid Levels in Type 2 Diabetes: A Meta-Analysis. PLoS One. 2015;10(10):e0139565. Published 2015 Oct 2. doi: 10.1371/journal.pone.0139565.

Chen CY, Huang WS, Chen HC, et al. Effect of a 90 g/day Low-Carbohydrate Diet on Glycaemic Control, Small, Dense Low-Density Lipoprotein and Carotid Intima-Media Thickness in Type 2 Diabetic Patients: An 18-Month Randomised Controlled Trial. PLoS One. 2020 Oct 5;15(10):e0240158. doi: 10.1371/journal.pone.0240158. PMID: 33017456; PMCID: PMC7535044.

Chen R, Ovbiagele B, Feng W. Diabetes and Stroke: Epidemiology, Pathophysiology, Pharmaceuticals and Outcomes. Am J Med Sci. 2016;351(4):380–86. doi: 10.1016/j.amjms.2016.01.011.

Chen S, Zhao X, Ran L, et al. Resveratrol Improves Insulin Resistance, Glucose and Lipid Metabolism in Patients with Non-Alcoholic Fatty Liver Disease: A Randomized Controlled Trial. Dig Liver Dis. 2015 Mar;47(3):226–32. doi: 10.1016/j.dld.2014.11.015. Epub 2014 Dec 16. PMID: 25577300.

Cheng CW, Villani V, Buono R, et al. Fasting-Mimicking Diet Promotes Ngn3-Driven β-Cell Regeneration to Reverse Diabetes. Cell. 2017;168(5):775–788.e12. doi: 10.1016/j.cell.2017.01.040.

Chödrön P. *Living Beautifully with Uncertainty and Change* (Shambhala Press, 2019).

Choi SW, Claycombe KJ, Martinez JA, et al. Nutritional Epigenomics: A Portal to Disease Prevention. Adv Nutr. 2013;4(5):530–32. Published 2013 Sep 1. doi: 10.3945/an.113.004168.

Choi YJ, et al. Impact of a Ketogenic Diet on Metabolic Parameters in Patients with Obesity or Overweight and With or Without Type 2 Diabetes: A Meta-Analysis of Randomized Controlled Trials. Nutrients. 2020 Jul 6;12(7):2005. doi: 10.3390/nu12072005.

Chondronikola M, Volpi E, Børsheim E, et al. Brown Adipose Tissue Improves Whole-Body Glucose Homeostasis and Insulin Sensitivity in Humans. Diabetes. 2014;63(12):4089–99. doi: 10.2337/db14-0746.

Chow CK, Ramasundarahettige C, Hu W, et al. Availability and Affordability of Essential Medicines for Diabetes Across High-Income, Middle-Income, and Low-Income Countries: A Prospective Epidemiological Study. Lancet Diab Endocrinol. 2018;6(10):798–808. doi: 10.1016/S2213-8587(18)30233-X.

Chowdhury R, Warnakula S, Kunutsor S, Crowe F, et al. Association of Dietary, Circulating, and Supplement Fatty Acids with Coronary Risk: A Systematic Review and Meta-Analysis. Ann Intern Med. 2014 Mar 18;160(6):398–406. doi: 10.7326/M13-1788. Published correction in Ann Intern Med. 2014 May 6;160(9):658. PMID: 24723079.

Christine PJ, Auchincloss AH, Bertoni AG, et al. Longitudinal Associations Between Neighborhood Physical and Social Environments and Incident Type 2 Diabetes Mellitus: The Multi-Ethnic Study of Atherosclerosis (MESA). JAMA Intern Med. 2015 Aug;175(8):1311–20. doi: 10.1001/jamainternmed.2015.2691. PMID: 26121402; PMCID: PMC4799846.

Chung HY, Kim DH, Bang E, Yu BP. Impacts of Calorie Restriction and Intermittent Fasting on Health and Diseases: Current Trends. Nutrients. 2020;12(10):2948. Published 2020 Sep 25. doi: 10.3390/nu12102948.

Ciechanowski PS, Katon WJ, Russo JE, Hirsch IB. The Relationship of Depressive Symptoms to Symptom Reporting, Self-Care and Glucose Control in Diabetes. Gen Hosp Psychiatry. 2003 Jul–Aug;25(4):246–52. doi: 10.1016/s0163-8343(03)00055-0. PMID: 12850656.

Cimons, Marlene. Chronic Inflammation Is Long Lasting, Insidious, Dangerous. *Washington Post.* 2020 Jan 20. https://washingtonpost.com/health.

Cito M, Pellegrini S, Piemonti L, Sordi V. The Potential and Challenges of Alternative Sources of β Cells for the Cure of Type 1 Diabetes. Endocr Connect. 2018;7(3):R114–R125. doi: 10.1530/EC-18-0012.

Cohen DE. Balancing Cholesterol Synthesis and Absorption in the Gastrointestinal Tract. J Clin Lipidol. 2008;2(2):S1–S3. doi: 10.1016/j.jacl.2008.01.004.

Cohn A, Sofia AM, Kupfer SS. Type 1 Diabetes and Celiac Disease: Clinical Overlap and New Insights into Disease Pathogenesis. Current Diab Rep. 2014;14(8):517. doi: 10.1007/s11892-014-0517-x.

Cohut M. Link Between Diabetes and Cancer Firmly Established. *Medical News Today.* 2018 Jul.

Colditz GA, Willett WC, Stampfer MJ, et al. Patterns of Weight Change and Their Relation to Diet in a Cohort of Healthy Women. Am J Clin Nutr. 1990 Jun;51(6):1100–05. doi: 10.1093/ajcn/51.6.1100. PMID: 2349925.

Coletta JM, Bell SJ, Roman AS. Omega-3 Fatty Acids and Pregnancy. Rev Obstet Gynecol. 2010;3(4):163–71.

Conner F, Pfiester E, Elliott J, Slama-Chaudhry A. Unaffordable Insulin: Patients Pay the Price. Lancet Diab Endocrinol. 2019 Oct;7(10):748. doi: 10.1016/S2213-8587(19)30260-8. PMID: 31535616.

Constant A, Moirand R, Thibault R, Val-Laillet D. Meeting of Minds Around Food Addiction: Insights from Addiction Medicine, Nutrition, Psychology, and Neurosciences. Nutrients. 2020;12(11):3564. Published 2020 Nov 20. doi: 10.3390/nu12113564.

Cousminer DL, Ahlqvist E, Mishra R, et al. First Genome-Wide Association Study of Latent Autoimmune Diabetes in Adults Reveals Novel Insights Linking Immune and Metabolic Diabetes. Diabetes Care. 2018;41:2396–403. doi: 10.2337/dc18 -1032.

Criscitelli K, Avena NM. The Neurobiological and Behavioral Overlaps of Nicotine and Food Addiction. Prev Med. 2016 Nov;92:82–89. doi: 10.1016/j.ypmed.2016.08.009 .Epub 2016 Aug 7. PMID: 27509870.

Cryan J, Dinan T. Mind-Altering Microorganisms: The Impact of the Gut Microbiota on Brain and Behaviour. Nat Rev Neurosci. 2012;13:701–12. doi: 10.1038 /nrn3346.

Daft JG, Lorenz RG. Role of the Gastrointestinal Ecosystem in the Development of Type 1 Diabetes. Pediatr Diab. 2015 Sep;16(6):407–18. doi: 10.1111/pedi.12282 .Epub 2015 May 8. PMID: 25952017; PMCID: PMC4534320.

Daghestani, MH. A Preprandial and Postprandial Plasma Levels of Ghrelin Hormone in Lean, Overweight and Obese Saudi Females. J King Saud University—Science. 2009;21(2):119–24, ISSN 1018-3647, doi: 10.1016/j.jksus.2009.05.001.

Daily Show. Sonia Sotomayor—"Just Ask!" & Life as a Supreme Court Justice. 2019 Sep 23.

Daley CA, Abbott A, Doyle PS, et al. A Review of Fatty Acid Profiles and Antioxidant Content in Grass-Fed and Grain-Fed Beef. Nutr J. 2010 Mar 10;9:10. doi: 10 .1186/1475-2891-9-10. PMID: 20219103; PMCID: PMC2846864.

Dantzer R, O'Connor JC, Freund GG, et al. From Inflammation to Sickness and Depression: When the Immune System Subjugates the Brain. Nat Rev Neurosci. 2008;9(1):46–56. doi: 10.1038/nrn2297.

Daugherty O. Colorado Becomes First State to Cap Out-of-Pocket Insulin Costs. *The Hill.* 2019 May 23.

David LA, Maurice CF, Carmody RN, et al. Diet Rapidly and Reproducibly Alters the Human Gut Microbiome. Nature. 2015;505(7484):559–63. doi: 10.1038 /nature12820.

davidji. *destressifying* (Hay House, 2015).

Davies M, Dahl D, Heise T, et al. Introduction of Biosimilar Insulins in Europe. Diab Med. 2017 Oct;34(10):1340–53. doi: 10.1111/dme.13400. Epub 2017 Jul 16. PMID: 28608570; PMCID: PMC5637898.

Dawkins M, Menon T, Myers AK. Examining the Causes and Consequences of Increasing Insulin Costs with Prospective Interventions. Am J Ther. 2020 Jan/ Feb;27(1):e115–e120. doi: 10.1097/MJT.0000000000001111. PMID: 31703009.

de Cabo R, Mattson MP. Effects of Intermittent Fasting on Health, Aging, and Disease. N Engl J Med. 2019 Dec 26;381(26):2541–51. doi: 10.1056/NEJMra1905136. Published correction in N Engl J Med. 2020 Jan 16;382(3):298. Published correction in N Engl J Med. 2020 Mar 5;382(10):978. PMID: 31881139.

de la Lastra CA, Villegas I. Resveratrol as an Antioxidant and Pro-Oxidant Agent: Mechanisms and Clinical Implications. Biochem Soc Trans. 2007 Nov;35(pt 5):1156–60. doi: 10.1042/BST0351156. PMID: 17956300.

de Vries SK, Meule A. Food Addiction and Bulimia Nervosa: New Data Based on the Yale Food Addiction Scale 2.0. Eur Eat Disord Rev. 2016 Nov;24(6):518–22. doi: 10.1002/erv.2470. Epub 2016 Aug 30. PMID: 27578243.

Dehghan M, Mente A, Zhang X, et al. Prospective Urban Rural Epidemiology (PURE) Study Investigators. Associations of Fats and Carbohydrate Intake with Cardiovascular Disease and Mortality in 18 Countries from Five Continents (PURE): A Prospective Cohort Study. Lancet. 2017 Nov 4;390(10107):2050–62. doi: 10.1016 /S0140-6736(17)32252-3. Epub 2017 Aug 29. PMID: 28864332.

Del Gobbo LC, et al. 2016. Polyunsaturated Fatty Acid Biomarkers and Coronary Heart Disease: Pooling Project of 19 Cohort Studies. JAMA Intern Med. 2016 Aug 1;176(8):1155–66.

den Braver NR, Lakerveld J, Rutters F, et al. Built Environmental Characteristics and Diabetes: A Systematic Review and Meta-Analysis. BMC Med. 2018 Jan 31;16(1):12. doi: 10.1186/s12916-017-0997-z. PMID: 29382337; PMCID: PMC5791730.

Denham J, O'Brien BJ, Harvey JT, Charchar FJ. Genome-Wide Sperm DNA Methylation Changes After 3 Months of Exercise Training in Humans. Epigenomics. 2015;7:717–31.

Di Francesco A, Di Germanio C, Bernier M, de Cabo R. A Time to Fast. Science. 2018 Nov 16;362(6416):770–75. doi: 10.1126/science.aau2095. PMID: 30442801.

Di Liberto D, Carlisi D, D'Anneo A, et al. Gluten Free Diet for the Management of Non Celiac Diseases: The Two Sides of the Coin. Healthcare (Basel). 2020 Oct 14;8(4):400. doi: 10.3390/healthcare8040400. PMID: 33066519; PMCID: PMC7712796.

DiabetesMine 2021. Why Is There No Generic Insulin? Healthline. September 14, 2021. https://www.healthline.com/diabetesmine/why-is-there-no-generic-insulin.

Diepvens K, Westerterp KR, Westerterp-Plantenga MS. Obesity and Thermogenesis Related to the Consumption of Caffeine, Ephedrine, Capsaicin, and Green Tea. Am J Physiol Regul Integr Comp Physiol. 2007 Jan;292(1):R77–R85. doi: 10.1152 /ajpregu.00832.2005. Epub 2006 Jul 13. PMID: 16840650.

Díez-Espino J, Basterra-Gortari FJ, Salas-Salvadó J, et al. Egg Consumption and Cardiovascular Disease According to Diabetic Status: The PREDIMED Study. Clin Nutr. 2017 Aug;36(4):1015–21. doi: 10.1016/j.clnu.2016.06.009. Epub 2016 Jun 29. PMID: 27448949.

DiFeliceantonio AG, Coppin G, Rigoux L, et al. Supra-Additive Effects of Combining Fat and Carbohydrate on Food Reward. Cell Metab. 2018 Jul 3;28(1):33–44.e3. doi: 10.1016/j.cmet.2018.05.018. Epub 2018 Jun 14. PMID: 29909968.

DiGruccio MR, Mawla AM, Donaldson CJ, et al. Comprehensive Alpha, Beta and Delta Cell Transcriptomes Reveal That Ghrelin Selectively Activates Delta Cells and Promotes Somatostatin Release from Pancreatic Islets. Mol Metab. 2016 May 3;5(7):449–58. doi: 10.1016/j.molmet.2016.04.007. PMID: 27408771; PMCID: PMC4921781.

Dimitrov V, White JH. Vitamin D Signaling in Intestinal Innate Immunity and Homeostasis. Mol Cell Endocrinol. 2017 Sep 15;453:68–78. doi: 10.1016/j.mce .2017.04.010. Epub 2017 Apr 12. PMID: 28412519.

Ding QY, Tian JX, Li M, et al. Interactions Between Therapeutics for Metabolic Disease, Cardiovascular Risk Factors, and Gut Microbiota. Front Cell Infect Microbiol. 2020 Oct 23;10:530160. doi: 10.3389/fcimb.2020.530160. PMID: 33194785; PMCID: PMC7644821.

DiNicolantonio JJ, Lucan SC, O'Keefe JH. The Evidence for Saturated Fat and for Sugar Related to Coronary Heart Disease. Prog Cardiovasc Dis. 2016 Mar–Apr;58(5):464–72. doi: 10.1016/j.pcad.2015.11.006. Epub 2015 Nov 14. PMID: 26586275; PMCID: PMC4856550.

Divers J, Mayer-Davis EJ, Lawrence JM, et al. Trends in Incidence of Type 1 and Type 2 Diabetes Among Youths—Selected Counties and Indian Reservations, United States, 2002–2015. MMWR Morb Mortal Wkly Rep 2020;69:161–65. doi: 10.15585/mmwr.mm6906a3.

Dobosz AM, Dziewulska A, Dobrzyń A. Spotlight on Epigenetics as a Missing Link Between Obesity and Type 2 Diabetes. Postepy Biochem. 2018;64(2):157–65. doi: 10.18388/pb.2018_126.

Donkin I, Barrès R. Sperm Epigenetics and Influence of Environmental Factors. Mol Metab. 2018;14:1–11.

Donofry SD, Erickson KI, Levine MD, et al. Relationship Between Dispositional Mindfulness, Psychological Health, and Diet Quality Among Healthy Midlife Adults. Nutrients. 2020;12(11):3414. Published 2020 Nov 6. doi: 10.3390/nu12113414.

Doucette ED, Salas J, Wang J, Scherrer JF. Insurance Coverage and Diabetes Quality Indicators Among Patients with Diabetes in the US General Population. Prim Care Diab. 2017 Dec;11(6):515–21. doi: 10.1016/j.pcd.2017.05.007. Epub 2017 Jun 12. PMID: 28619242.

Drexler AJ, Robertson C. Therapy of Type 1 Diabetes Mellitus. In Poretsky L (ed). *Principles of Diabetes Mellitus* (Springer, 2004). doi: 10.1007/978-1-4757-6260-0_31.

Drouin-Chartier JP, Brassard D, Tessier-Grenier M, et al. Systematic Review of the Association Between Dairy Product Consumption and Risk of Cardiovascular-Related Clinical Outcomes. Adv Nutr. 2016 Nov 15;7(6):1026–40. doi: 10.3945/an.115.011403. PMID: 28140321; PMCID: PMC5105032.

Dupuis ML, Pagano MT, Pierdominici M, Ortona E. The Role of Vitamin D in Autoimmune Diseases: Could Sex Make the Difference? Biol Sex Differ. 2021 Jan 12;12(1):12. doi: 10.1186/s13293-021-00358-3. PMID: 33436077; PMCID: PMC7802252.

Dutta D, et al. Vitamin-D Supplementation in Prediabetes Reduced Progression to Type 2 Diabetes and Was Associated with Decreased Insulin Resistance and Systemic Inflammation: An Open Label Randomized Prospective Study from Eastern India. Diab Res Clin Pract. 2014. doi: 10.1016/j.diabres.2013.12.044.

Edelman S, Polonsky WH, Parkin CG. Biosimilar Insulins Are Coming: What They Are, What You Need to Know. Curr Med Res Opin. 2014 Nov;30(11):2217–22. doi: 10.1185/03007995.2014.952718. Epub 2014 Aug 20. PMID: 25105307.

Egan S. *Devoured: How What We Eat Defines Who We Are* (HarperCollins, 2017).

El-Sheikh AA, Morsy MA, Okasha AM. Inhibition of NF-κB/TNF-α Pathway May Be Involved in the Protective Effect of Resveratrol Against Cyclophosphamide-Induced Multi-Organ Toxicity. Immunopharmacol Immunotoxicol. 2017 Aug;39(4):180–87. doi: 10.1080/08923973.2017.1318913. Epub 2017 May 2. PMID: 28463035.

Epel E, Lapidus R, McEwen B, Brownell K. Stress May Add Bite to Appetite in Women: A Laboratory Study of Stress-Induced Cortisol and Eating Behavior.

Psychoneuroendocrinology. 2001 Jan;26(1):37–49. doi: 10.1016/s0306-4530 (00)00035-4. PMID: 11070333.

Ericson U, Hellstrand S, Brunkwall L, et al. Food Sources of Fat May Clarify the Inconsistent Role of Dietary Fat Intake for Incidence of Type 2 Diabetes. Am J Clin Nutr. 2015 May;101(5):1065–80. doi: 10.3945/ajcn.114.103010. Epub 2015 Apr 1. PMID: 25832335.

Evangelou E, Ntritsos G, Chondrogiorgi M, et al. Exposure to Pesticides and Diabetes: A Systematic Review and Meta-Analysis. Environment International. 2016;91:60–68.

Evans GW, Kantrowitz E. Socioeconomic Status and Health: The Potential Role of Environmental Risk Exposure. Annual Rev Public Health. 2002;23(1):303–31.

Ewen M, Lepeska M, Beran D. Addressing the Challenge and Constraints of Insulin Sources and Supply (ACCISS) Study. ACCISS-Fact Sheet 1. 2015 Nov. Health Action International Food.

Faghihzadeh F, Adibi P, Rafiei R, Hekmatdoost A. Resveratrol Supplementation Improves Inflammatory Biomarkers in Patients with Nonalcoholic Fatty Liver Disease. Nutr Res. 2014 Oct;34(10):837–43. doi: 10.1016/j.nutres.2014.09.005. Epub 2014 Sep 23. PMID: 25311610.

Fan R, Koehler K, Chung S. Adaptive Thermogenesis by Dietary n-3 Polyunsaturated Fatty Acids: Emerging Evidence and Mechanisms. Biochim Biophys Acta Mol Cell Biol Lipids. 2019;1864(1):59–70. doi: 10.1016/j.bbalip.2018.04.012.

Fang Y, Zhang C, Shi H, et al. Characteristics of the Gut Microbiota and Metabolism in Patients with Latent Autoimmune Diabetes in Adults: A Case-Control Study. Diabetes Care. 2021 Dec;44(12):2738–46. doi: 10.2337/dc20-2975.

Farzi A, Hassan AM, Zenz G, Holzer P. Diabesity and Mood Disorders: Multiple Links Through the Microbiota-Gut-Brain Axis. Mol Aspects Med. 2019 Apr;66:80–93. doi: 10.1016/j.mam.2018.11.003. Epub 2018 Dec 13. PMID: 30513310.

Fatahia S, Matin SS, Sohouli MH, et al. Association of Dietary Fiber and Depression Symptom: A Systematic Review and Meta-Analysis of Observational Studies. Complement Ther Med. 2021 Jan;56:102621.

FDA. 2022 Nov 17. FDA Approves First Drug That Can Delay Onset of Type 1 Diabetes. https://www.fda.gov/news-events/press-announcements/fda-approves-first-drug-can -delay-onset-type-1-diabetes.

Fée N. *How to Save the World for Free* (Laurence King Publishing, 2021).

Felix KM, Tahsin S, Wu HJ. Host-Microbiota Interplay in Mediating Immune Disorders. Ann N Y Acad Sci. 2018 Apr;1417(1):57–70. doi: 10.1111/nyas.13508. Epub 2017 Oct 6. PMID: 28984367; PMCID: PMC5889363.

Felman A, Martinez, K. Everything You Need to Know About Inflammation. *Medical News Today*. 2020 Apr 13. https://medicalnewstoday.com/articles/248423.

Fernandez-Twinn DS, Hjort L, Novakovic B, et al. Intrauterine Programming of Obesity and Type 2 Diabetes. Diabetologia. 2019 Oct;62(10):1789–801. doi: 10.1007 /s00125-019-4951-9. Epub 2019 Aug 27. PMID: 31451874; PMCID: PMC6731191.

Figlewicz DP, Benoit SC. Insulin, Leptin, and Food Reward: Update 2008. Am J Physiol Regul Integr Comp Physiol. 2009;296(1):R9–R19. doi: 10.1152/ajpregu.90725.2008.

Fisher L, Chesla CA, Mullan JT, et al. Contributors to Depression in Latino and European-American Patients with Type 2 Diabetes. Diabetes Care. 2001 Oct;24(10):1751–57. doi: 10.2337/diacare.24.10.1751. PMID: 11574437.

Fletcher, Jenna. Anti-Inflammatory Diet: What to Know. *Medical News Today.* 2020 Jan 3. https://medicalnewstoday.com/articles/320233.

Food, Inc. 2008 documentary. Directed and produced by Robert Kenner, narrated by Michael Pollan and Eric Schlosser.

Foretz M, Guigas B, Viollet B. Understanding the Glucoregulatory Mechanisms of Metformin in Type 2 Diabetes Mellitus. Nat Rev Endocrinol. 2019 Oct;15(10):569–89. doi: 10.1038/s41574-019-0242-2. Epub 2019 Aug 22. PMID: 31439934.

Forslund K, Hildebrand F, Nielsen T, et al. Disentangling Type 2 Diabetes and Metformin Treatment Signatures in the Human Gut Microbiota. Nature. 2015 Dec 10;528(7581):262–66. doi: 10.1038/nature15766. Epub 2015 Dec 2. Published correction in Nature. 2017 May 3;545(7652):116. PMID: 26633628; PMCID: PMC4681099.

Forsythe CE, Phinney SD, Feinman RD, et al. Limited Effect of Dietary Saturated Fat on Plasma Saturated Fat in the Context of a Low Carbohydrate Diet. Lipids. 2010 Oct;45(10):947–62. doi: 10.1007/s11745-010-3467-3. Epub 2010 Sep 7. PMID: 20820932; PMCID: PMC2974193.

Fortmann AL, Savin KL, Clark TL, et al. Innovative Diabetes Interventions in the US Hispanic Population. Diab Spectr. 2019;32(4):295–301. doi: 10.2337/ds19-0006.

Fourlanos S, Dotta F, Greenbaum CJ, et al. Latent Autoimmune Diabetes in Adults (LADA) Should Be Less Latent. Diabetologia. 2005;48(11):2206–12. doi: 10.1007/s00125-005-1960-7.

Fowler SP, Williams K, Resendez RG, et al. Fueling the Obesity Epidemic? Artificially Sweetened Beverage Use and Long-Term Weight Gain. Obesity (Silver Spring). 2008 Aug;16(8):1894–900. doi: 10.1038/oby.2008.284. Epub 2008 Jun 5. PMID: 18535548.

Francisco V, Pino J, Campos-Cabaleiro V, et al. Obesity, Fat Mass and Immune System: Role for Leptin. Front Physiol. 2018;9:640. Published 2018 Jun 1. doi: 10.3389/fphys.2018.00640.

Franck C, Grandi SM, Eisenberg MJ. Agricultural Subsidies and the American Obesity Epidemic. Am. J. Preventive Med. 2013;45:327–333.

Fuhri Snethlage CM, Nieuwdorp M, van Raalte DH, et al. Auto-Immunity and the Gut Microbiome in Type 1 Diabetes: Lessons from Rodent and Human Studies. Best Pract Res Clin Endocrinol Metab. 2021 May;35(3):101544.

Furmli S, Elmasry R, Ramos M, Fung J. Therapeutic Use of Intermittent Fasting for People with Type 2 Diabetes as an Alternative to Insulin. BMJ Case Rep. 2018 Oct 9. doi: 10.1136/bcr-2017-221854.

Gale EAM. Latent Autoimmune Diabetes in Adults: A Guide for the Perplexed. Diabetologia. 2005;48:2195–99. doi: 10.1007/s00125-005-1954-5.

Gavard JA, Lustman PJ, Clouse RE. Prevalence of Depression in Adults with Diabetes. An Epidemiological Evaluation. Diabetes Care. 1993 Aug;16(8):1167–78. doi: 10.2337/diacare.16.8.1167. PMID: 8375247.

Gay R. *Hunger: A Memoir of (My) Body* (HarperCollins, 2018).

Gearhardt A, Roberts M, Ashe M. If Sugar Is Addictive . . . What Does It Mean for the Law? J Law Med Ethics. 2013 Mar;41(Suppl 1):46–49. doi: 10.1111/jlme.12038. PMID: 23590740.

Gearhardt AN, White MA, Masheb RM, et al. An Examination of the Food Addiction Construct in Obese Patients with Binge Eating Disorder. Int J Eat Disord. 2012;45:657–63.

Geiker NRW, Larsen ML, Dyerberg J, et al. [Eggs Do Not Increase the Risk of Cardiovascular Disease and Can Be Safely Consumed.] Ugeskr Laeger. 2017 May 15;179(20):V11160792. Danish. PMID: 28504636.

Geiker NRW, Larsen ML, Dyerberg J, et al. Egg Consumption, Cardiovascular Diseases and Type 2 Diabetes. Eur J Clin Nutr. 2018 Jan;72(1):44–56. doi: 10.1038 /ejcn.2017.153. Epub 2017 Sep 27. PMID: 28952608.

Gelman L. 13 Signs You're Obsessed with Food. Prevention.com. 2012 Dec 14. https://www .prevention.com/weight-loss/a20433766/different-food-obsessions-and-treatment.

Gershuni VM, et al. Nutritional Ketosis for Weight Management and Reversal of Metabolic Syndrome. Curr Nutr Rep. 2018;7(3):97–106. doi: 10.1007/s13668-018 -0235-0.

Ghorbani Y, Schwenger KJP, Allard JP. Manipulation of Intestinal Microbiome as Potential Treatment for Insulin Resistance and Type 2 Diabetes. Eur J Nutr. 2021 Mar 2. doi: 10.1007/s00394-021-02520-4. Epub ahead of print. PMID: 33651137.

Gijsbers L, Ding EL, Malik VS, et al. Consumption of Dairy Foods and Diabetes Incidence: A Dose-Response Meta-Analysis of Observational Studies. Am J Clin Nutr. 2016 Apr;103(4):1111–24. doi: 10.3945/ajcn.115.123216. Epub 2016 Feb 24. PMID: 26912494.

Gilbert J, Blaser M, Caporaso J, et al. Current Understanding of the Human Microbiome. Nat Med. 2018;24:392–400. doi: 10.1038/nm.4517.

Giwa AM, Ahmed R, Omidian Z, et al. Current Understandings of the Pathogenesis of Type 1 Diabetes: Genetics to Environment. World J Diab. 2020; 11(1):13–25. doi: 10.4239/wjd.v11.i1.13.

Golbidi S, Daiber A, Korac B, et al. Health Benefits of Fasting and Caloric Restriction. Curr Diab Rep. 2017 Oct 23;17(12):123. doi: 10.1007/s11892-017-0951-7. PMID: 29063418.

Goodwin G. Type 1 Diabetes Mellitus and Celiac Disease: Distinct Autoimmune Disorders That Share Common Pathogenic Mechanisms. Horm Res Paediatr. 2019;92(5):285–92. doi: 10.1159/000503142. Epub 2019 Oct 8. PMID: 31593953.

Gordon EL, Ariel-Donges AH, Bauman V, Merlo LJ. What Is the Evidence for "Food Addiction"? A Systematic Review. Nutrients. 2018 Apr 12;10(4):477. doi: 10.3390 /nu10040477. PMID: 29649120; PMCID: PMC5946262.

Gower BA, Goss AM. A Lower-Carbohydrate, Higher-Fat Diet Reduces Abdominal and Intermuscular Fat and Increases Insulin Sensitivity in Adults at Risk of Type 2 Diabetes. J Nutr. 2015 Jan;145(1):177S–183S. doi: 10.3945/jn.114.195065. Epub 2014 Dec 3. PMID: 25527677; PMCID: PMC4264021.

Gradisteanu Pircalabioru G, Corcionivoschi N, Gundogdu O, et al. Dysbiosis in the Development of Type I Diabetes and Associated Complications: From Mechanisms to Targeted Gut Microbes Manipulation Therapies. Int J Mol Sci. 2021 Mar 9;22(5):2763. doi: 10.3390/ijms22052763. PMID: 33803255; PMCID: PMC7967220.

Grajower MM, Horne BD. Clinical Management of Intermittent Fasting in Patients with Diabetes Mellitus. Nutrients. 2019 Apr 18;11(4):873. doi: 10.3390 /nu11040873. PMID: 31003482; PMCID: PMC6521152.

Greenberg P. *The Climate Diet: 50 Simple Ways to Trim Your Carbon Footprint* (Penguin, 2021).

Greene JA, Riggs KR. Why Is There No Generic Insulin? Historical Origins of a Modern Problem. N Engl J Med. 2015 Mar 19;372(12):1171–75. doi: 10.1056/NEJMms1411398. PMID: 25785977.

Grill V, Åsvold BO. A Form of Autoimmune Diabetes in Adults Named LADA—An Update on Essential Features and Controversies. Curr Diab Rev. 2019;15(3):172–73. doi: 10.2174/1573399814666180716152342. PMID: 30009712.

Grisel J. *Never Enough: The Neuroscience and Experience of Addiction* (Anchor, 2020).

Groh KJ, Backhaus T, Carney-Almroth B, et al. Overview of Known Plastic Packaging-Associated Chemicals and Their Hazards. Sci Total Env. 2019;651:3253–68.

Groop L, Bottazzo GF, Doniach D. Islet Cell Antibodies Identify Latent Type 1 Diabetes in Patients Aged 35–75 Years at Diagnosis. Diabetes. 1986;35:237–41.

Groop L, Tuomi T, Rowley M, et al. Latent Autoimmune Diabetes in Adults (LADA)—More than a Name. Diabetologia. 2006;49:1996–98. doi: 10.1007/s00125-006-0345-x.

Gross LS, Li L, Ford ES, Liu S. Increased Consumption of Refined Carbohydrates and the Epidemic of Type 2 Diabetes in the United States: An Ecologic Assessment. Am J Clin Nutr. 2004 May;79(5):774–79. doi: 10.1093/ajcn/79.5.774. PMID: 15113714.

Grunberger G. Insulin Analogs—Are They Worth It? Yes! Diabetes Care. 2014 Jun;37(6):1767–70. doi: 10.2337/dc14-0031.

Gucciardi E, Vahabi M, Norris N, et al. The Intersection Between Food Insecurity and Diabetes: A Review. Curr Nutr Rep. 2014;3(4):324–32. doi: 10.1007/s13668-014-0104-4. PMID: 25383254; PMCID: PMC4218969.

Gucciardi E, Yang A, Cohen-Olivenstein K, et al. Emerging Practices Supporting Diabetes Self-Management Among Food Insecure Adults and Families: A Scoping Review. PLoS One. 2019;14(11):e0223998. doi: 10.1371/journal.pone.0223998.

Guglielmi C, Palermo A, Pozzilli P. Latent Autoimmune Diabetes in the Adults (LADA) in Asia: From Pathogenesis and Epidemiology to Therapy. Diab Metab Res Rev. 2012;28:40–46. doi: 10.1002/dmrr.2345.

Guo TL, Chen Y, Xu HS, et al. Gut Microbiome in Neuroendocrine and Neuroimmune Interactions: The Case of Genistein. Toxicol Appl Pharmacol. 2020 Sep 1;402:115130. doi: 10.1016/j.taap.2020.115130. Epub 2020 Jul 14. PMID: 32673657; PMCID: PMC7398836.

Gupta RS, Springston EE, Warrier MR, et al. The Prevalence, Severity, and Distribution of Childhood Food Allergy in the United States. Pediatrics. 2011 Jul;128(1):e9–e17. doi: 10.1542/peds.2011-0204.

Gupta RS, Warren CM, Smith BM, et al. Prevalence and Severity of Food Allergies Among US Adults. JAMA Netw Open. 2019;2(1):e185630. doi: 10.1001/jamanetworkopen.2018.5630.

Hafermann M. Personal communication with author. 2021 Jun 17.

Hallberg SJ, Gershuni VM, Hazbun TL, Athinarayanan SJ. Reversing Type 2 Diabetes: A Narrative Review of the Evidence. Nutrients. 2019 Apr 1;11(4):766. doi: 10.3390/nu11040766. PMID: 30939855; PMCID: PMC6520897.

Hals IK. Treatment of Latent Autoimmune Diabetes in Adults: What is Best? Curr Diab Rev. 2019;15(3):188–93. doi: 10.2174/1573399814666180716144429.

Hamilton-Williams EE, Lorca GL, Norris JM, Dunne JL. A Triple Threat? The Role of Diet, Nutrition, and the Microbiota in T1D Pathogenesis. Front Nutr. 2021;8:600756. Published 2021 Apr 1. doi: 10.3389/fnut.2021.600756.

Han H, Li Y, Fang J, et al. Gut Microbiota and Type 1 Diabetes. Int J Mol Sci. 2018;19(4):995. Published 2018 Mar 27. doi: 10.3390/ijms19040995.

Hanh TN. *Peace Is Every Step: The Path of Mindfulness in Everyday Life* (Random House, 1992).

Harrar S. Latent Autoimmune Diabetes in Adults: How to Diagnose and Treat LADA. Ontrackdiabetes.com. 2016.

Harris L, Hamilton S, Azevedo LB, Olajide J, et al. Intermittent Fasting Interventions for Treatment of Overweight and Obesity in Adults: A Systematic Review and Meta-Analysis. JBI Database System Rev Implement Rep. 2018 Feb;16(2):507–47. doi: 10.11124/JBISRIR-2016-003248. PMID: 29419624.

Harris ML, Loxton D, Sibbritt DW, Byles JE. The Influence of Perceived Stress on the Onset of Arthritis in Women: Findings from the Australian Longitudinal Study on Women's Health. Ann Behav Med. 2013 Aug;46(1):9–18. doi: 10.1007/s12160-013 -9478-6. PMID: 23436274.

Harris ML, Oldmeadow C, Hure A, et al. Stress Increases the Risk of Type 2 Diabetes Onset in Women: A 12-Year Longitudinal Study Using Causal Modelling. PLoS One. 2017;12(2):e0172126. Published 2017 Feb 21. doi: 10.1371/journal.pone.0172126.

Harjo J. *Poet Warrior: A Memoir* (WW Norton, 2001).

Hartle JC, Navas-Acien A, Lawrence RS. 2016. The Consumption of Canned Food and Beverages and Urinary Bisphenol A Concentrations in NHANES 2003–2008. Env Res. 2016;150:375–82.

Hartweg J, Perera R, Montori V, et al. Omega-3 Polyunsaturated Fatty Acids (PUFA) for Type 2 Diabetes Mellitus. Cochrane Database Syst Rev. 2008;(1):CD003205. PMID: 18254017.

Harvard Health Letter. April 2006. Harvard Medical School.

Harvard Medical School. Harvard Health Publishing. Foods That Fight Inflammation. Published 2014 Jun; updated 2018 Nov 7. Health.harvard.edu.

Harvard Medical School. Harvard Health Publishing. Inflammation: A Unifying Theory of Disease? 2020 May 8. Health.harvard.edu.

Harvard Medical School. Harvard Health Publishing. Maturity Onset Diabetes of the Young (MODY): What Is It? 2019 Apr.

Harvard Medical School. Harvard Health Publishing. No Need to Avoid Healthy Omega-6 Fats. Updated 2019 Aug 20. https://www.health.harvard.edu/newsletter _article/no-need-to-avoid-healthy-omega-6-fats.

Hashmi AM, Butt Z, Umair M. Is Depression an Inflammatory Condition? A Review of Available Evidence. J Pak Med Assoc. 2013;63(7):899–906.

Haug LS, Huber S, Becher G, Thomsen C. Characterisation of Human Exposure Pathways to Perfluorinated Compounds—Comparing Exposure Estimates with Biomarkers of Exposure. Environ Int. 2011 May;37(4):687–93. doi: 10.1016/j .envint.2011.01.011. Epub 2011 Feb 18. PMID: 21334069.

Hawa MI, Kolb H, Schloot N, et al. Adult-Onset Autoimmune Diabetes in Europe Is Prevalent with a Broad Clinical Phenotype: Action LADA 7 Diabetes Care. 2013;36(4):908–13. doi: 10.2337/dc12-0931. Published correction in Diabetes Care. 2014 May;37(5):1494.

He C, Shan Y, Song W. Targeting Gut Microbiota as a Possible Therapy for Diabetes. Nutr Res. 2015 May;35(5):361–67. doi: 10.1016/j.nutres.2015.03.002. Epub 2015 Mar 14. PMID: 25818484.

Heath C, Heath D. *Switch: How to Change Things When Change Is Hard* (Penguin Random House, 2010).

Heijmans BT, Tobi EW, Stein AD, et al. Persistent Epigenetic Differences Associated with Prenatal Exposure to Famine in Humans. Proc Natl Acad Sci USA. 2008;105(44):17046–49. doi: 10.1073/pnas.0806560105.

Heinemann L, Baughman R, Boss A, Hompesch M. Pharmacokinetic and Pharmacodynamic Properties of a Novel Inhaled Insulin. J Diab Sci Tech. 2017;11(1):148–56. doi: 10.1177/1932296816658055.

Heinemann L, Parkin CG. Rethinking the Viability and Utility of Inhaled Insulin in Clinical Practice. J Diab Res. 2018 Mar 7;2018:4568903. doi: 10.1155/2018/4568903. PMID: 29707584; PMCID: PMC5863311.

Heneberg P, Kocková L, Čecháková M, et al. Autoimmunity-Associated PTPN22 Polymorphisms in Latent Autoimmune Diabetes of the Adult Differ from Those of Type 1 Diabetes Patients. Int Arch Allergy Immunol. 2018;177(1):57–68. doi: 10.1159/000489225.

Herkert D, Vijayakumar P, Luo J, et al. Cost-Related Insulin Underuse Among Patients with Diabetes. JAMA Intern Med. 2019;179(1):112–14. doi: 10.1001/jamainternmed.2018.5008.

Hernández M, Mauricio D. Latent Autoimmune Diabetes in Adults: A Review of Clinically Relevant Issues. Adv Exp Med Biol. 2021;1307:29–41. doi: 10.1007/5584_2020_533. PMID: 32424495.

Herron KL, Vega-Lopez S, Conde K, et al. Men Classified as Hypo- or Hyperresponders to Dietary Cholesterol Feeding Exhibit Differences in Lipoprotein Metabolism. J Nutr. 2003 Apr;133(4):1036–42. doi: 10.1093/jn/133.4.1036. PMID: 12672915.

Hill-Briggs F, Adler NE, Berkowitz SA, et al. Social Determinants of Health and Diabetes: A Scientific Review. Diabetes Care. 2021 Jan 1;44(1):258–79. doi: 10.2337/dci20-0053.

Hirsch IB. Glycemic Variability and Diabetes Complications: Does It Matter? Of Course It Does! Diabetes Care 2015;38:1610–14.

Hirsch IB. Introduction: History of Glucose Monitoring. In *Role of Continuous Glucose Monitoring in Diabetes Treatment* (American Diabetes Association; 2018 Aug). Available from https://www.ncbi.nlm.nih.gov/books/NBK538968. doi: 10.2337/db20181-1.

Hjort L, Martino D. Gestational Diabetes and Maternal Obesity Are Associated with Epigenome-Wide Methylation Changes in Children. JCI Insight. 2018;3

Hjort R, Ahlqvist E, Alfredsson L, et al. Physical Activity and the Risk of LADA: Results from a Swedish Case-Control Study and the Norwegian HUNT Study. Diabetologia. 2018a;61(Suppl 1):S1–S620. doi: 10.1007/s00125-018-4596-0.

Hjort R, Ahlqvist E, Carlsson PO, et al. Overweight, Obesity and the Risk of LADA: Results from a Swedish Case-Control Study and the Norwegian HUNT Study. Diabetologia. 2018b;61:1333–43. doi: 10.1007/s00125-018-4596-0.

Hjort R, Alfredsson L, Andersson T, et al. Family History of Type 1 and Type 2 Diabetes and Risk of Latent Autoimmune Diabetes in Adults (LADA). Diab Metab. 2017;43(6):536–42. doi: 10.1016/j.diabet.2017.05.010.

Hjort R, Löfvenborg JE, Ahlqvist E, et al. Interaction Between Overweight and Genotypes of HLA, TCF7L2, and FTO in Relation to the Risk of Latent Autoimmune Diabetes in Adults and Type 2 Diabetes. J Clin Endocrinol Metab. 2019 Oct;104(10):4815–26. PMID: 31125083; PMCID: PMC6735731.

Ho KY, Veldhuis JD, Johnson ML, et al. Fasting Enhances Growth Hormone Secretion and Amplifies the Complex Rhythms of Growth Hormone Secretion in Man. J Clin Invest. 1988;81(4):968–75.

Hoch T, Kreitz S, Gaffling S, Pischetsrieder M, Hess A. Fat/Carbohydrate ratio but Not Energy Density Determines Snack Food Intake and Activates Brain Reward Areas. Sci Rep. 2015 May 14;5:10041. doi: 10.1038/srep10041. PMID: 25973686; PMCID: PMC4431128.

Holt RI, de Groot M, Golden SH. Diabetes and Depression. Curr Diab Rep. 2014 Jun;14(6):491. doi: 10.1007/s11892-014-0491-3. PMID: 24743941; PMCID: PMC4476048.

Horne BD, Muhlestein JB, May HT, et al. Intermountain Heart Collaborative Study Group. Relation of Routine, Periodic Fasting to Risk of Diabetes Mellitus, and Coronary Artery Disease in Patients Undergoing Coronary Angiography. Am J Cardiol. 2012 Jun 1;109(11):1558–62. doi: 10.1016/j.amjcard.2012.01.379. Epub 2012 Mar 16. PMID: 22425331.

Hostalek U. Global Epidemiology of Prediabetes—Present and Future Perspectives. Clin Diab endocrinol. 2019 May 9;5:5. doi: 10.1186/s40842-019-0080-0.

Hu MD, Lawrence KG, Bodkin MR, et al. Neighborhood Deprivation, Obesity, and Diabetes in Residents of the US Gulf Coast. Am J Epidemiol. 2021 Feb 1;190(2):295–304. doi: 10.1093/aje/kwaa206. PMID: 33524122; PMCID: PMC7850038.

Hua L, Lei M, Xue S, et al. Effect of Fish Oil Supplementation Combined with High-Intensity Interval Training in Newly Diagnosed Non-Obese Type 2 Diabetes: A Randomized Controlled Trial. J Clin Biochem Nutr. 2020;66(2):146–51. doi: 10.3164/jcbn.19-64.

Hua X, Carvalho N, Tew M, et al. Expenditures and Prices of Antihyperglycemic Medications in the United States: 2002–2013. JAMA. 2016;315(13):1400–02. doi: 10.1001/jama.2016.0126.

Huang G, Yin M, Xiang Y, et al. Persistence of Glutamic Acid Decarboxylase Antibody (GADA) Is Associated with Clinical Characteristics of Latent Autoimmune Diabetes in Adults: A Prospective Study with 3-Year Follow-Up. Diab Metab Res Rev. 2016 Sep;32(6):615–22. doi: 10.1002/dmrr.2779. Epub 2016 Mar 3. PMID: 26787598.

Huang J, Pearson J, Wong F, et al. Innate Immunity in Latent Autoimmune Diabetes in Adults (LADA). Diab Metab Res Rev. 2022 Jan;38(1):e3480. doi: 10.1002/dmrr.3480.

Huang R, Wang K, Hu J. Effect of Probiotics on Depression: A Systematic Review and Meta-Analysis of Randomized Controlled Trials. Nutrients. 2016;8(8):483. Published 2016 Aug 6. doi: 10.3390/nu8080483.

Huetteman E. 2019. Klobuchar Wants to Stop "Pay-For-Delay" Deals That Keep Drug Prices High. Kaiser Health News. April 26, 2019. https://khn.org/news/klobuchar-wants-to-stop-pay-for-delay-deals-that-keep-drug-prices-high/.

Huizen J. Soluble and Insoluble Fiber: What Is the Difference? *Medical News Today*. 2017 Aug 31. https://medicalnewstoday.com/articles/319176.

Hussain TA, Mathew TC, Dashti AA, et al. Effect of Low-Calorie Versus Low-Carbohydrate Ketogenic Diet in Type 2 Diabetes. Nutrition. 2012 Oct;28(10):1016–21. doi: 10.1016/j.nut.2012.01.016. Epub 2012 Jun 5. PMID: 22673594.

Hwang JJ, Jiang L, Sanchez Rangel E, et al. Glycemic Variability and Brain Glucose Levels in Type 1 Diabetes. Diabetes. 2019;68(1):163–71. doi: 10.2337/db18-0722.

Hwang SW, Bugeja AL. Barriers to Appropriate Diabetes Management Among Homeless People in Toronto. CMAJ. 2000;163(2):161–65.

Hwangbo DS, Lee HY, Abozaid LS, Min KJ. Mechanisms of Lifespan Regulation by Calorie Restriction and Intermittent Fasting in Model Organisms. Nutrients. 2020;12(4):1194. Published 2020 Apr 24. doi: 10.3390/nu12041194.

Hyman M. *Food: What the Heck Should I Eat?* (Little, Brown, 2018).

Iavicoli I, Fontana L, Bergamaschi A. The Effects of Metals as Endocrine Disruptors. J Toxicol Environ Health B Crit Rev. 2009 Mar;12(3):206–23. doi: 10.1080/10937400902902062. PMID: 19466673.

Imamura F, Micha R, Wu JHY, et al. Effects of Saturated Fat, Polyunsaturated Fat, Monounsaturated Fat, and Carbohydrate on Glucose-Insulin Homeostasis: A Systematic Review and Meta-Analysis of Randomised Controlled Feeding Trials. PLoS Med. 2016;13(7):e1002087. doi: 10.1371/journal.pmed.1002087.

Innis SM. Dietary Omega 3 Fatty Acids and the Developing Brain. Brain Res. 2008 Oct 27;1237:35–43. doi: 10.1016/j.brainres.2008.08.078. Epub 2008 Sep 9. PMID: 18789910.

Iwen KA, Backhaus J, Cassens M, et al. Cold-Induced Brown Adipose Tissue Activity Alters Plasma Fatty Acids and Improves Glucose Metabolism in Men. J Clin Endocrinol Metab. 2017;102(11):4226–34. doi: 10.1210/jc.2017-01250.

Jain AP, Aggarwal KK, Zhang P-Y. 2015. Omega-3 Fatty Acids and Cardiovascular Disease. Eur Rev Med Pharmacol Sci. 2015;19(3):441–45.

Jamison L. *The Recovering: Intoxication and Its Aftermath* (Back Bay Books, 2018).

Jang KM. Maturity-Onset Diabetes of the Young: Update and Perspectives on Diagnosis and Treatment. Yeungnam Univ J Med. 2020;37(1):13–21. doi: 10.12701/yujm.2019.00409.

Jeon EJ. Diabetes and Depression. Yeungnam Univ J Med. 2018 Jun;35(1):27–35. doi: 10.12701/yujm.2018.35.1.27. Epub 2018 Jun 30. PMID: 31620567; PMCID: PMC6784677.

Jeromson S, Gallagher IJ, Galloway SD, Hamilton DL. Omega-3 Fatty Acids and Skeletal Muscle Health. Mar Drugs. 2015 Nov 19;13(11):6977–7004. doi: 10.3390/md13116977. PMID: 26610527; PMCID: PMC4663562.

Jialal I, Singh G. Management of Diabetic Dyslipidemia: An Update. World J Diab. 2019;10(5):280–90.

Jiménez-Murcia S, Agüera Z, Paslakis G, et al. Food Addiction in Eating Disorders and Obesity: Analysis of Clusters and Implications for Treatment. Nutrients 2019;11:2633. doi: 10.3390/nu11112633.

Jin D, Wu S, Zhang YG, et al. Lack of Vitamin D Receptor Causes Dysbiosis and Changes the Functions of the Murine Intestinal Microbiome. Clin Ther. 2015 May 1;37(5):996–1009.e7. doi: 10.1016/j.clinthera.2015.04.004. PMID: 26046242.

Johnson KVA, Foster KR. Why Does the Microbiome Affect Behaviour? Microbiol. 2018 Oct;16:647–55.

Jørgensen SW, Brøns C, Bluck L, et al. Metabolic Response to 36 Hours of Fasting in Young Men Born Small vs Appropriate for Gestational Age. Diabetologia. 2015;58:178–87.

Jörns A, Wedekind D, Jähne J, Lenzen S. Pancreas Pathology of Latent Autoimmune Diabetes in Adults (LADA) in Patients and in a LADA Rat Model Compared with Type 1 Diabetes. Diabetes. 2020 Apr;69(4):624-633. doi: 10.2337/db19-0865. Epub 2020 Jan 23. PMID: 31974139.

Joubert M, Reznik Y. Personal Continuous Glucose Monitoring (CGM) in Diabetes Management: Review of the Literature and Implementation for Practical Use. Diab Res Clin Pract. 2012;96(3):294–305. doi: 10.1016/j.diabres.2011.12.010.

Juszczak A, Pryse R, Schuman A, Owen KR. When to Consider a Diagnosis of MODY at the Presentation of Diabetes: Aetiology Matters for Correct Management. Br J Gen Pract. 2016;66(647):e457–e459. doi: 10.3399/bjgp16X685537.

Kaati G, Bygren LO, Edvinsson S. Cardiovascular and Diabetes Mortality Determined by Nutrition During Parents' and Grandparents' Slow Growth Period. Eur J Hum Genet. 2002;10:682–88.

Kahleova H, Belinova L, Malinska H, et al. Eating Two Larger Meals a Day (Breakfast and Lunch) Is More Effective than Six Smaller Meals in a Reduced-Energy Regimen for Patients with Type 2 Diabetes: A Randomised Crossover Study Diabetologia. 2014;57(8):1552–60. doi: 10.1007/s00125-014-32535. Published correction in Diabetologia. 2015 Jan;58(1):205.

Kaisanlahti A, Glumoff T. Browning of White Fat: Agents and Implications for Beige Adipose Tissue to Type 2 Diabetes. J Physiol Biochem. 2019;75(1):1–10. doi: 10.1007/s13105-018-0658-5.

Kalra S, Jena BN, Yeravdekar R. Emotional and Psychological Needs of People with Diabetes. Indian J Endocrinol Metab. 2018 Sep–Oct;22(5):696–704. doi: 10.4103/ijem.IJEM_579_17. PMID: 30294583; PMCID: PMC6166557.

Kang H, Lobo JM, Kim S, Sohn M-W. Cost-Related Medication Non-Adherence Among US Adults with Diabetes. Diabetes Res Clin Pract 2018;143:24–33.

Kaplan, K. Half of Americans Have Diabetes or a High Risk for It—and Many of Them Are Unaware. *LA Times.* 2017 Jul 18.

Karges B, Schwandt A, Heidtmann B, et al. Association of Insulin Pump Therapy vs Insulin Injection Therapy with Severe Hypoglycemia, Ketoacidosis, and Glycemic Control Among Children, Adolescents, and Young Adults with Type 1 Diabetes. JAMA. 2017;318(14):1358–66.

Karlovitch S. Biosimilar Insulin Could Offer Patients Cost-Saving Options. Am J Manag Care. 2019 Sep 1;25(10 Spec No.):88172. PMID: 31860243.

Katon WJ, Rutter C, Simon G, et al. The Association of Comorbid Depression with Mortality in Patients with Type 2 Diabetes. Diabetes Care. 2005 Nov;28(11):2668–72. doi: 10.2337/diacare.28.11.2668. PMID: 16249537.

Kaur N, Bhadada SK, Minz RW, et al. Interplay Between Type 1 Diabetes Mellitus and Celiac Disease: Implications in Treatment. Dig Dis. 2018;36(6):399–408. doi: 10.1159/000488670. Epub 2018 Jul 25. PMID: 30045024.

Kessler DA. 2020. Fast Carbs, Slow Carbs: The Simple Truth About Food, Weight, and Disease. Harper Collins.

Kiecolt-Glaser JK, Belury MA, Andridge R, Malarkey WB, Glaser R. Omega-3 Supplementation Lowers Inflammation and Anxiety in Medical Students: A Randomized Controlled Trial. Brain Behav Immun. 2011;25(8):1725–34. doi: 10.1016/j.bbi.2011.07.229.

Kim K, Yang WH, Jung YS, Cha JH. A New Aspect of an Old Friend: The Beneficial Effect of Metformin on Anti-Tumor Immunity. BMB Rep. 2020 Nov;53(10):512–20. doi: 10.5483/BMBRep.2020.53.10.149. PMID: 32731915; PMCID: PMC7607149.

Kim Y, Je Y. Dairy Consumption and Risk of Metabolic Syndrome: A Meta-Analysis. Diab Med. 2016 Apr;33(4):428–40. doi: 10.1111/dme.12970. Epub 2015 Oct 27. PMID: 26433009.

Kirwan H. New Study Finds More Omega-3s in Milk from Grass-Fed Cows. Wisconsin Public Radio. 2018 Mar 2.

Kissileff HR, Thornton JC, Torres MI, et al. Leptin Reverses Declines in Satiation in Weight-Reduced Obese Humans. Am J Clin Nutr. 2012 Feb;95(2):309–17. doi: 10.3945/ajcn.111.012385. Epub 2012 Jan 11. PMID: 22237063; PMCID: PMC3260066.

Klatzkin RR, Baldassaro A, Hayden E. The Impact of Chronic Stress on the Predictors of Acute Stress-Induced Eating in Women. Appetite. 2018 Apr 1;123:343–51. doi: 10.1016/j.appet.2018.01.007. Epub 2018 Jan 5. PMID: 29309852.

Kobayashi T, Maruyama T, Shimada A, et al. Insulin Intervention to Preserve Beta Cells in Slowly Progressive Insulin-Dependent (Type 1) Diabetes Mellitus. Ann N Y Acad Sci. 2002 Apr;958:117–30. doi: 10.1111/j.1749-6632.2002.tb02954.x.PMID: 12021091.

Kolb H, Kempf K, Röhling M, et al. Insulin: Too Much of a Good Thing Is Bad. BMC Med. 2020;18(1):224. doi: 10.1186/s12916-020-01688-6.

Kolb H, Martin S. Environmental/Lifestyle Factors in the Pathogenesis and Prevention of Type 2 Diabetes. BMC Med. 2017 Jul 19;15(1):131. doi: 10.1186/s12916-017-0901-x. PMID: 28720102; PMCID: PMC5516328.

Kondo Y, Goto A, Noma H, Iso H, et al. Effects of Coffee and Tea Consumption on Glucose Metabolism: A Systematic Review and Network Meta-Analysis. Nutrients. 2018 Dec 27;11(1):48. doi: 10.3390/nu11010048. PMID: 30591664; PMCID: PMC6356434.

Kos E, Liszek MJ, Emanuele MA, et al. Effect of Metformin Therapy on Vitamin D and Vitamin B_{12} Levels in Patients with Type 2 Diabetes Mellitus. Endocr Pract. 2012 Mar–Apr;18(2):179–84. doi: 10.4158/EP11009.OR. PMID: 21940283.

Kosinski C, Jornayvaz FR. Effects of Ketogenic Diets on Cardiovascular Risk Factors: Evidence from Animal and Human Studies. Nutrients. 2017 May 19;9(5):517. doi: 10.3390/nu9050517. PMID: 28534852; PMCID: PMC5452247.

Krebs JD, Bell D, Hall R, et al. Improvements in Glucose Metabolism and Insulin Sensitivity with a Low-Carbohydrate Diet in Obese Patients with type 2 Diabetes. J Am Coll Nutr. 2013;32(1):11-17. doi: 10.1080/07315724.2013.767630. PMID: 24015695.

Krebs JD, Parry Strong A, Cresswell P, et al. A Randomised Trial of the Feasibility of a Low Carbohydrate Diet vs Standard Carbohydrate Counting in Adults with Type 1 Diabetes Taking Body Weight into Account. Asia Pac J Clin Nutr. 2016;25(1):78–84. doi: 10.6133/apjcn.2016.25.1.11. PMID: 26965765.

Kriz KLM. The Efficacy of Overeaters Anonymous in Fostering Abstinence in Binge-Eating Disorder and Bulimia Nervosa.Virginia Polytechnic Institute and State University doctoral dissertation, 2002.

Kuchkuntla AR, Shah M, Velapati S, et al. Ketogenic Diet: An Endocrinologist Perspective. Curr Nutr Rep. 2019 Dec;8(4):402–10. doi: 10.1007/s13668-019-00297-x .PMID: 31705484.

Kumar M, Kumar SD, Swasti S, et al. 2020. Environmental Endocrine-Disrupting Chemical Exposure: Role in Non-Communicable Diseases. Front Public Health. 2020 Sep 24;8:553850. doi: 10.3389/fpubh.2020.553850.

Kumar S, Subhakumari KN. Role of Anti-GAD, Anti-IA2 Antibodies and C-Peptide in Differentiating Latent Autoimmune Diabetes in Adults from Type 2 Diabetes Mellitus. Int J Diabetes Dev Ctries. 2016;36:313–319. doi: 10.1007/s13410-015-0351-y.

Kuwahara A, Matsuda K, Kuwahara Y, et al. Microbiota-Gut-Brain Axis: Enteroendocrine Cells and the Enteric Nervous System Form an Interface Between the Microbiota and the Central Nervous System. Biomed Res. 2020;41(5):199–216. doi: 10.2220/biomedres.41.199. PMID: 33071256.

Kyriachenko Y, Falalyeyeva T, Korotkyi O, et al. Crosstalk Between Gut Microbiota and Antidiabetic Drug Action. World J Diab. 2019 Mar 15;10(3):154–68. doi: 10.4239/ wjd.v10.i3.154. PMCID: PMC6422856. PMID: 30891151.

Laaksonen MA, Knekt P, Rissanen H, et al. The Relative Importance of Modifiable Potential Risk Factors of Type 2 Diabetes: A Meta-Analysis of Two Cohorts. Eur J Epidemiol. 2010 Feb;25(2):115–24. doi: 10.1007/s10654-009-9405-0. Epub 2009 Dec 13. PMID: 20012885.

Lach G, Schellekens H, Dinan TG, Cryan JF. Anxiety, Depression, and the Microbiome: A Role for Gut Peptides. Neurotherapeutics. 2018 Jan;15(1):36–59. doi: 10.1007/s13311-017-0585-0. PMID: 29134359; PMCID: PMC5794698.

Lacourt TE, Vichaya EG, Chiu GS, et al. The High Costs of Low-Grade Inflammation: Persistent Fatigue as a Consequence of Reduced Cellular-Energy Availability and Non-Adaptive Energy Expenditure. Front Behav Neurosci. 2018;12:78. Published 2018 Apr 26. doi: 10.3389/fnbeh.2018.00078.

Lancet Diabetes Endocrinology. The Bare Essentials: Ensuring Affordable Access to Insulin. Lancet Diab Endocrinol. 2017 Mar;5(3):151. doi: 10.1016/S2213 -8587(17)30038-4. Epub 2017 Feb 9. PMID: 28189655.

Lappé FM. Frances Moore Lappé interview with Annie B. Copps. 2020 Feb 2.

Laugesen E, Østergaard JA, Leslie RD. Latent Autoimmune Diabetes of the Adult: Current Knowledge and Uncertainty. Diabet Med. 2015;32(7):843–52. doi: 10.1111 /dme.12700.lin.

Laverty AA, Magee L, Monteiro CA, Saxena S, Millett C. Sugar and Artificially Sweetened Beverage Consumption and Adiposity Changes: National Longitudinal Study.

Int J Behav Nutr Phys Act. 2015 Oct 26;12:137. doi: 10.1186/s12966-015-0297-y .PMID: 26503493; PMCID: PMC4624385.

Laymon K. *Heavy: An American Memoir* (Scribner, 2019).

Lean ME, Leslie WS, Barnes AC, et al. Primary Care-Led Weight Management for Remission of Type 2 Diabetes (DiRECT): An Open-Label, Cluster-Randomised Trial. Lancet. 2018 Feb 10;391(10120):541–51. doi: 10.1016/S0140-6736(17)33102-1. Epub 2017 Dec 5. PMID: 29221645.

Lean MEJ, Leslie WS, Barnes AC, et al. Durability of a Primary Care-Led Weight-Management Intervention for Remission of Type 2 Diabetes: 2-Year Results of the DiRECT Open-Label, Cluster-Randomised Trial. Lancet Diab Endocrinol. 2019 May;7(5):344–55. doi: 10.1016/S2213-8587(19)30068-3. Epub 2019 Mar 6. PMID: 30852132.

Lee DY, Li H, Lim HJ, et al. Anti-Inflammatory Activity of Sulfur-Containing Compounds from Garlic. J Medicinal Food. 2012;15(11):992–99. doi: 10.1089 /jmf.2012.2275.

Lee S, Lee DY. Glucagon-Like Peptide-1 and Glucagon-Like Peptide-1 Receptor Agonists in the Treatment of Type 2 Diabetes. Ann Pediatr Endocrinol Metab. 2017;22(1):15–26. doi: 10.6065/apem.2017.22.1.15.

Leigh SJ, Morris MJ. The Role of Reward Circuitry and Food Addiction in the Obesity Epidemic: An Update. Biol Psychol. 2018 Jan;131:31–42. doi: 10.1016/j .biopsycho.2016.12.013. Epub 2016 Dec 21. PMID: 28011401.

Leighton E, Sainsbury CA, Jones GC. A Practical Review of C-Peptide Testing in Diabetes. Diabetes Ther. 2017 Jun;8(3):475–487. doi: 10.1007/s13300-017-0265-4. Epub 2017 May 8. PMID: 28484968; PMCID: PMC5446389.

Lemieux P, Weisnagel SJ, Caron AZ, et al. Effects of 6-Month Vitamin D Supplementation on Insulin Sensitivity and Secretion: A Randomised, Placebo-Controlled Trial. Eur J Endocrinol. 2019 Sep;181(3):287–99. doi: 10.1530/EJE-19-0156. PMID: 31344685.

Lennerz B, Alsop DC, Holsen LM, et al. Effects of Dietary Glycemic Index on Brain Regions Related to Reward and Craving in Men. Am J Clin Nutr. 2013 Sep;98(3):641–47. doi: 10.3945/ajcn.113.064113.

Lennerz B, Lennerz JK. Food Addiction, High-Glycemic-Index Carbohydrates, and Obesity. Clin Chem. 2018 Jan;64(1):64–71. doi: 10.1373/clinchem.2017.273532 .Epub 2017 Nov 20. PMID: 29158252; PMCID: PMC5912158.

Lennerz BS, Barton A, Bernstein RK, et al. Management of Type 1 Diabetes with a Very Low-Carbohydrate Diet. Pediatrics. 2018;141(6):e20173349.

Leonard MM, Vasagar B. US Perspective on Gluten-Related Diseases. Clin Exp Gastroenterol. 2014;7:25–37. doi: 10.2147/CEG.S54567.

Leow ZZX, Guelfi KJ, Davis EA, et al. The Glycaemic Benefits of a Very-Low-Carbohydrate Ketogenic Diet in Adults with Type 1 Diabetes Mellitus May Be Opposed by Increased Hypoglycaemia Risk and Dyslipidaemia. Diabet Med. 2018 May 8. doi: 10.1111/dme.13663. Epub ahead of print. PMID: 29737587.

Leslie I. The Sugar Conspiracy. *Guardian*. 2016 Apr 7.

Leung CW, Epel ES, Willett WC, et al. Household Food Insecurity Is Positively Associated with Depression Among Low-Income Supplemental Nutrition Assistance Program Participants and Income-Eligible Nonparticipants. J Nutr. 2015;145:622–27.

Leung PS. The Potential Protective Action of Vitamin D in Hepatic Insulin Resistance and Pancreatic Islet Dysfunction in Type 2 Diabetes Mellitus. Nutrients. 2016;8(3):147. Published 2016 Mar 5. doi: 10.3390/nu8030147.

Levy M, Kolodziejczyk AA, Thaiss CA, Elinav E. Dysbiosis and the Immune System. Nat Rev Immunol. 2017 Apr;17(4):219–32. doi: 10.1038/nri.2017.7. Epub 2017 Mar 6. PMID: 28260787.

Li H, Wu G, Zhao L, Zhang M. Suppressed Inflammation in Obese Children Induced by a High-Fiber Diet Is Associated with the Attenuation of Gut Microbial Virulence Factor Genes. Virulence. 2021 Dec;12(1):1754–70. doi: 10.1080/21505594.2021.1948252. PMID: 34233588; PMCID: PMC8274444.

Li X, Atkinson MA. The Role for Gut Permeability in the Pathogenesis of Type 1 Diabetes—a Solid or Leaky Concept? Pediatr Diab. 2015 Nov;16(7):485–92. doi: 10.1111/pedi.12305. Epub 2015 Aug 13. PMID: 26269193; PMCID: PMC4638168.

Li X, Chen Y, Xie Y, et al. Decline Pattern of Beta-Cell Function in Adult-Onset Latent Autoimmune Diabetes: An 8-Year Prospective Study. J Clin Endocrinol Metab. 2020 Jul 1;105(7):dgaa205. doi: 10.1210/clinem/dgaa205.

Li X, Liao L, Yan X, et al. Protective Effects of 1-Alpha-Hydroxyvitamin D_3 on Residual Beta-Cell Function in Patients with Adult-Onset Latent Autoimmune Diabetes (LADA). Diab Metab Res Rev. 2009;25(5):411–16.

Li X, Yang L, Zhou Z, et al. Glutamic Acid Decarboxylase 65 Autoantibody Levels Discriminate Two Subtypes of Latent Autoimmune Diabetes in Adults. Chin Med J (Engl). 2003 Nov;116(11):1728–32. PMID: 14642146.

Li Y, Wang C, Huai Q, et al. Effects of Tea or Tea Extract on Metabolic Profiles in Patients with Type 2 Diabetes Mellitus: A Meta-Analysis of Ten Randomized Controlled Trials. Diab Metab Res Rev. 2016 Jan;32(1):2–10. doi: 10.1002/dmrr.2641. Epub 2015 Apr 21. PMID: 25689396.

Lichtash C, Fung J, Ostoich KC, Ramos M. Therapeutic Use of Intermittent Fasting and Ketogenic Diet as an Alternative Treatment for Type 2 Diabetes in a Normal Weight Woman: A 14-Month Case Study. BMJ Case Rep. 2020;13(7):e234223. Published 2020 Jul 7. doi: 10.1136/bcr-2019-234223.

Lin J, Thompson TJ, Cheng YJ, et al. Projection of the Future Diabetes Burden in the United States Through 2060. Popul Health Metrics. 2018 Jun 15;16(1):9. doi: 10.1186/s12963-018-0166-4.

Lindblom M. New Washington State Law Now Caps Monthly Insulin Copay at $100. *Seattle Times.* 2021 Jan 2.

Ling C, Rönn T. Epigenetics in Human Obesity and Type 2 Diabetes. Cell Metab. 2019;29(5):1028–44. doi: 10.1016/j.cmet.2019.03.009.

Link CL, McKinlay JB. Disparities in the Prevalence of Diabetes: Is It Race/Ethnicity or Socioeconomic Status? Results from the Boston Area Community Health (BACH) Survey. Ethn Dis. 2009;19(3):288–92.

Lipman F, Claro D. *The New Health Rules: Simple Changes to Achieve Whole-Body Wellness* (Artisan, 2014).

Liu B, Xiang Y, Liu Z, Zhou Z. Past, Present and Future of Latent Autoimmune Diabetes in Adults. Diabetes Metab Res Rev. 2020 Jan;36(1):e3205. doi: 10.1002/dmrr.3205. Epub 2019 Jul 31. PMID: 31318117.

Liu HQ, Qiu Y, Mu Y, et al. A High Ratio of Dietary n-3/n-6 Polyunsaturated Fatty Acids Improves Obesity-Linked Inflammation and Insulin Resistance Through Suppressing Activation of TLR4 in SD Rats. Nutr Res. 2013 Oct;33(10):849–58. doi: 10.1016/j.nutres.2013.07.004. Epub 2013 Aug 9. PMID: 24074743.

Liu K, Zhou R, Wang B, et al. Effect of Green Tea on Glucose Control and Insulin Sensitivity: A Meta-Analysis of 17 Randomized Controlled Trials. Am J Clin Nutr. 2013 Aug;98(2):340–48. doi: 10.3945/ajcn.112.052746. Epub 2013 Jun 26. PMID: 23803878.

Liu K, Zhou R, Wang B, Mi MT. Effect of Resveratrol on Glucose Control and Insulin Sensitivity: A Meta-Analysis of 11 Randomized Controlled Trials. Am J Clin Nutr. 2014 Jun;99(6):1510–19. doi: 10.3945/ajcn.113.082024. Epub 2014 Apr 2. PMID: 24695890.

Liu L, Li X, Xiang Y, et al. LADA China Study Group. Latent Autoimmune Diabetes in Adults with Low-Titer GAD Antibodies: Similar Disease Progression with Type 2 Diabetes: A Nationwide, Multicenter Prospective Study (LADA China Study 3). Diabetes Care. 2015 Jan;38(1):16–21. doi: 10.2337/dc14-1770. Epub 2014 Oct 21. PMID: 25336751.

Liu YZ, Wang YX, Jiang CL. Inflammation: The Common Pathway of Stress-Related Diseases. Front Hum Neurosci. 2017;11:316. Published 2017 Jun 20. doi: 10.3389/fnhum.2017.00316.

Live Science. 1 in 3 Americans Will Have Diabetes by 2050, CDC Says. Live Science. 2010 Oct 22. https://www.livescience.com/10195-1-3-americans-diabetes-2050-cdc.html.

Lloyd CE, Dyer PH, Barnett AH. Prevalence of Symptoms of Depression and Anxiety in a Diabetes Clinic Population. Diabet Med. 2000 Mar;17(3):198–202. doi: 10.1046/j.1464-5491.2000.00260.x. PMID: 10784223.

Locklear M. 2022. Insulin Is an Extreme Financial Burden for over 14% of Americans Who Use It. Yale News, July 5, 2022. https://news.yale.edu/2022/07/05/insulin-extreme-financial-burden-over-14-americans-who-use-it.

Löfvenborg JE, Ahlqvist E, Alfredsson L, et al. 2020a. Genotypes of HLA, TCF7L2, and FTO as Potential Modifiers of the Association Between Sweetened Beverage Consumption and Risk of LADA and Type 2 Diabetes. Eur J Nutr. 2020 Feb;59(1):127–35. doi: 10.1007/s00394-019-01893-x. Epub 2019 Jan 17. PMID: 30656477; PMCID: PMC7000500.

Löfvenborg JE, Ahlqvist E, Alfredsson L, et al. 2020b. Consumption of Red Meat, Genetic Susceptibility, and Risk of LADA and Type 2 Diabetes. Eur J Nutr. 2021 Mar;60(2): 769–79. doi: 10.1007/s00394-020-02285-2. Epub 2020 May 22. PMID: 32444887.

Löfvenborg JE, Andersson T, Carlsson PO, Dorkhan M, Groop L, Martinell M, Rasouli B, Storm P, Tuomi T, Carlsson S. Coffee Consumption and the Risk of Latent Autoimmune Diabetes in Adults—Results from a Swedish Case-Control Study. Diab Med. 2014 Jul;31(7):799–805. doi: 10.1111/dme.12469. Epub 2014 May 2. PMID: 24750356.

Löfvenborg JE, Andersson T, Carlsson PO, Dorkhan M, Groop L, Martinell M, Tuomi T, Wolk A, Carlsson S. Sweetened Beverage Intake and Risk of Latent Autoimmune Diabetes in Adults (LADA) and Type 2 Diabetes. Eur J Endocrinol. 2016 Dec;175(6):605-614. doi: 10.1530/EJE-16-0376. PMID: 27926472.

Logan SL, Spriet LL. Omega-3 Fatty Acid Supplementation for 12 Weeks Increases Resting and Exercise Metabolic Rate in Healthy Community-Dwelling Older Females. PLoS One. 2015 Dec 17;10(12):e0144828. doi: 10.1371/journal.pone.0144828. PMID: 26679702; PMCID: PMC4682991.

Loh M, Zhou L, Ng HK, Chambers JC. Epigenetic Disturbances in Obesity and Diabetes: Epidemiological and Functional Insights. Mol Metab. 2019 Sep;27S(Suppl):S33–S41. doi: 10.1016/j.molmet.2019.06.011. PMID: 31500829; PMCID: PMC6768506.

López L, Tan-McGrory A, Horner G, Betancourt JR. Eliminating Disparities Among Latinos with Type 2 Diabetes: Effective eHealth Strategies. J Diab Complicats. 2016;30(3):554–60. doi: 10.1016/j.jdiacomp.2015.12.003.

Loxton NJ, Tipman RJ. Reward Sensitivity and Food Addiction in Women. Appetite. 2017 Aug 1;115:28–35. doi: 10.1016/j.appet.2016.10.022. Epub 2016 Oct 15. PMID: 27756640.

Lucan SC, DiNicolantonio JJ. How Calorie-Focused Thinking About Obesity and Related Diseases May Mislead and Harm Public Health. An Alternative. Public Health Nutr. 2015 Mar;18(4):571–81. doi: 10.1017/S1368980014002559. Epub 2014 Nov 24. PMID: 25416919.

Ludwig DS. The Ketogenic Diet: Evidence for Optimism but High-Quality Research Needed. J Nutr. 2020;150(6):1354–59. doi: 10.1093/jn/nxz308.

Ludwig DS, Ebbeling CB. The Carbohydrate-Insulin Model of Obesity: Beyond "Calories In, Calories Out." JAMA Intern Med. 2018;178(8):1098–103.

Ludwig DS, Friedman MI. Increasing Adiposity: Consequence or Cause of Overeating? JAMA. 2014;311(21):2167–68.

Luo J, Gellad WF. Origins of the Crisis in Insulin Affordability and Practical Advice for Clinicians on Using Human Insulin. Curr Diab Rep. 2020 Jan 29;20(1):2. doi: 10.1007/s11892-020-1286-3. PMID: 31997036.

Lyssenko V, Laakso M. Genetic Screening for the Risk of Type 2 Diabetes: Worthless or Valuable? Diabetes Care. 2013 Aug;36(Suppl 2):S120–26. doi: 10.2337/dcS13-2009. PMID: 23882036; PMCID: PMC3920800.

Maahs DM, West NA, Lawrence JM, Mayer-Davis EJ. Epidemiology of Type 1 Diabetes. Endocrinol Metab Clin North Am. 2010;39(3):481–97. doi: 10.1016/j.ecl.2010.05.011.

Macedo RC, Vieira A, Marin DP, Otton R. Effects of Chronic Resveratrol Supplementation in Military Firefighters Undergo a Physical Fitness Test—A Placebo-Controlled, Double Blind Study. Chem Biol Interact. 2015 Feb 5;227:89–95. doi: 10.1016/j.cbi.2014.12.033. Epub 2015 Jan 5. PMID: 25572586.

Mackinnon E. Candy Not Corn for Cows in Drought. Live Science. 2012 Aug 23.

Maddaloni E, Moretti C, Mignogna C, Buzzetti R. Adult-Onset Autoimmune Diabetes in 2020: An Update. Maturitas. 2020 Jul;137:37–44. doi: 10.1016/j.maturitas.2020.04.014.

Malik VS, Popkin BM, Bray GA, et al. Sugar-Sweetened Beverages and Risk of Metabolic Syndrome and Type 2 Diabetes: A Meta-Analysis. Diabetes Care. 2010 Nov;33(11):2477–83. doi: 10.2337/dc10-1079. Epub 2010 Aug 6. PMID: 20693348; PMCID: PMC2963518.

Mallone R, Eizirik DL. Presumption of Innocence for Beta Cells: Why Are They Vulnerable Autoimmune Targets in Type 1 Diabetes? Diabetologia. 2020 Oct;63(10):1999–2006. doi: 10.1007/s00125-020-05176-7. Epub 2020 Sep 7. PMID: 32894310.

Mancini JG, Filion KB, Atallah R, Eisenberg MJ. Systematic Review of the Mediterranean Diet for Long-Term Weight Loss. Am J Med. 2016;129(4):407–15.e4.

Mao QQ, Xu XY, Cao SY, et al. Bioactive Compounds and Bioactivities of Ginger (*Zingiber officinale* Roscoe). Foods (Basel). 2019;8(6):185. doi: 10.3390/foods8060185.

Martínez-Fernández L, Laiglesia LM, Huerta AE, et al. Omega-3 Fatty Acids and Adipose Tissue Function in Obesity and Metabolic Syndrome. Prostaglandins Other Lipid Mediat. 2015 Sep;121(pt A):24–41. doi: 10.1016/j.prostaglandins.2015.07.003. Epub 2015 Jul 26. PMID: 26219838.

Maruyama T, Tanaka S, Shimada A, et al. Insulin Intervention in Slowly Progressive Insulin-Dependent (Type 1) Diabetes Mellitus. J Clin Endocrinol Metab. 2008;93(6):2115–21. doi: 10.1210/jc.2007-2267.

Marventano S, Kolacz P, Castellano S, et al. A Review of Recent Evidence in Human Studies of n-3 and n-6 PUFA Intake on Cardiovascular Disease, Cancer, and Depressive Disorders: Does the Ratio Really Matter? Int J Food Sci Nutr. 2015;66(6):611–22. doi: 10.3109/09637486.2015.1077790. Epub 2015 Aug 26. PMID: 26307560.

Mason SM, Flint AJ, Field AE, et al. Abuse Victimization in Childhood or Adolescence and Risk of Food Addiction in Adult Women. Obesity (Silver Spring). 2013 Dec;21(12):E775–81. doi: 10.1002/oby.20500. Epub 2013 Jul 29. PMID: 23637085; PMCID: PMC3855159.

Mattson MP, Allison DB, Fontana L, et al. Meal Frequency and Timing in Health and Disease. Proc Natl Acad Sci USA. 2014 Nov 25;111(47):16647–53. doi: 10.1073/pnas.1413965111. Epub 2014 Nov 17. PMID: 25404320; PMCID: PMC4250148.

Mattson MP, Longo VD, Harvie M. Impact of Intermittent Fasting on Health and Disease Processes. Ageing Res Rev. 2017 Oct;39:46-58. doi: 10.1016/j.arr.2016.10.005. Epub 2016 Oct 31. PMID: 27810402; PMCID: PMC5411330.

Mayo Clinic website. https//www.mayoclinic.org.

McDonald TJ, Ellard S. Maturity Onset Diabetes of the Young: Identification and Diagnosis. Ann Clin Biochem. 2013;50(pt 5):403–15. doi: 10.1177/0004563213483458.

McGhee H. *The Sum of Us: What Racism Costs Everyone and How We Can Prosper Together* (Penguin Random House, 2021).

McGill JB, Peters A, Buse JB, et al. Comprehensive Pulmonary Safety Review of Inhaled Technosphere® Insulin in Patients with Diabetes Mellitus. Clin Drug Investig. 2020 Oct;40(10):973–83. doi: 10.1007/s40261-020-00958-8. PMID: 32720187; PMCID: PMC7511468.

McNamara DJ. Dietary Cholesterol and the Optimal Diet for Reducing Risk of Atherosclerosis. Can J Cardiol. 1995 Oct;11(Suppl G):123G–126G. PMID: 7585286.

Mejía-León ME, Barca AM. Diet, Microbiota and Immune System in Type 1 Diabetes Development and Evolution. Nutrients. 2015 Nov 6;7(11):9171–84. doi: 10.3390/nu7115461. PMID: 26561831; PMCID: PMC4663589.

Melitas C, Meiselman M. Metabolic Pancreatitis: Pancreatic Steatosis, Hypertriglyceridemia, and Associated Chronic Pancreatitis in 3 Patients with Metabolic Syndrome. Case Rep Gastroenterol. 2018 Jun 25;12(2):331–36. doi: 10.1159/000490042. PMID: 30022925; PMCID: PMC6047553.

Mena-Sánchez G, Becerra-Tomás N, Babio N, Salas-Salvadó J. Dairy Product Consumption in the Prevention of Metabolic Syndrome: A Systematic Review and Meta-Analysis of Prospective Cohort Studies. Adv Nutr. 2019 May 1;10(Suppl 2):S144–S153. doi: 10.1093/advances/nmy083. PMID: 31089736; PMCID: PMC6518129.

Mendenhall E, Norris SA, Shidhaye R, Prabhakaran D. Depression and Type 2 Diabetes in Low- and Middle-Income Countries: A Systematic Review. Diabetes Res Clin Pract. 2014 Feb;103(2):276–85. doi: 10.1016/j.diabres.2014.01.001. Epub 2014 Jan 13. PMID: 24485858; PMCID: PMC3982306.

Mendes AF, Cruz MT, Gualillo O. Editorial: The Physiology of Inflammation—The Final Common Pathway to Disease. Front Physiol. 2018 Dec 4;9:1741. doi: 10.3389/fphys.2018.01741.

Meng JM, Cao SY, Wei XL, et al. Effects and Mechanisms of Tea for the Prevention and Management of Diabetes Mellitus and Diabetic Complications: An Updated Review. Antioxidants (Basel). 2019 Jun 10;8(6):170. doi: 10.3390/antiox8060170. PMID: 31185622; PMCID: PMC6617012.

Mensink RP, World Health Organization. *Effects of Saturated Fatty Acids on Serum Lipids and Lipoproteins: A Systematic Review and Regression Analysis* (World Health Organization, 2016). https://apps.who.int/iris/handle/10665/246104.

Messerly M. First Diabetes Drug Transparency Report Reveals Profits, Costs Associated with Treating the Disease. *Nevada Independent.* 2019 Mar 13.

Meule A. How Prevalent Is "Food Addiction"? Front Psychiatry. 2011 Nov 3;2:61. doi: 10.3389/fpsyt.2011.00061. PMID: 22065960; PMCID: PMC3207274.

Meule A. The Psychology of Food Cravings: The Role of Food Deprivation. Curr Nutr Rep. 2020;9(3):251–57. doi: 10.1007/s13668-020-00326-0.

Meza-Perez S, Randall TD. Belly Fat Has a Role to Play in Fighting Infections. *The Scientist.* 2018 Oct.

Micha R, Wallace SK, Mozaffarian D. Red and Processed Meat Consumption and Risk of Incident Coronary Heart Disease, Stroke, and Diabetes Mellitus: A Systematic Review and Meta-Analysis. Circulation. 2010 Jun 1;121(21):2271–83. doi: 10.1161/CIRCULATIONAHA.109.924977. Epub 2010 May 17. PMID: 20479151; PMCID: PMC2885952.

Mikhail N. Safety of Technosphere Inhaled Insulin. Curr Drug Saf. 2017;12(1):27–31. doi: 10.2174/1574886311666160829144240. PMID: 27572546.

Miles K. "Radical Communion: An Interview with Camille T. Dungy." Terrain.org. 11 May 2022.

Minhaj H. How America Is Causing Global Obesity. *The Patriot Act.* Netflix. 2019 Dec 22.

Minihane AM, Armah CK, Miles EA, et al. Consumption of Fish Oil Providing Amounts of Eicosapentaenoic Acid and Docosahexaenoic Acid That Can Be Obtained from the Diet Reduces Blood Pressure in Adults with Systolic Hypertension: A Retrospective Analysis. J Nutr. 2016 Mar;146(3):516–23. doi: 10.3945/jn.115.220475. Epub 2016 Jan 27. PMID: 26817716.

Minihane AM, Vinoy S, Russell WR, et al. Low-Grade Inflammation, Diet Composition and Health: Current Research Evidence and Its Translation. Br J Nutr. 2015;114(7):999–1012. doi: 10.1017/S0007114515002093.

Mirhosseini N, Vatanparast H, Mazidi M, Kimball SM. The Effect of Improved Serum 25-Hydroxyvitamin D Status on Glycemic Control in Diabetic Patients: A Meta-Analysis. J Clin Endocrinol Metab. 2017 Sep 1;102(9):3097–110. doi: 10.1210/jc.2017-01024. PMID: 28957454.

Mirror Mirror website. https://mirror-mirror.org.

Mishra R, Åkerlund M, Cousminer DL, et al. Genetic Discrimination Between LADA and Childhood-Onset Type 1 Diabetes Within the MHC. Diabetes Care. 2020 Feb;43(2):418–25. doi: 10.2337/dc19-0986. Epub 2019 Dec 16. PMID: 31843946; PMCID: PMC6971787.

Mishra R, Chesi A, Cousminer DL, et al. Relative Contribution of Type 1 and Type 2 Diabetes Loci to the Genetic Etiology of Adult-Onset, Non-Insulin-Requiring Autoimmune Diabetes. BMC Med. 2017 Apr 25;15(1):88. doi: 10.1186/s12916-017-0846-0. PMID: 28438156; PMCID: PMC5404312.

Mitri J, Muraru MD, Pittas AG. Vitamin D and Type 2 Diabetes: A Systematic Review. Eur J Clin Nutr. 2011 Sep;65(9):1005–15. doi: 10.1038/ejcn.2011.118. Epub 2011 Jul 6. PMID: 21731035; PMCID: PMC4066381.

Moffa S, Mezza T, Cefalo C, et al. The Interplay Between Immune System and Microbiota in Diabetes. Mediators Inflamm. 2019 Dec 30:9367404. doi: 10.1155/2019/9367404.

Monneret C. What Is an Endocrine Disruptor? C R Biol. 2017 Sep–Oct;340(9–10):403–05. doi: 10.1016/j.crvi.2017.07.004. PMID: 29126512.

Moore CJ, Cunningham SA. Social Position, Psychological Stress, and Obesity: A Systematic Review. J Acad Nutr Diet. 2012 Apr;112(4):518–26. doi: 10.1016/j.jand.2011.12.001. PMID: 22709702.

Morales I, Berridge KC. "Liking" and "Wanting" in Eating and Food Reward: Brain Mechanisms and Clinical Implications. Physiol Behav. 2020 Dec 1;227:113152. doi: 10.1016/j.physbeh.2020.113152. Epub 2020 Aug 23. PMID: 32846152; PMCID: PMC7655589.

Morio B, Fardet A, Legrand P, Lecerf JM. Involvement of Dietary Saturated Fats, from All Sources or of Dairy Origin Only, in Insulin Resistance and Type 2 Diabetes. Nutr Rev. 2016 Jan;74(1):33–47. doi: 10.1093/nutrit/nuv043. Epub 2015 Nov 5. PMID: 26545916.

Morland KB, Evenson KR. Obesity Prevalence and the Local Food Environment. Health Place. 2009 Jun;15(2):491–95. doi: 10.1016/j.healthplace.2008.09.004. Epub 2008 Oct 7. PMID: 19022700; PMCID: PMC4964264.

Morstein M. *Master Your Diabetes: A Comprehensive, Integrative Approach for Both Type 1 and Type 2 Diabetes* (Chelsea Green Publishing, 2017).

Moss M. Hooked: *Food, Free Will, and How the Food Giants Exploit Our Addictions* (Random House Publishing Group, 2021).

Moyer AE, Rodin J, Grilo CM, et al. Stress-Induced Cortisol Response and Fat Distribution in Women. Obes Res. 1994 May;2(3):255–62. doi: 10.1002/j.1550-8528.1994.tb00055.x. PMID: 16353426.

Mozaffarian D. Dietary and Policy Priorities for Cardiovascular Disease, Diabetes, and Obesity: A Comprehensive Review. Circulation. 2016;133(2):187–225. doi: 10.1161/CIRCULATIONAHA.115.018585.

Mozaffarian D, Rimm EB. Fish Intake, Contaminants, and Human Health: Evaluating the Risks and the Benefits. JAMA. 2006;296:1885–99.

Mullaney JA, Stephens JE, Costello ME, et al. Type 1 Diabetes Susceptibility Alleles Are Associated with Distinct Alterations in the Gut Microbiota. Microbiome. 2018 Feb 17;6(1):35. doi: 10.1186/s40168-018-0417-4.

Musso G, Gambino R, Cassader M. Interactions Between Gut Microbiota and Host Metabolism Predisposing to Obesity and Diabetes. Annu Rev Med. 2011;62:361–80. doi: 10.1146/annurev-med-012510-175505. PMID: 21226616.

Nabhan GP. *Coming Home to Eat: The Pleasures and Politics of Local Food* (WW Norton, 2009).

Nagao T, Hase T, Tokimitsu I. A Green Tea Extract High in Catechins Reduces Body Fat and Cardiovascular Risks in Humans. Obesity (Silver Spring). 2007 Jun;15(6):1473–83. doi: 10.1038/oby.2007.176. PMID: 17557985.

Naik RG, Brooks-Worrell BM, Palmer JP. Latent Autoimmune Diabetes in Adults. J Clin Endocrinol Metab. 2009;94(12):4635–44. doi: 10.1210/jc.2009-1120.

Nakamura M, Sadoshima J. Cardiomyopathy in Obesity, Insulin Resistance and Diabetes. J Physiol. 2020;598:2977–93. doi: 10.1113/JP276747.

Nania R. Pastor Blends Faith, Farms to End Food Insecurity in Black Churches. WTOP News. 2019 Feb 4.

National Academies of Sciences, Engineering, and Medicine. *Environmental Chemicals, the Human Microbiome, and Health Risk: A Research Strategy* (National Academies Press, 2018).

Neel BA, Sargis RM. The Paradox of Progress: Environmental Disruption of Metabolism and the Diabetes Epidemic. Diabetes. 2011;60(7):1838–48. doi: 10.2337/db11-0153.

Nelder M, Cahill F, Zhang H, et al. The Association Between an Addictive Tendency Toward Food and Metabolic Characteristics in the General Newfoundland Population. Front Endocrinol (Lausanne). 2018 Nov 9;9:661. doi: 10.3389/fendo .2018.00661. PMID: 30473679; PMCID: PMC6237829.

Nelson M, Bhandari N, Wener J. Sitagliptin-Induced Pancreatitis—A Longer Road than Expected. Clin Case Rep. 2014 Aug;2(4):149–52. doi: 10.1002/ccr3.83. Epub 2014 Jun 6. PMID: 25356274; PMCID: PMC4184652.

Ng SF, Lin RC, Laybutt DR, et al. Chronic High-Fat Diet in Fathers Programs Beta-Cell Dysfunction in Female Rat Offspring. Nature. 2010;467:963–66.

Nguyen VK, Kahana A, Heidt J, et al. A Comprehensive Analysis of Racial Disparities in Chemical Biomarker Concentrations in United States Women, 1999–2014. Env Int. 2020;137:105496.

Nhoung HK, Goyal M, Cacciapuoti M, et al. Food Insecurity and Insulin Use in Hyperglycemic Patients Presenting to the Emergency Department. West J Emerg Med. 2020;21(4):959–63. Published 2020 Jul 3. doi: 10.5811/westjem.2020.4.45918.

Nicolucci A, Ceriello A, Di Bartolo P, et al. Rapid-Acting Insulin Analogues Versus Regular Human Insulin: A Meta-Analysis of Effects on Glycemic Control in Patients with Diabetes. Diabetes Ther. 2020 Mar;11(3):573–84. doi: 10.1007/s13300-019 -00732-w. Epub 2019 Dec 23. PMID: 31873857; PMCID: PMC7048883.

Nishimura A, Matsumura K, Kikuno S, et al. Slowly Progressive Type 1 Diabetes Mellitus: Current Knowledge and Future Perspectives. Diabetes Metab Syndr Obes. 2019;12:2461–77. Published 2019 Nov 28. doi: 10.2147/DMSO.S191007.

Northwest Medicine Healthbeat website. https://www.nm.org/healthbeat.

Nwadiugwu MC, Bastola DR, Haas C, Russell D. Identifying Glycemic Variability in Diabetes Patient Cohorts and Evaluating Disease Outcomes. J Clin Med. 2021 Apr 2;10(7):1477. doi: 10.3390/jcm10071477. PMID: 33918347; PMCID: PMC8038275.

Ohkuma T, Peters SAE, Woodward M. Sex Differences in the Association Between Diabetes and Cancer: A Systematic Review and Meta-Analysis of 121 Cohorts Including 20 Million Individuals and One Million Events. Diabetologia. 2018;61:2140–54. doi: 10.1007/s00125-018-4664-5.

Oken E, et al. 2008. Maternal Fish Intake During Pregnancy, Blood Mercury Levels, and Child Cognition at Age 3 Years in a US Cohort. Am J Epidemiol. 2008 May 15;167(10):1171–81.

Okla M, Kim J, Koehler K, Chung S. Dietary Factors Promoting Brown and Beige Fat Development and Thermogenesis. Adv Nutr. 2017;8(3):473–83. Published 2017 May 15. doi: 10.3945/an.116.014332.

Oleck J, Kassam S, Goldman JD. Commentary: Why Was Inhaled Insulin a Failure in the Market? Diabetes Spectr. 2016;29(3):180–84. doi: 10.2337/diaspect.29.3.180.

Omran F, Christian M. Inflammatory Signaling and Brown Fat Activity. Front Endocrinol (Lausanne). 2020;11:156. Published 2020 Mar 24. doi: 10.3389/fendo.2020.00156.

O'Neal KS, Johnson JL, Panak RL. Recognizing and Appropriately Treating Latent Autoimmune Diabetes in Adults. Diab Spectr. 2016;29(4):249–52. doi: 10.2337/ds15-0047.

Ong SE, Koh JJK, Toh SES, et al. Assessing the Influence of Health Systems on Type 2 Diabetes Mellitus Awareness, Treatment, Adherence, and Control: A Systematic Review. PLoS One. 2018;13(3):e0195086. Published 2018 Mar 29. doi: 10.1371/journal.pone.0195086.

Oram RA, Sims EK, Evans-Molina C. Beta Cells in Type 1 Diabetes: Mass and Function; Sleeping or Dead? Diabetologia. 2019 Apr;62(4):567–77. doi: 10.1007/s00125-019-4822-4. Epub 2019 Feb 14. PMID: 30767048; PMCID: PMC6688846.

Orr CJ, Keyserling TC, Ammerman AS, Berkowitz SA. Diet Quality Trends Among Adults with Diabetes by Socioeconomic Status in the US: 1999–2014. BMC Endocr Disord. 2019 May 31;19(1):54. doi: 10.1186/s12902-019-0382-3. PMID: 31151439; PMCID: PMC6544994.

Ortega MA, Fraile-Martínez O, Naya I, et al. Type 2 Diabetes Mellitus Associated with Obesity (Diabesity). The Central Role of Gut Microbiota and Its Translational Applications. Nutrients. 2020;12(9):2749. Published 2020 Sep 9. doi: 10.3390/nu12092749.

O'Sullivan TE, Rapp M, Fan X, et al. Adipose-Resident Group 1 Innate Lymphoid Cells Promote Obesity-Associated Insulin Resistance. Immunity. 2016;45(2):428–41. doi: 10.1016/j.immuni.2016.06.016.

Ota M, Matsuo J, Ishida I, et al. Effects of a Medium-Chain Triglyceride-Based Ketogenic Formula on Cognitive Function in Patients with Mild-to-Moderate Alzheimer's Disease. Neurosci Lett. 2019;690:232–36.

Out M, Top WMC, Lehert P, et al. Long-Term Treatment with Metformin in Type 2 Diabetes and Vitamin D Levels: A Post-Hoc Analysis of a Randomized Placebo-Controlled Trial. Diabetes Obes Meab. 2018 Aug;20(8):1951–56. doi: 10.1111/dom.13327. Epub 2018 May 14. PMID: 29667290.

Ovalle F, Grimes T, Xu G, et al. Verapamil and Beta Cell Function in Adults with Recent-Onset Type 1 Diabetes. Nat Med. 2018 Aug;24(8):1108–12. doi: 10.1038/s41591-018-0089-4. Epub 2018 Jul 9. PMID: 29988125; PMCID: PMC6092963.

Owens DR. Clinical Evidence for the Earlier Initiation of Insulin Therapy in Type 2 Diabetes. Diabetes Technol Ther. 2013;15(9):776–85. doi: 10.1089/dia.2013.0081.

Pannett R and Roubein R. "The GOP Blocked an Insulin Price Cap: What It Means for Diabetics." Washington Post. August 8, 2022, updated August 9, 2022.

Paoli A, Tinsley G, Bianco A, Moro T. The Influence of Meal Frequency and Timing on Health in Humans: The Role of Fasting. Nutrients. 2019 Mar 28;11(4):719. doi: 10.3390/nu11040719. PMID: 30925707; PMCID: PMC6520689.

Parker HM, Johnson NA, Burdon CA, et al. Omega-3 Supplementation and Non-Alcoholic Fatty Liver Disease: A Systematic Review and Meta-Analysis. J Hepatol. 2012 Apr;56(4):944–51. doi: 10.1016/j.jhep.2011.08.018. Epub 2011 Oct 21. PMID: 22023985.

Patel MR, Piette JD, Resnicow K, et al. Social Determinants of Health, Cost-Related Non-Adherence, and Cost-Reducing Behaviors Among Adults with Diabetes: Findings from the National Health Interview Survey. Med Care 2016;54:796–803.

Patel R. Foreword. In Wise TA. Eating Tomorrow: Agribusiness, Family Farmers, and the Battle for the Future of Food (New Press, 2019).

Patterson R, McNamara E, Tainio M, et al. Sedentary Behaviour and Risk of All-Cause, Cardiovascular and Cancer Mortality, and Incident Type 2 Diabetes: A Systematic Review and Dose Response Meta-Analysis. Eur J Epidemiol. 2018 Sep;33(9):811–29. doi: 10.1007/s10654-018-0380-1. Epub 2018 Mar 28. PMID: 29589226; PMCID: PMC6133005.

Patterson RE, Sears DD. Metabolic Effects of Intermittent Fasting. Annu Rev Nutr. 2017 Aug 21;37:371–93. doi: 10.1146/annurev-nutr-071816-064634. Epub 2017 Jul 17. PMID: 28715993.

Paun A, Danska JS. Modulation of Type 1 and Type 2 Diabetes Risk by the Intestinal Microbiome. Pediatr Diab. 2016 Nov;17(7):469–77. doi: 10.1111/pedi.12424. Epub 2016 Aug 3. PMID: 27484959.

Paun A, Yau C, Danska JS. The Influence of the Microbiome on Type 1 Diabetes. J Immunol. 2017 Jan 15;198(2):590–95. doi: 10.4049/jimmunol.1601519. PMID: 28069754.

Perrin C, Ewen M, Beran D. The Role of Biosimilar Manufacturers in Improving Access to Insulin Globally. Lancet Diab Endocrinol. 2017 Aug;5(8):578. doi: 10.1016/S2213-8587(17)30218-8. Epub 2017 Jun 16. PMID: 28629907.

Peterson W. A Billion Dollars a Day: The Economics and Politics of Agricultural Subsidies. 2009. Wiley-Blackwell.

Phillips SM, Chevalier S, Leidy HJ. Protein "Requirements" Beyond the RDA: Implications for Optimizing Health. Appl Physiol Nutr Metab. 2016;41(5):565–72. doi: 10.1139/apnm-2015-0550.

Piette JD, Wagner TH, Potter MB, Schillinger D. Health Insurance Status, Cost-Related Medication Underuse, and Outcomes Among Diabetes Patients in Three Systems of Care. Med Care 2004;42:102–09.

Pilkington K, Kirkwood G, Rampes H, Richardson J. Yoga for Depression: The Research Evidence. J Affect Disord. 2005 Dec;89(1–3):13–24. doi: 10.1016/j.jad.2005.08.013. Epub 2005 Sep 26. PMID: 16185770.

Poitelon Y, Kopec AM, Belin S. Myelin Fat Facts: An Overview of Lipids and Fatty Acid Metabolism. Cells. 2020;9(4):812. doi: 10.3390/cells9040812.

Pollan M. *Food Rules: An Eater's Manual* (Penguin, 2009).

Pollan M. *The Omnivore's Dilemma: A Natural History of Four Meals* (Penguin, 2007).

Ponnampalam EN, Mann NJ, Sinclair AJ. Effect of Feeding Systems on Omega-3 Fatty Acids, Conjugated Linoleic Acid and Trans Fatty Acids in Australian Beef Cuts: Potential Impact on Human Health. Asia Pac J Clin Nutr. 2006;15(1):21–29. PMID: 16500874.

Pozzilli P, Pieralice S. Latent Autoimmune Diabetes in Adults: Current Status and New Horizons. Endocrinol Metab. 2018 Jun;33(2):147–59.

Prasad R. The Human Cost of Insulin in America. BBC News. 2019 Mar 14. https://bbc.com/news.

Prieto J, Singh KB, Nnadozie MC, et al. New Evidence in the Pathogenesis of Celiac Disease and Type 1 Diabetes Mellitus: A Systematic Review. Cureus. 2021 Jul 29;13(7):e16721. doi: 10.7759/cureus.16721. PMID: 34513356; PMCID: PMC8405172.

Puckrein GA, Egan BM, Howard G. Social and Medical Determinants of Cardiometabolic Health: The Big Picture. Ethn Dis. 2015;25(4):521–24. Published 2015 Nov 5. doi: 10.18865/ed.25.4.521.

Pursey KM, Stanwell P, Gearhardt AN, et al. The Prevalence of Food Addiction as Assessed by the Yale Food Addiction Scale: A Systematic Review. Nutrients. 2014 Oct 21;6(10):4552–90. doi: 10.3390/nu6104552. PMID: 25338274; PMCID: PMC4210934.

Püschel GP, Henkel J. Dietary Cholesterol Does Not Break Your Heart but Kills Your Liver. Porto Biomed J. 2019;3(1):e12. doi: 10.1016/j.pbj.0000000000000012.

Quigley F. Making Insulin Affordable: Its Cost Is Creating a Crisis. Foreign Affairs. 2017 Mar 13. https://www.foreignaffairs.com/articles/world/2017-03-13/making-insulin-affordable.

Raevuori A, Suokas J, Haukka J, et al. Highly Increased Risk of Type 2 Diabetes in Patients with Binge Eating Disorder and Bulimia Nervosa. Int J Eat Disord. 2015 Sep;48(6):555–62. doi: 10.1002/eat.22334. Epub 2014 Jul 25. PMID: 25060427.

Rajkumar V and Levine SN. Latent Autoimmune Diabetes. [Updated 2022 Jun 21] In StatPearls [Internet]. Treasure Island (FL): StatPearls Publishing, 2022 Jan. https://www.ncbi.nlm.nih.gov/books/NBK557897/.

Ramdath DD, Padhi EM, Sarfaraz S, et al. Beyond the Cholesterol-Lowering Effect of Soy Protein: A Review of the Effects of Dietary Soy and Its Constituents on Risk Factors for Cardiovascular Disease. Nutrients. 2017;9(4):324. doi: 10.3390/nu9040324.

Ramel A, Martinéz A, Kiely M, et al. Beneficial Effects of Long-Chain n-3 Fatty Acids Included in an Energy-Restricted Diet on Insulin Resistance in Overweight and Obese European Young Adults. Diabetologia. 2008 Jul;51(7):1261–68. doi: 10.1007/s00125-008-1035-7. Epub 2008 May 20. PMID: 18491071.

Ramsey L. There's Something Odd About the Way Insulin Prices Change. *Business Insider Australia*. 2016 Sep 18.

Ramu D, Perumal V, Paul SFD. Association of Common Type 1 and Type 2 Diabetes Gene Variants with Latent Autoimmune Diabetes in Adults: A Meta-Analysis. J Diabetes. 2019;11(6):484–96. doi: 10.1111/1753-0407.12879.

Randall L, Begovic J, Hudson M, et al. Recurrent Diabetic Ketoacidosis in Inner-City Minority Patients: Behavioral, Socioeconomic, and Psychosocial Factors. Diabetes Care. 2011;34(9):1891–96. doi: 10.2337/dc11-0701.

Raskin P, Heller S, Honka M, et al. Pulmonary Function Over 2 Years in Diabetic Patients Treated with Prandial Inhaled Technosphere Insulin or Usual Antidiabetes Treatment: A Randomized Trial. Diabetes Obes Metab. 2012 Feb;14(2):163–73. doi: 10.1111/j.1463-1326.2011.01500.x. Epub 2011 Nov 3. PMID: 21951325.

Ravussin E, Beyl RA, Poggiogalle E, et al. Early Time-Restricted Feeding Reduces Appetite and Increases Fat Oxidation But Does Not Affect Energy Expenditure in Humans. Obesity (Silver Spring). 2019 Aug;27(8):1244–54. doi: 10.1002/oby.22518. PMID: 31339000; PMCID: PMC6658129.

Rewers M, Ludvigsson J. Environmental Risk Factors for Type 1 Diabetes. Lancet. 2016;387:2340–48. doi: 10.1016/S0140-6736(16)30507-4.

Richard C, Cristall L, Fleming E, et al. Impact of Egg Consumption on Cardiovascular Risk Factors in Individuals with Type 2 Diabetes and at Risk for Developing Diabetes: A Systematic Review of Randomized Nutritional Intervention Studies. Can J Diab. 2017 Aug;41(4):453–63. doi: 10.1016/j.jcjd.2016.12.002. Epub 2017 Mar 27. PMID: 28359773.

Roberfroid M, Gibson GR, Hoyles L, et al. Prebiotic Effects: Metabolic and Health Benefits. Br J Nutr. 2010 Aug;104(Suppl 2):S1–63. doi: 10.1017/S0007114510003363 .PMID: 20920376.

Rodricks J, Huang Y, Mantus E, Shubat P. Do Interactions Between Environmental Chemicals and the Human Microbiome Need to Be Considered in Risk Assessments? Risk Anal. 2019;39(11):2353–58. doi: 10.1111/risa.13316.

Rodríguez-García C, Sánchez-Quesada C, Toledo E, et al. Naturally Lignan-Rich Foods: A Dietary Tool for Health Promotion? Molecules (Basel). 2019;24(5):917. doi: 10.3390/molecules24050917.

Roep BO, Thomaidou S, van Tienhoven R, Zaldumbide A. Type 1 Diabetes Mellitus as a Disease of the β-Cell (Do Not Blame the Immune System?). Nat Rev Endocrinol. 2021 Mar;17(3):150–61. doi: 10.1038/s41574-020-00443-4. Epub 2020 Dec 8. PMID: 33293704; PMCID: PMC7722981.

Rohrmann S, Overvad K, Bueno-de-Mesquita HB, et al. Meat Consumption and Mortality—Results from the European Prospective Investigation into Cancer and Nutrition. BMC Med. 2013 Mar 7;11:63. doi: 10.1186/1741-7015-11-63. PMID: 23497300; PMCID: PMC3599112.

Rosário PW, Reis JS, Fagundes TA, et al. Latent Autoimmune Diabetes in Adults (LADA): Usefulness of Anti-GAD Antibody Titers and Benefit of Early Insulinization. Arq Bras Endocrinol Metab. 2007;51(1):52–58. doi: 10.1590/s0004-27302007000100009.

Roseboom T. Epidemiological Evidence for the Developmental Origins of Health and Disease: Effects of Prenatal Undernutrition in Humans, J Endocrinol. 2019;242(1):T135–T144.

Rosenfeld CS. Gut Dysbiosis in Animals Due to Environmental Chemical Exposures. Front Cell Infect Microbiol. 2017 Sep 8;7:396. doi: 10.3389/fcimb.2017.00396.

Rosenthal E. When High Prices Mean Needless Death. JAMA Intern Med. 2019;179:114–15.

Roth G. *This Messy Magnificent Life: A Field Guide to Mind, Body, and Soul* (Scribner, 2019).

Roth G. *Women, Food, and God: An Unexpected Path to Almost Everything* (Scribner, 2011).

Rowland C. "A Group of Hospitals Has a Plan to Get Around Congress's Refusal to Lower the Cost of Insulin." *Washington Post*, March 3, 2022.

Rowley ER, Elliott JA, Conner F, et al. Access to Insulin: Patients Will Pave the Way. Lancet Diab Endocrinol. 2017 Jun;5(6):419. doi: 10.1016/S2213-8587(17) 30149-3.

Ruhl J. *Blood Sugar 101: What They Don't Tell You About Diabetes*. 2nd edition (Technion Books, 2015).

Ruhl J. *Your Diabetes Questions Answered: Practical Solutions That Work and Keep on Working* (Technion Books, 2017).

Sable-Smith B. "We're Fighting for Our Lives": Patients Protest Sky-High Insulin Prices. *Morning Edition*. NPR. 2018 Dec 10.

Sainsbury E, Kizirian NV, Partridge SR, et al. Effect of Dietary Carbohydrate Restriction on Glycemic Control in Adults with Diabetes: A Systematic Review and Meta-Analysis. Diab Res Clin Pract. 2018 May;139:239–52. doi: 10.1016/j .diabres.2018.02.026. Epub 2018 Mar 6. PMID: 29522789.

Salehi B, Mishra AP, Nigam M, et al. Resveratrol: A Double-Edged Sword in Health Benefits. Biomedicines. 2018;6(3):91. doi: 10.3390/biomedicines6030091.

Salleh MR. Life Event, Stress and Illness. Malays J Med Sci. 2008;15(4):9–18.

Sallis JF, Floyd MF, Rodríguez DA, Saelens BE. Role of Built Environments in Physical Activity, Obesity, and Cardiovascular Disease. Circulation. 2012 Feb 7;125(5):729–37. doi: 10.1161/CIRCULATIONAHA.110.969022. PMID: 22311885; PMCID: PMC3315587.

Sanllorente A, Lassale C, Soria-Florido MT, et al. Modification of High-Density Lipoprotein Functions by Diet and Other Lifestyle Changes: A Systematic Review of Randomized Controlled Trials. J Clin Med. 2021 Dec 15;10(24):5897. doi: 10.3390/jcm10245897. PMID: 34945193; PMCID: PMC8707678.

Sartorius N. Depression and Diabetes. Dialogues Clin Neurosci. 2018;20(1):47–52. doi: 10.31887/DCNS.2018.20.1/nsartorius.

Saydah S, Imperatore G, Cheng Y, et al. Disparities in Diabetes Deaths Among Children and Adolescents—United States, 2000–2014. MMWR Morb Mortal Wkly Rep. 2017;66:502–05. doi: 10.15585/mmwr.mm6619a4.

Scarpellini E, Tack J. Obesity and Metabolic Syndrome: An Inflammatory Condition. Dig Dis. 2012;30(2):148–53. doi: 10.1159/000336664.

Schecter A, Haffner D, Colacino J, et al. Polybrominated Diphenyl Ethers (PBDEs) and Hexabromocyclodecane (HBCD) in Composite US Food Samples. Environ Health Perspect. 2010 Mar;118(3):357–62. doi: 10.1289/ehp.0901345. Epub 2009 Oct 28. PMID: 20064778; PMCID: PMC2854763.

Schecter A, Päpke O, Tung KC, et al. Polybrominated Diphenyl Ethers Contamination of United States Food. Environ Sci Technol. 2004 Oct 15;38(20):5306–11. doi: 10.1021/es0490830. PMID: 15543730.

Scheen AJ, Van Gaal LF. Le médicament du mois. Sitagliptine (Januvia): incrétino-potentiateur indiqué comme insulinosécrétagogue dans le traitement du diabète de type 2 [Sitagliptine (Januvia): Incretin Enhancer Potentiating Insulin Secretion for the Treatment of Type 2 Diabetes]. Rev Med Liege. 2008 Feb;63(2):105–09. French. PMID: 18372550.

Scheer R, Moss D. "How Does Mercury Get into Fish?" *Scientific American*. Dec 2011.

Scheiner G. *Think Like a Pancreas: A Practical Guide to Managing Diabetes with Insulin*. Revised edition (Da Capo Press, 2011).

Scheithauer TPM, Rampanelli E, Nieuwdorp M, et al. Gut Microbiota as a Trigger for Metabolic Inflammation in Obesity and Type 2 Diabetes. Front Immunol. 2020 Oct 16;11:571731. doi: 10.3389/fimmu.2020.571731. PMID: 33178196; PMCID: PMC7596417.

Schernthaner G, Hink S, Kopp HP, et al. Progress in the Characterization of Slowly Progressive Autoimmune Diabetes in Adult Patients (LADA or Type 1.5 Diabetes). Exp Clin Endocrinol Diabetes. 2001;109(Suppl 2):S94–108. doi: 10.1055/s-2001-18573. PMID: 11460597.

Schmidt, C. Thinking from the Gut. Nature. 2015;518(7540):S12–S14. doi: 10.1038/518S13a.

Schug TT, Janesick A, Blumberg B, Heindel JJ. Endocrine Disrupting Chemicals and Disease Susceptibility. J Steroid Biochem Mol Biol. 2011;127(3–5), 204–15. doi: 10.1016/j.jsbmb.2011.08.007.

Schulte EM, Avena NM, Gearhardt AN. Which Foods May Be Addictive? The Roles of Processing, Fat Content, and Glycemic Load. PLoS One. 2015;10:e0117959.

Schulte EM, Gearhardt AN. Associations of Food Addiction in a Sample Recruited to Be Nationally Representative of the United States. Eur Eat Disord Rev. 2018 Mar;26(2):112–19. doi: 10.1002/erv.2575. Epub 2017 Dec 21. PMID: 29266583.

Schulte EM, Yokum S, Potenza MN, Gearhardt AN. Neural Systems Implicated in Obesity as an Addictive Disorder: From Biological to Behavioral Mechanisms. Prog Brain Res. 2016;223:329–46. doi: 10.1016/bs.pbr.2015.07.011. Epub 2015 Oct 23. PMID: 26806784.

Schultz R. 2017. Feeding Candy to Cows Is Sweet for Their Digestion. *Wisconsin State Journal*. 2017 Jan 29.

Schulz LO, Bennett PH, Ravussin E, et al. Effects of Traditional and Western Environments on Prevalence of Type 2 Diabetes in Pima Indians in Mexico and the US. Diabetes Care. 2006;29(8):1866–71. doi: 10.2337/dc06-0138.

Schwingshackl L, Hoffmann G, Lampousi AM, et al. Food Groups and Risk of Type 2 Diabetes Mellitus: A Systematic Review and Meta-Analysis of Prospective Studies. Eur J Epidemiol. 2017 May;32(5):363–75. doi: 10.1007/s10654-017-0246-y. Epub 2017 Apr 10. PMID: 28397016; PMCID: PMC5506108.

Seligman HK, Lyles C, Marshall MB, Prendergast K, Smith MC, Headings A, Bradshaw G, Rosenmoss S, Waxman E. A Pilot Food Bank Intervention Featuring Diabetes-Appropriate Food Improved Glycemic Control Among Clients in Three States.

Health Aff (Millwood). 2015 Nov;34(11):1956–63. doi: 10.1377/hlthaff.2015.0641 .PMID: 26526255.

Seligman HK, Smith M, Rosenmoss S, Marshall MB, Waxman E. Comprehensive Diabetes Self-Management Support from Food Banks: A Randomized Controlled Trial. Am J Public Health. 2018 Sep;108(9):1227–34. doi: 10.2105/AJPH.2018 .304528. Epub 2018 Jul 19. PMID: 30024798; PMCID: PMC6085038.

Shanahan F, Sheehan D. Microbial Contributions to Chronic Inflammation and Metabolic Disease. Curr Opin Clin Nutr Metab Care. 2016 Jul;19(4):257–62. doi: 10.1097/MCO.0000000000000282. PMID: 27097361.

Shang M, Sun J. Vitamin D/VDR, Probiotics, and Gastrointestinal Diseases. Curr Med Chem. 2017;24(9):876–87. doi: 10.2174/0929867323666161202150008. PMID: 27915988; PMCID: PMC5457364.

Sharma A, Barrett MS, Cucchiara AJ, et al. A Breathing-Based Meditation Intervention for Patients with Major Depressive Disorder Following Inadequate Response to Antidepressants: A Randomized Pilot Study. J Clin Psychiatry. 2017;78(1):e59–e63. doi: 10.4088/JCP.16m10819.

Sharma S, Tripathi P. Gut Microbiome and Type 2 Diabetes: Where We Are and Where to Go? J Nutr Biochem. 2019 Jan;63:101–08. doi: 10.1016/j.jnutbio.2018.10.003. Epub 2018 Oct 11. PMID: 30366260.

Sharp GC, Lawlor DA, Richmond RC, et al. Maternal Pre-Pregnancy BMI and Gestational Weight Gain, Offspring DNA Methylation and Later Offspring Adiposity: Findings from the Avon Longitudinal Study of Parents and Children. Int J Epidemiol. 2015;44:1288–1304.

Sharp GC, Salas LA, Monnereau C, et al. Maternal BMI at the Start of Pregnancy and Offspring Epigenome-Wide DNA Methylation: Findings from the Pregnancy and Childhood Epigenetics (PACE) Consortium. Hum Mol Genet. 2017;26:4067–85.

Shiva V. *Soil Not Oil: Environmental Justice in an Age of Climate Crisis* (North Atlantic Books, 2015).

Shoelson SE, Lee J, Goldfine AB. Inflammation and Insulin Resistance J Clin Invest. 2006;116(7):1793–801. doi: 10.1172/JCI29069. Published correction in J Clin Invest. 2006 Aug;116(8):2308.

Sia HK, Tu ST, Liao PY, et al. A Convenient Diagnostic Tool for Discriminating Adult-Onset Glutamic Acid Decarboxylase Antibody-Positive Autoimmune Diabetes from Type 2 Diabetes: A Retrospective Study. PeerJ. 2020 Feb 14;8:e8610. doi: 10.7717/peerj.8610. PMID: 32095379; PMCID: PMC7025710.

Siddiqui NI. Incretin Mimetics and DPP-4 Inhibitors: New Approach to Treatment of Type 2 Diabetes Mellitus. Mymensingh Med J. 2009 Jan;18(1):113–24. PMID: 19182763.

Siegel K. Yes, There's Such a Thing as Eating Too Healthy. Greatist.com. 2017 Sep 20.

Siegler B. 2005. Halle Berry: My Battle with Diabetes. *Daily Mail.* 2005 Dec 14. https:// dailymail.co.uk.

Silverman J, Krieger J, Kiefer M, et al. The Relationship Between Food Insecurity and Depression, Diabetes Distress and Medication Adherence Among Low-Income Patients with Poorly-Controlled Diabetes. J Gen Intern Med. 2015;30:1476–1480.

Simon MC, Strassburger K, Nowotny B, et al. Intake of *Lactobacillus reuteri* Improves Incretin and Insulin Secretion in Glucose-Tolerant Humans: A Proof of Concept.

Diabetes Care. 2015 Oct;38(10):1827–34. doi: 10.2337/dc14-2690. Epub 2015 Jun 17. PMID: 26084343.

Singh S, Chang HY, Richards TM, et al. Glucagonlike Peptide 1-Based Therapies and Risk of Hospitalization for Acute Pancreatitis in Type 2 Diabetes Mellitus: A Population-Based Matched Case-Control Study. JAMA Intern Med. 2013 Apr 8;173(7):534–39. doi: 10.1001/jamainternmed.2013.2720. PMID: 23440284.

Siri-Tarino PW, Sun Q, Hu FB, Krauss RM. Saturated Fatty Acids and Risk of Coronary Heart Disease: Modulation by Replacement Nutrients. Curr Atheroscler Rep. 2010 Nov;12(6):384–90. doi: 10.1007/s11883-010-0131-6. PMID: 20711693; PMCID: PMC2943062.

Skyler JS. Primary and Secondary Prevention of Type 1 Diabetes. Diabet Med. 2013;30(2):161–69. doi: 10.1111/dme.12100.

Smith LL, Mosley JF 2nd, Parke C, et al. Dulaglutide (Trulicity): The Third Once-Weekly GLP-1 Agonist. P T. 2016;41(6):357–60.

Smith T. Colorado Becomes First State to Pass Bill Capping Insulin Costs. 2019 May 23. Beyondtype1.org.

Snel M, Jonker JT, Schoones J, et al. Ectopic Fat and Insulin Resistance: Pathophysiology and Effect of Diet and Lifestyle Interventions. Int J Endocrinol. 2012;2012:983814. doi: 10.1155/2012/983814. Epub 2012 May 24. PMID: 22675355; PMCID: PMC3366269.

Socal MP, Greene JA. Interchangeable Insulins—New Pathways for Safe, Effective, Affordable Diabetes Therapy. N Engl J Med. 2020 Mar 12;382(11):981–83. doi: 10.1056/NEJMp1916387. PMID: 32160658.

Song Y, Chou EL, Baecker A, et al. Endocrine-Disrupting Chemicals, Risk of Type 2 Diabetes, and Diabetes-Related Metabolic Traits: A Systematic Review and Meta-Analysis. J Diabetes 2016;8:516–32.

Soota K, Telfah M, Ramesh N, et al. Dipeptidyl Peptidase-4 Inhibitor-Induced Acute Pancreatitis: A Complication Well Documented but Under Recognized. Am J Gastroenterol. 2013 Oct;108:S262.

Spadaro L, Magliocco O, Spampinato D, et al. Effects of n-3 Polyunsaturated Fatty Acids in Subjects with Nonalcoholic Fatty Liver Disease. Dig Liver Dis. 2008 Mar;40(3): 194–99. doi: 10.1016/j.dld.2007.10.003. Epub 2007 Dec 4. PMID: 18054848.

Springmann M and Freund F. Options for Reforming Agricultural Subsidies from Health, Climate, and Economic Perspectives. Nat Commun. 2022 13; 82. https://doi.org/10.1038/s41467-021-27645-2.

Stanley T. Life, Death and Insulin. *Washington Post Magazine*. January 7, 2019.

Steinbrecher A, Morimoto Y, Heak S, et al. The Preventable Proportion of Type 2 Diabetes by Ethnicity: The Multiethnic Cohort. Ann Epidemiol. 2011 Jul;21(7):526–35. doi: 10.1016/j.annepidem.2011.03.009. Epub 2011 Apr 16. PMID: 21497517; PMCID: PMC3109209.

Stellman SD, Garfinkel L. Artificial Sweetener Use and One-Year Weight Change Among Women. Prev Med. 1986 Mar;15(2):195–202. doi: 10.1016/0091-7435(86)90089-7. PMID: 3714671.

Stenström G, Gottsäter A, Bakhtadze E, et al. Latent Autoimmune Diabetes in Adults: Definition, Prevalence, Beta-Cell Function, and Treatment. Diabetes. 2005 Dec;54(Suppl 2):S68–72. doi: 10.2337/diabetes.54.suppl_2.s68. PMID: 16306343.

Steur M, Johnson L, Sharp SJ, et al. Dietary Fatty Acids, Macronutrient Substitutions, Food Sources and Incidence of Coronary Heart Disease: Findings From the EPIC–CVD Case–Cohort Study Across Nine European Countries. J Am Heart Assoc. 2021;10:e019814 doi: 10.1161/JAHA.120.019814.

Stratton IM, Adler AI, Neil HA, et al. Association of Glycaemia with Macrovascular and Microvascular Complications of Type 2 Diabetes (UKPDS 35): Prospective Observational Study. BMJ. 2000 Aug 12;321(7258):405–12. doi: 10.1136/bmj.321.7258.405. PMID: 10938048; PMCID: PMC27454.

Street ME, Angelini S, Bernasconi S, et al. Current Knowledge on Endocrine Disrupting Chemicals (EDCs) from Animal Biology to Humans, from Pregnancy to Adulthood: Highlights from a National Italian Meeting. Int J Mol Sci. 2018;19(6):1647. doi: 10.3390/ijms19061647.

Sutton EF, Beyl R, Early KS, et al. Early Time-Restricted Feeding Improves Insulin Sensitivity, Blood Pressure, and Oxidative Stress Even Without Weight Loss in Men with Prediabetes. Cell Metab. 2018 Jun 5;27(6):1212–21.e3. doi: 10.1016/j.cmet.2018.04.010. Epub 2018 May 10. PMID: 29754952; PMCID: PMC5990470.

Szymczak-Pajor I, Drzewoski J, Śliwińska A. The Molecular Mechanisms by Which Vitamin D Prevents Insulin Resistance and Associated Disorders. Int J Mol Sci. 2020;21(18):6644. Published 2020 Sep 11. doi: 10.3390/ijms21186644.

T1International website. https://www.t1international.com.

T1International. Costs and Rationing of Insulin and Diabetes Supplies: Findings from the 2018 T1 International Patient Survey. https://www.t1international.com/media/assets/file/T1International_Report_-_Costs_and_Rationing_of_Insulin__Diabetes_Supplies_2.pdf.

Tabesh M, Azadbakht L, Faghihimani E, et al. Effects of Calcium-Vitamin D Co-Supplementation on Metabolic Profiles in Vitamin D Insufficient People with Type 2 Diabetes: A Randomised Controlled Clinical Trial. Diabetologia. 2014 Oct;57(10):2038–47. doi: 10.1007/s00125-014-3313-x. Epub 2014 Jul 10. PMID: 25005333.

Talib WH, Mahmod AI, Abuarab SF, et al. Diabetes and Cancer: Metabolic Association, Therapeutic Challenges, and the Role of Natural Products. Molecules. 2021 Apr 10;26(8):2179. doi: 10.3390/molecules26082179. PMID: 33920079; PMCID: PMC8070467.

Tao S, Yuan Q, Mao L, et al. Vitamin D Deficiency Causes Insulin Resistance by Provoking Oxidative Stress in Hepatocytes. Oncotarget. 2017;8(40):67605–13. Published 2017 Jun 28. doi: 10.18632/oncotarget.18754.

Tara S. *The Secret Life of Fat: The Science Behind the Body's Least-Understood Organ and What It Means for You* (WW Norton, 2017).

Tay J, Luscombe-Marsh ND, Thompson CH, et al. Comparison of Low- and High-Carbohydrate Diets for Type 2 Diabetes Management: A Randomized Trial. Am J Clin Nutr. 2015 Oct;102(4):780-90. doi: 10.3945/ajcn.115.112581. Epub 2015 Jul 29. PMID: 26224300.

Taylor MK, Sullivan DK, Mahnken JD, et al. Feasibility and Efficacy Data from a Ketogenic Diet Intervention in Alzheimer's Disease. Alzheimers Dement (NY). 2018;4:28–36.

Teare K. One in Four Patients Say They've Skimped on Insulin Because of High Cost. *YaleNews.* 2018 Dec 3.

Temple NJ. Fat, Sugar, Whole Grains and Heart Disease: 50 Years of Confusion. Nutrients. 2018 Jan 4;10(1):39. doi: 10.3390/nu10010039. PMID: 29300309; PMCID: PMC5793267.

Thayer KA, Heindel JJ, Bucher JR, Gallo MA. Role of Environmental Chemicals in Diabetes and Obesity: A National Toxicology Program Workshop Review. Env Health Perspect. 2012;120(6): 779–89.

Thompson PA, Khatami M, Baglole CJ, et al. Environmental Immune Disruptors, Inflammation and Cancer Risk. Carcinogenesis. 2015;36(Suppl 1):S232–S253. doi: 10.1093/carcin/bgv038.

Thompson PJ, Shah A, Ntranos V, et al. Targeted Elimination of Senescent Beta Cells Prevents Type 1 Diabetes. Cell Metab. 2019 May 7;29(5):1045–60.e10. doi: 10.1016/j.cmet.2019.01.021. Epub 2019 Feb 21. PMID: 30799288.

Thornley S, McRobbie H, Eyles H, et al. The Obesity Epidemic: Is Glycemic Index the Key to Unlocking a Hidden Addiction? Med Hypotheses. 2008 Nov;71(5):709–14. doi: 10.1016/j.mehy.2008.07.006. Epub 2008 Aug 13. PMID: 18703288.

Time. The Science of Nutrition: Special *Time* Edition. 2020 May.

Tobias DK, Chen M, Manson JE, et al. Effect of Low-Fat Diet Interventions Versus Other Diet Interventions on Long-Term Weight Change in Adults: A Systematic Review and Meta-Analysis. Lancet Diab Endocrinol. 2015;3(12):968–79.

Tolbert J, Orgera K, Damico A. Key Facts About the Uninsured Population. Kaiser Family Foundation. November 6, 2020. https://www.kff.org/uninsured/issue-brief/key-facts-about-the-uninsured-population/.

Tomiyama AJ, Mann T, Vinas D, et al. Low Calorie Dieting Increases Cortisol. Psychosom Med. 2010;72(4):357–64. doi: 10.1097/PSY.0b013e3181d9523c.

Toni G, Berioli MG, Cerquiglini L, et al. Eating Disorders and Disordered Eating Symptoms in Adolescents with Type 1 Diabetes. Nutrients. 2017;9(8):906. doi: 10.3390/nu9080906.

Tousen Y, Ichimaru R, Kondo T, et al. The Combination of Soy Isoflavones and Resveratrol Preserve Bone Mineral Density in Hindlimb-Unloaded Mice. Nutrients. 2020;12(7):2043. Published 2020 Jul 9. doi: 10.3390/nu12072043.

Trinity College Dublin. Scientists Unearth Vital Link Between Fat, Immunity and Heat Regulation. *Science Daily.* 2018 Apr.

Tromba V, Silvestri F. Vegetarianism and Type 1 Diabetes in Children. Metabol Open. 2021;11100099. doi: 10.1016/j.metop.2021.100099.

Tsao JP, Liu CC, Wang HF, et al. Oral Resveratrol Supplementation Attenuates Exercise-Induced Interleukin-6 but Not Oxidative Stress After a High Intensity Cycling Challenge in Adults. Int J Med Sci. 2021 Mar 18;18(10):2137–45. doi: 10.7150/ijms.55633. PMID: 33859520; PMCID: PMC8040419.

Turner R, Stratton I, Horton V, et al. UKPDS 25: Autoantibodies to Islet-Cell Cytoplasm and Glutamic Acid Decarboxylase for Prediction of Insulin Requirement in Type 2 Diabetes. Lancet. 1997 Nov 1;350(9087):1288–93. doi: 10.1016/s0140-6736(97)03062-6. Published correction in Lancet. 1998 Jan 31;351(9099):376.

UN. World Diabetes Day, Ban Urges Greater Access to Health Foods, Physical Activity. UN News Centre. 2013 Nov 14.

University of Michigan Health System. Sugar Shock: Insulin Costs Tripled in 10 Years, Study Finds: Both Yearly Spending by People with Diabetes, and Cost per Milliliter, up Sharply—Outpacing Costs for Other Blood Sugar Medications. *ScienceDaily*. 2016 Apr 5. https://www.sciencedaily.com/releases/2016/04/160405122030.htm.

University of Texas Medical Branch at Galveston. Brown Fat Protects Against Diabetes, Obesity in Humans. *ScienceDaily*. 2014 Jul 23.

Upreti V, Maitri V, Dhull P, et al. Effect of Oral Vitamin D Supplementation on Glycemic Control in Patients with Type 2 Diabetes Mellitus with Coexisting Hypovitaminosis D: A Parallel Group Placebo Controlled Randomized Controlled Pilot Study. Diab Metab Syndr. 2018 Jul;12(4):509–12. doi: 10.1016/j.dsx.2018.03.008. Epub 2018 Mar 16. PMID: 29580871.

US Bureau of Labor Statistics website. Accessed September 1, 2022. https://www.bls.gov/opub/ted/2017/employment-population-ratio-and-labor-force-participation-rate-by-age.htm.

US Environmental Protection Agency. https://www.epa.gov/international-cooperation/mercury-emissions-global-context. Accessed 2022 Oct 23.

US Geological Survey. https://www.usgs.gov/mission-areas/water-resources/science/mercury. Accessed 23 Oct 2022.

Vaarala O, Atkinson MA, Neu J. The "Perfect Storm" for Type 1 Diabetes: The Complex Interplay Between Intestinal Microbiota, Gut Permeability, and Mucosal Immunity. Diabetes. 2008 Oct;57(10):2555–62. doi: 10.2337/db08-0331. PMID: 18820210; PMCID: PMC2551660.

Vallianou NG, Stratigou T, Tsagarakis S. Metformin and Gut Microbiota: Their Interactions and Their Impact on Diabetes. Hormones (Athens). 2019 Jun;18(2):141–44. doi: 10.1007/s42000-019-00093-w. Epub 2019 Feb 4. PMID: 30719628.

Vallianou NG, Stratigou T, Tsagarakis S. Microbiome and Diabetes: Where Are We Now? Diabetes Res Clin Pract. 2018 Dec;146:111–18. doi: 10.1016/j.diabres.2018.10.008. Epub 2018 Oct 18. PMID: 30342053.

Valsdottir TD, Henriksen C, Odden N, et al. Effect of a Low-Carbohydrate High-Fat Diet and a Single Bout of Exercise on Glucose Tolerance, Lipid Profile and Endothelial Function in Normal Weight Young Healthy Females. Front Physiol. 2019;10:1499. Published 2019 Dec 19. doi: 10.3389/fphys.2019.01499.

Varshavsky JR, Morello-Frosch R, Woodruff TJ, Zota AR. Dietary Sources of Cumulative Phthalates Exposure Among the US General Population in NHANES 2005–2014. Env Int. 2018;115:417–29.

Vecchio I, Tornali C, Bragazzi NL, Martini M. The Discovery of Insulin: An Important Milestone in the History of Medicine. Front Endocrinol (Lausanne). 2018;9:613. Published 2018 Oct 23. doi: 10.3389/fendo.2018.00613.

Vieira G. Dealing with Diabetes Burnout: How to Recharge and Get Back on Track When You Feel Frustrated and Overwhelmed Living with Diabetes. 2014 Demos Medical Publishing.

Vijay-Kumar M, Aitken JD, Carvalho FA. Metabolic Syndrome and Altered Gut Microbiota in Mice Lacking Toll-Like Receptor 5. Science. 2010;328(5975):228–31.

Viollet B, Foretz M. Revisiting the Mechanisms of Metformin Action in the Liver. Ann Endocrinol (Paris). 2013 May;74(2):123–29. doi: 10.1016/j.ando.2013.03.006. Epub 2013 Apr 10. PMID: 23582849.

Viollet B, Guigas B, Sanz Garcia N, et al. Cellular and Molecular Mechanisms of Metformin: An Overview. Clin Sci (London). 2012;122(6):253–70. doi: 10.1042/CS20110386.

Vohl MC, Malagón MM, Ramos-Molina B. Editorial: Dietary Factors, Epigenetics and Their Implications for Human Obesity. Front Endocrinol (Lausanne). 2020;11:601. Published 2020 Aug 28. doi: 10.3389/fendo.2020.00601.

Volk BM, Kunces LJ, Freidenreich DJ, et al. Effects of Step-Wise Increases in Dietary Carbohydrate on Circulating Saturated Fatty Acids And Palmitoleic Acid in Adults with Metabolic Syndrome. PLoS One. 2014;9(11):e113605. Published 2014 Nov 21. doi: 10.1371/journal.pone.0113605.

Volkow ND, Wang GJ, Fowler JS, et al. Food and Drug Reward: Overlapping Circuits in Human Obesity and Addiction. Curr Top Behav Neurosci. 2012;11:1–24.

Volkow ND, Wise RA, Baler R. The Dopamine Motive System: Implications for Drug and Food Addiction. Nat Rev Neurosci. 2017 Nov 16;18(12):741–52. doi: 10.1038/nrn.2017.130. PMID: 29142296.

Vrieze A, Van Nood E, Holleman F. Transfer of Intestinal Microbiota from Lean Donors Increases Insulin Sensitivity in Individuals with Metabolic Syndrome. Gastroenterology. 2012;143(4):913–16.e7.

Walker RJ, Garacci E, Campbell JA, Egede LE. The Influence of Daily Stress on Glycemic Control and Mortality in Adults with Diabetes. J Behav Med. 2020 Oct;43(5):723–31. doi: 10.1007/s10865-019-00109-1. Epub 2019 Oct 15. PMID: 31617047; PMCID: PMC7156304.

Wall R, Ross RP, Fitzgerald GF, Stanton C. Fatty Acids from Fish: The Anti-Inflammatory Potential of Long-Chain Omega-3 Fatty Acids. Nutr Rev. 2010 May;68(5):280–89. doi: 10.1111/j.1753-4887.2010.00287.x. PMID: 20500789.

Walls HL, Johnston D, Tak M, et al. The Impact of Agricultural Input Subsidies on Food and Nutrition Security: A Systematic Review. Food Security. 2018 10;1425–1436.

Wang F, Baden MY, Rexrode KM, Hu FB. 2021. Dietary Fat Intake and the Risk of Stroke: Results from Two Prospective Cohort Studies. J Am Heart Assoc. Abstract 9343. Originally published Circulation. 2021 Nov 8;144:A9343.

Wang LL, Wang Q, Hong Y, Ojo O, et al. The Effect of Low-Carbohydrate Diet on Glycemic Control in Patients with Type 2 Diabetes Mellitus. Nutrients. 2018 May 23;10(6):661. doi: 10.3390/nu10060661. PMID: 29882884; PMCID: PMC6024764.

Wang Q, Liang X, Wang L, et al. Effect of Omega-3 Fatty Acids Supplementation on Endothelial Function: A Meta-Analysis of Randomized Controlled Trials. Atherosclerosis. 2012 Apr;221(2):536–43. doi: 10.1016/j.atherosclerosis.2012.01.006. Epub 2012 Jan 20. PMID: 22317966.

Wang X, Zhao X, Dorje T, et al. Glycemic Variability Predicts Cardiovascular Complications in Acute Myocardial Infarction Patients with Type 2 Diabetes Mellitus. Int J Cardiol. 2014 Mar 15;172(2):498–500. doi: 10.1016/j.ijcard.2014.01.015. Epub 2014 Jan 21. PMID: 24529823.

Wang Z, Klipfell E, Bennett BJ. Gut Flora Metabolism of Phosphatidylcholine Promotes Cardiovascular Disease. Nature. 2011;472(7341):57–63.

Wei Q, Qi L, Lin H, et al. Pathological Mechanisms in Diabetes of the Exocrine Pancreas: What's Known and What's to Know. Front Physiol. 2020;11:570276. Published 2020 Oct 28. doi: 10.3389/fphys.2020.570276.

Wenclewska S, Szymczak-Pajor I, Drzewoski J, et al. Vitamin D Supplementation Reduces Both Oxidative DNA Damage and Insulin Resistance in the Elderly with Metabolic Disorders. Int J Mol Sci. 2019 Jun 13;20(12):2891. doi: 10.3390/ijms20122891. PMID: 31200560; PMCID: PMC6628266.

Wenxia Lu, Sainan Li, Jingjing Li, et al. Effects of Omega-3 Fatty Acid in Nonalcoholic Fatty Liver Disease: A Meta-Analysis. Gastroenterol Res Pract. 2016;2016:1459790. doi: 10.1155/2016/1459790.

Wessels I, Rink L. Micronutrients in Autoimmune Diseases: Possible Therapeutic Benefits of Zinc and Vitamin D. J Nutr Biochem. 2020 Mar;77:108240. doi: 10.1016/j.jnutbio.2019.108240. Epub 2019 Oct 30. PMID: 31841960.

Westman EC, Tondt J, Maguire E, Yancy WS Jr. Implementing a Low-Carbohydrate, Ketogenic Diet to Manage Type 2 Diabetes Mellitus. Expert Rev Endocrinol Metab. 2018 Sep;13(5):263–72. doi: 10.1080/17446651.2018.1523713. PMID: 30289048.

Whiteman H. Type 1 Diabetes: Does the Gut Hold the Key to Prevention? *Medical News Today.* 2018 Feb 20.

Wilkin TJ. The Accelerator Hypothesis: Weight Gain as the Missing Link Between Type I and Type II Diabetes. Diabetologia. 2001 Jul;44(7):914–22. doi: 10.1007/s001250100548. PMID: 11508279.

Williamson G, Sheedy K. Effects of Polyphenols on Insulin Resistance. Nutrients. 2020 Oct 14;12(10):3135. doi: 10.3390/nu12103135. PMID: 33066504; PMCID: PMC7602234.

Willner S, Whittemore R, Keene D. "Life or Death": Experiences of Insulin Insecurity Among Adults with Type 1 Diabetes in the United States. SSM Popul Health. 2020;11:100624. Published 2020 Jun 27. doi: 10.1016/j.ssmph.2020.100624.

Wilson P. Death of the Calorie. *The Economist: 1843.* 2019 Apr–May.

Wimalawansa SJ. Associations of Vitamin D with Insulin Resistance, Obesity, Type 2 Diabetes, and Metabolic Syndrome. J Steroid Biochem Mol Biol. 2018 Jan;175:177–89. doi: 10.1016/j.jsbmb.2016.09.017. Epub 2016 Sep 20. PMID: 27662816.

Wiss DA, Avena N, Rada P. Sugar Addiction: From Evolution to Revolution. Front Psychiatry. 2018;9:545. Published 2018 Nov 7. doi: 10.3389/fpsyt.2018.00545.

Wiss DA, Brewerton TD. Incorporating Food Addiction into Disordered Eating: The Disordered Eating Food Addiction Nutrition Guide (DEFANG). Eat Weight Disord. 2017 Mar;22(1):49–59. doi: 10.1007/s40519-016-0344-y. Epub 2016 Dec 10. PMID: 27943202; PMCID: PMC5334442.

Wiss DA, Brewerton T. Separating the Signal from the Noise: How Psychiatric Diagnoses Can Help Discern Food Addiction from Dietary Restraint. Nutrients. 2020 Sep 25;12(10):2937. doi: 10.3390/nu12102937. PMID: 32992768; PMCID: PMC7600542.

World Health Organization website. https://www.who.int. Accessed 2021 Mar.

World Health Organization. Aflatoxins. Food Safety Digest. 2018 Feb. Ref no. WHO/NHM/FOS/RAM/18.1.

Wu G. Dietary Protein Intake and Human Health. Food Funct. 2016;7;3:1251–65. doi: 10.1039/c5fo01530h.

Wu GD, Chen J, Hoffmann C, et al. Linking Long-Term Dietary Patterns with Gut Microbial Enterotypes. Science. 2011;334(6052):105–08. doi: 10.1126/science.1208344.

Wu L, Piotrowski K, Rau T, et al. Walnut-Enriched Diet Reduces Fasting Non-HDL-Cholesterol and Apolipoprotein B in Healthy Caucasian Subjects: A Randomized Controlled Cross-Over Clinical Trial. Metabolism. 2014 Mar;63(3):382–91. doi: 10.1016/j.metabol.2013.11.005.

Xu F, Liu J, Na L, Chen L. Roles of Epigenetic Modifications in the Differentiation and Function of Pancreatic β-Cells. Front Cell Dev Biol. 2020;8:748. Published 2020 Aug 28. doi: 10.3389/fcell.2020.00748.

Xu H, Liu M, Cao J, et al. The Dynamic Interplay Between the Gut Microbiota and Autoimmune Diseases. J Immunol Res. 2019 Oct 27;2019:7546047. doi: 10.1155/2019/7546047. PMID: 31772949; PMCID: PMC6854958.

Xu R, Bai Y, Yang K, Chen G. Effects of Green Tea Consumption on Glycemic Control: A Systematic Review and Meta-Analysis of Randomized Controlled Trials. Nutr Metab (London). 2020 Jul 10;17:56. doi: 10.1186/s12986-020-00469-5. PMID: 32670385; PMCID: PMC7350188.

Yamada T, Kamata R, Ishinohachi K, et al. Biosimilar vs Originator Insulins: Systematic Review and Meta-Analysis. Diabetes Obes Metab. 2018 Jul;20(7):1787–92. doi: 10.1111/dom.13291. Epub 2018 Apr 17. PMID: 29536603.

Yamada Y, Uchida J, Izumi H, et al. A Non-Calorie-Restricted Low-Carbohydrate Diet Is Effective as an Alternative Therapy for Patients with Type 2 Diabetes. Intern Med. 2014;53(1):13–19. doi: 10.2169/internalmedicine.53.0861. PMID: 24390522.

Yamamoto EA, Jørgensen TN. Relationships Between Vitamin D, Gut Microbiome, and Systemic Autoimmunity. Front Immunol. 2020 Jan 21;10:3141. doi: 10.3389/fimmu.2019.03141. PMID: 32038645; PMCID: PMC6985452.

Yan J, Zhao Y, Zhao B. Green Tea Catechins Prevent Obesity Through Modulation of Peroxisome Proliferator-Activated Receptors. Sci China Life Sci. 2013 Sep;56(9):804–10. doi: 10.1007/s11427-013-4512-2. Epub 2013 Jul 12. PMID: 23864528.

Yan K. Medicaid and CGM: Who's Covered? DiaTribe.org. 2019 Nov 21. https://diatribe.org/medicaid-cgm.

Yang F, Liu A, Li Y, et al. Food Addiction in Patients with Newly Diagnosed Type 2 Diabetes in Northeast China. Front Endocrinol (Lausanne). 2017;8:218. Published 2017 Aug 30. doi: 10.3389/fendo.2017.00218.

Yang O, Kim HL, Weon JI, Seo YR. Endocrine-Disrupting Chemicals: Review of Toxicological Mechanisms Using Molecular Pathway Analysis. Journal Cancer Prev. 2015;20(1):12–24. doi: 10.15430/JCP.2015.20.1.12.

Yang Q. Gain Weight by "Going Diet"? Artificial Sweeteners and the Neurobiology of Sugar Cravings. Yale J Biol Med. 2010;83(2):101–08.

Yang SN, Hsieh CC, Kuo HF, et al. The Effects of Environmental Toxins on Allergic Inflammation. Allergy Asthma Immunol Res. 2014;6(6):478–84. doi: 10.4168/aair.2014.6.6.478.

Yap YA, Mariño E. An Insight into the Intestinal Web of Mucosal Immunity, Microbiota, and Diet in Inflammation. Front Immunol. 2018 Nov 20;9:2617. doi: 10.3389/fimmu.2018.02617. PMID: 30532751; PMCID: PMC6266996.

Yingling L, Allen NA, Litchman ML, et al. An Evaluation of Digital Health Tools for Diabetes Self-Management in Hispanic Adults: Exploratory Study. JMIR Diabetes. 2019;4(3):e12936. Published 2019 Jul 16. doi: 10.2196/12936.

Yoo JY, Groer M, Dutra SVO, et al. Gut Microbiota and Immune System Interactions. Microorganisms. 2020 Oct 15;8(10):1587. doi: 10.3390/microorganisms8101587. PMID: 33076307; PMCID: PMC7602490. Published correction in Microorganisms. 2020 Dec 21;8(12).

Yu E, Hu FB. Dairy Products, Dairy Fatty Acids, and the Prevention of Cardiometabolic Disease: A Review of Recent Evidence. Current Atheroscler Rep. 2018;20(5):24. doi: 10.1007/s11883-018-0724-z.

Yu R, Y-Hua L, Hong L. Depression in Newly Diagnosed Type 2 Diabetes. Int J Diabetes Dev Ctries. 2010;30(2):102–04. doi: 10.4103/0973-3930.62601.

Zampetti S, Campagna G, Tiberti C, et al. High GADA Titer Increases the Risk of Insulin Requirement in LADA Patients: A 7-Year Follow-Up (NIRAD Study 7). Eur J Endocrinol. 2014 Dec;171(6):697–704. doi: 10.1530/EJE-14-0342. Epub 2014 Sep 11. PMID: 25213702.

Zampetti S, Capizzi M, Spoletini M, et al. GADA Titer-Related Risk for Organ-Specific Autoimmunity in LADA Subjects Subdivided According to Gender (NIRAD Study 6). J Clin Endocrinol Metab. 2012 Oct;97(10):3759–65. doi: 10.1210/jc.2012-2037. Epub 2012 Aug 3. PMID: 22865904.

Zeevi D, Korem T, Zmora N, et al. Personalized Nutrition by Prediction of Glycemic Responses. Cell. 2015 Nov 19;163(5):1079–94. doi: 10.1016/j.cell.2015.11.001. PMID: 26590418.

Zhao Y, Yang L, Xiang Y, et al. Dipeptidyl Peptidase 4 Inhibitor Sitagliptin Maintains β-Cell Function in Patients with Recent-Onset Latent Autoimmune Diabetes in Adults: One Year Prospective Study. J Clin Endocrinol Metab. 2014 May 1;99(5):E876–E880. doi: 10.1210/jc.2013-3633.

Zhong T, Tang R, Gong S, et al. The Remission Phase in Type 1 Diabetes: Changing Epidemiology, Definitions, and Emerging Immuno-Metabolic Mechanisms. Diabetes Metab Res Rev. 2020 Feb;36(2):e3207. doi: 10.1002/dmrr.3207. Epub 2019 Aug 13. PMID: 31343814.

Zhou H, Sun L, Zhang S, et al. Evaluating the Causal Role of Gut Microbiota in Type 1 Diabetes and Its Possible Pathogenic Mechanisms. Front Endocrinol. 2020;11. doi: 10.3389/fendo.2020.00125.

Zhou Z, Xia L. [Latent Autoimmune Diabetes in Adults: An Update.] Acta Academiae Medicinae Sinicae. 2003;25(5):630–34.

Zhu X, Han Y, Du J, et al. Microbiota-Gut-Brain Axis and the Central Nervous System. Oncotarget. 2017 May 10;8(32):53829–38. doi: 10.18632/oncotarget.17754. PMID: 28881854; PMCID: PMC5581153.

Zota AR, Calafat AM, Woodruff TJ. Temporal Trends in Phthalate Exposures: Findings from the National Health and Nutrition Examination Survey, 2001–2010. Env Health Perspect. 2014;122(3):235–41. doi: 10.1289/ehp.1306681.

Zota AR, Phillips CA, Mitro SD. 2016. Recent Fast Food Consumption and Bisphenol A and Phthalates Exposures Among the US Population in NHANES, 2003–2010. Env Health Perspect. 2016;124(10):1521–28.

Zubrzycki A, Cierpka-Kmiec K, Kmiec Z, Wronska A. The Role of Low-Calorie Diets and Intermittent Fasting in the Treatment of Obesity and Type-2 Diabetes. J Physiol Pharmacol. 2018 Oct;69(5). doi: 10.26402/jpp.2018.5.02. Epub 2019 Jan 21. PMID: 30683819.

NOTES

PART I.

CHAPTER ONE: WHAT THE HECK IS LADA?

1. Hernández 2021, O'Neal 2016, Laugesen 2015
2. Liu 2020, Carlsson 2019a, Nishimura 2019, Pozzilli 2018, Buzzetti 2017, Groop 2006, Zhou 2003
3. Fourlanos 2005
4. Rajkumar 2022
5. Hawa 2013
6. Huang 2021, Groop 1986
7. Rajkumar 2022, Jörns 2020, Naik 2009, Fourlanos 2005
8. Pozzilli 2018, O'Neal 2016, Calsolari 2008
9. Hostalek 2019, Lin 2018, Boyle 2010, Live Science 2010

CHAPTER TWO: DIABETES? INCONCEIVABLE!

1. O'Neal 2016
2. Vecchio 2018

CHAPTER THREE: WHY ARE THERE MANY TYPES OF DIABETES?

1. Gale 2005
2. Guglielmi 2012
3. Carlsson 2019a, Nishimura 2019, O'Neal 2016, Zhou 2003
4. Jang 2020, Harvard Medical School 2019, Juszczak 2016, McDonald 2013
5. Maddaloni 2020
6. Owens 2013, Maruyama 2008, Rosário 2007, Zhou 2003
7. See chapter 12 and also Pozzilli 2018, Harrar 2016, O'Neal 2016, Brophy 2008, Calsolari 2008

CHAPTER FOUR: FROM BURNOUT TO HOPE

1. Schernthaner 2001
2. Sia 2020
3. Hals 2019
4. Jeon 2018, Kalra 2018, Sartorius 2018, Holt 2014, Mendenhall 2014, Yu 2010, Katon 2005, Ciechanowski 2003, Fisher 2001, Lloyd 2000, Gavard 1993
5. Vieira 2014 is a fun, insightful resource; there are many support services for depression, anxiety, or anger, some free or covered by insurance; in a mental health crisis we can dial 988.
6. Carré 2021, Roep 2021, Mallone 2020, Oram 2019, Thompson 2019
7. Roep 2021
8. Buzzetti 2020

CHAPTER FIVE: SYMPTOMS? WHAT SYMPTOMS?

1. Harrar 2016
2. O'Neal 2016
3. *Charlotte Observer* 2008
4. Siegler 2005

CHAPTER SIX: CAN I CURE MY DIABETES?

1. Ling 2019
2. Carlsson 2019a
3. Kolb 2020
4. Nakamura 2020
5. Nakamura 2020, Jialal 2019
6. Harvard Medical School 2020
7. Bungau 2020, CDC 2020, Morstein 2017
8. Jialal 2019
9. Nakamura 2020
10. Buzzetti 2017
11. Morstein 2017
12. Scheiner 2011
13. Mayo Clinic website
14. Morstein 2017
15. ADA 2020, Chen 2016
16. CDC 2020
17. Morstein 2017
18. Cohut 2018, Ohkuma 2018
19. ACCORD 2008
20. Morstein 2017
21. Morstein 2017
22. Bernstein 2011
23. Stratton 2000

24. Nwadiugwu 2021, Hwang 2019, Cardoso 2018, Hirsch 2015, Wang 2014
25. Hirsch 2015
26. Ruhl 2017, Standards 2014
27. Carlsson 2019a, Hjort R 2018b, Wilkin 2001
28. Naik 2009
29. Wei 2020
30. Morstein 2017

CHAPTER SEVEN: IS THIS MY FAULT?

1. Andersen 2019
2. Attia 2013
3. Rewers 2016
4. Carlsson 2019a, Steinbrecher 2011, Laaksonen 2010
5. Mishra 2020, Andersen 2019, Carlsson 2019a, Cousminer 2018, Hjort R 2018b, Hjort R 2017
6. Andersen 2020, Heneberg 2018
7. Heneberg 2018
8. Mishra 2017
9. Mishra 2020, Andersen 2019, Carlsson 2019a, Mishra 2017
10. Carlsson 2019a, Hjort R 2017
11. Loh 2019
12. Carlsson 2019a, Loh 2019, Dobosz 2018
13. Lyssenko 2013
14. Mishra 2020, Carlsson 2019a, Mishra 2017
15. Löfvenborg 2020, Hjort R 2019, Ramu 2019
16. Andersen 2020, Heneberg 2018
17. Vohl 2020, Carlsson 2019a, Fernandez-Twinn 2019, Ling 2019, Loh 2019, Roseboom 2019, Donkin 2018, Hjort L 2018, Hjort R 2018b, Sharp 2017, Allard 2015, Denham 2015, Jorgensen 2015, Sharp 2015, Choi 2013, Ng 2010, Heijmans 2008, Kaati 2002
18. Xu 2020, Ling 2019, Loh 2019, Dobosz 2018
19. Löfvenborg 2021, Giwa 2020, Löfvenborg 2020, Carlsson 2019a, Hjort R 2018a, Patterson 2018, Chen 2017, Kolb 2017, Morstein 2017, Schwingshackl 2017, Shanahan 2016, Smith 2016, Biswas 2015, Daft 2015, Li 2015, Laaksonen 2010, Gross 2004
20. Rewers 2016
21. Giwa 2020, Carlsson 2019a, Rewers 2016, Skyler 2013
22. Carlsson 2019a, Carlsson 2019b, Dobosz 2018, Schwingshackl 2017, Smith 2016
23. Liu 2015
24. Al-Goblan 2014
25. Kaplan 2017
26. Ruhl 2017
27. Hill-Briggs 2021, Hu 2021, CDC 2020, Divers 2020, Babar 2019, Beran 2018b, Fortmann 2019, Chow 2018, den Braver 2018, CDC 2017, Saydah 2017, Beran 2016, López 2016, Link 2009, Schulz 2006, Hwang 2000

PART II.

CHAPTER EIGHT: OUR DIABETIC SUPERPOWER

1. Miles 2022
2. Carlsson 2019a
3. Barnard 2007
4. Morstein 2017
5. Ruhl 2017
6. Hirsch 2018, Joubert 2012, Bailey 2007
7. Bolla 2019
8. Morstein 2017
9. Morstein 2017

BIG PICTURE 2

1. Hu 2021, CDC 2020, Wilner 2020, Babar 2019, Fortmann 2019, Stanley 2019, Yingling 2019, Beran 2018a, den Braver 2018, Wiss 2018, CDC 2017, Quigley 2017, Saydah 2017, Beran 2016, López 2016, Christine 2015, Puckrein 2015, Link 2009, Morland 2009
2. Hill-Briggs 2021, Hu 2021, Divers 2020, Burke 2019, den Braver 2018, Wiss 2018, Doucette 2017, Saydah 2017, Beckles 2016, Christine 2015, Puckrein 2015

CHAPTER NINE: ROAD MAP, NOT REPORT CARD

1. Ruhl 2015
2. Scheiner 2011
3. Morstein 2017
4. Bernstein 2011
5. Scheiner 2011

CHAPTER TEN: WHY DO WE HAVE FAT?

1. Omran 2020
2. Wilson 2019
3. Ludwig 2018, Mozaffarian 2016
4. Attia 2013, Snel 2012
5. Omran 2020, Snel 2012
6. Hjort R 2019, Scheiner 2011
7. Carlsson 2019a, Hjort R 2018b
8. Al-Goblan 2014
9. Schulz 2006
10. Meza-Perez 2018
11. Al-Goblan 2014
12. Omran 2020, Kaisanlahti 2019, Trinity College Dublin 2018, Okla 2017, Chondronikola 2014
13. University of Texas 2014

14. Omran 2020, Kaisanlahti 2019, Iwen 2017, Okla 2017
15. Tara 2017
16. Melitas 2018, Snel 2012
17. Tara 2017
18. Chaurasia 2020
19. Tara 2017

CHAPTER ELEVEN: TEND THE INNER GARDEN

1. Guo 2020
2. Yap 2018
3. Scheithauer 2020, Yoo 2020, Francisco 2018, Gilbert 2018, Vallianou 2018, O'Sullivan 2016, Shanahan 2016, Scarpellini 2012
4. Cimons 2020, Felman 2020, Lacourt 2018, Mendes 2018, Bonaccio 2016
5. Castelblanco 2018
6. Scarpellini 2012, Shoelson 2006
7. Harvard Medical School 2020
8. Minihane 2015
9. *Harvard Health Letter* 2006
10. *Harvard Health Letter* 2006
11. Farzi 2019, Johnson 2018, Huang 2016, Cryan 2012
12. Gilbert 2018
13. Bielka 2022
14. Gilbert 2018
15. Gilbert 2018
16. Bibbò 2017
17. Zhou 2020, Han 2018
18. Fuhri Snethlage 2021, Ghorbani 2021, Gradisteanu Pircalabioru 2021, Sharma 2019, Han 2018, Bibbò 2017, Brunkwall 2017, Paun 2017, Paun 2016, He 2015, Mejía-León 2015
19. Zhou 2020, Bibbò 2017
20. Whiteman 2018
21. Bielka 2022
22. Fang 2021
23. Al Theyab 2020, Ding 2020, Ortega 2020, Roberfroid 2020, Caesar 2019, Kyriachenko 2019, Xu 2019, Vallianou 2018, Breit 2018, Felix 2018, Mullaney 2018, Levy 2017, Forslund 2015, Musso 2011
24. Hamilton-Williams 2021
25. Bremner 2020, Kuwahara 2020, Farzi 2019, Bliss 2018, Chen 2017, Zhu 2017, Carabotti 2015
26. Forslund 2015
27. Li 2021, Zeevi 2015, David 2014, Wu 2011
28. Moffa 2019, Vrieze 2012, Wang 2011, Vijay-Kumar 2010
29. Aguirre 2015
30. Gilbert 2018
31. Gilbert 2018

32. Blaser 2017
33. Gilbert 2018
34. Huizen 2017
35. Bellerba 2021, Akimbekov 2020, Battistini 2020, Yamamoto 2020, Dimitrov 2017, Jin 2015

CHAPTER TWELVE: THE SKINNY ON MEDS

1. Pozzilli 2018
2. Foretz 2019
3. Viollet 2013
4. Ding 2020, Kim 2020, Caesar 2019, Kyriachenko 2019, Foretz 2019, Vallianou 2019, Forslund 2015
5. Ding 2020, Kim 2020, Kyriachenko 2019, Viollet 2012
6. Kyriachenko 2019
7. Beysel 2018
8. Kos 2012
9. Out 2018
10. Pozzilli 2018
11. Pozzilli 2018, Brophy 2011, Kobayashi 2002
12. Kyriachenko 2019, Siddiqui 2009
13. Pozzilli 2018, Lee 2017, Laugesen 2015, Zhao 2014, Aaboe 2010, Siddiqui 2009, Scheen 2008
14. Akimbekov 2020, Alkayali 2020, Buse 2017, Nelson 2014, Singh 2013, Soota 2013
15. Smith 2016
16. Kyriachenko 2019
17. Dupuis 2021, Abboud 2020, Shang 2017
18. Bellan 2020, Szymczak-Pajor 2020, Wessels 2020, Wenclewska 2019, Upreti 2018, Berridge 2017, Mirhosseini 2017, Tao 2017, Al-Shoumer 2015, Al-Goblan 2014, Dutta 2014, Tabesh 2014, Brophy 2011, Mitri 2011, Maahs 2010
19. Wimalawansa 2018
20. Leung 2016
21. Li 2009
22. Bellan 2020, Giwa 2020, Beysel 2018
23. Lemieux 2019
24. Abboud 2020, Shang 2017
25. Abboud 2020
26. Szymczak-Pajor 2020
27. Tara 2017
28. O'Neal 2016

CHAPTER THIRTEEN: EMBRACING INSULIN

1. Stenström 2005
2. Pozzilli 2018
3. Morstein 2017

4. Owens 2013
5. Brophy 2011, Maruyama 2008, Rosario 2007, Stenström 2005, Kobayashi 2002
6. Rajkumar 2022, Leighton 2017, Kumar 2016
7. Rosário 2007, Kobayashi 2002
8. Buzzetti 2020
9. Scheiner 2011
10. Nicolucci 2020, Grunberger 2014, Scheiner 2011
11. Oleck 2016, Raskin 2012
12. McGill 2020
13. Mikhail 2017, Oleck 2016
14. Mikhail 2017
15. Heinemann 2018, Heinemann 2017
16. Mikhail 2017
17. Mikhail 2017
18. Karges 2017, Scheiner 2011
19. Scheiner 2011
20. Morstein 2017
21. Scheiner 2011
22. Scheiner 2011
23. Drexler 2004
24. Morstein 2017
25. *Daily Show* 2019

CHAPTER FOURTEEN: MIND THE MIND

1. Farzi 2019
2. *Daily Show* 2019
3. Walker 2020, Harris 2017, Liu 2017, Harris 2013, Salleh 2008, Black 2006, Black 2002
4. Klatzkin 2018, Moore 2012, Moyer 1994
5. Fatahia 2021, Bear 2020, Bremner 2020, Cimons 2020, Breit 2018, Lach 2018, Huang 2016, Hashmi 2013, Dantzer 2008
6. davidji 2015
7. Bolte 2009
8. Donofry 2020, Breit 2018, Sharma 2017, Hashmi 2013, Pilkington 2005
9. *Time* 2020

PART III.

CHAPTER FIFTEEN: MY JOURNEY TO CRAFTY

1. Morstein 2017

CHAPTER SIXTEEN: CARB-CRAFT FUNDAMENTALS

1. Mozaffarian 2016
2. Imamura 2016, Rohrmann 2013, Micha 2010
3. Löfvenborg 2021

4. Kessler 2020
5. Bittman 2021
6. Gross 2004
7. Lennerz 2013
8. Scheiner 2011
9. Di Francesco 2018
10. Chung 2020, de Cabo 2020, Hwangbo 2020, Lichtash 2020, Anton 2019, Grajower 2019, Paoli 2019, Ravussin 2019, Di Francesco 2018, Furmli 2018, Harris 2018, Sutton 2018, Zubrzycki 2018, Cheng 2017, Golbidi 2017, Mattson 2017, Patterson 2017, Brandhorst 2015, Kahleova 2015, Mattson 2014, Horne 2012
11. Anton 2019, Paoli 2019, Anton 2018, Di Francesco 2018
12. Paoli 2018, Sutton 2018
13. Anton 2019, Ravussin 2019, Kahleova 2015
14. Ho 1988
15. Sutton 2018
16. Cheng 2017, Brandhorst 2015
17. Cheng 2017
18. Grajower 2019
19. Tara 2017
20. Anton 2019
21. Anton 2019
22. Wilson 2019
23. Wilson 2019, Ludwig 2018, Wiss 2018, Camacho 2017, Mozaffarian 2016, Lucan 2015
24. Ludwig 2018
25. Camacho 2017
26. Mozaffarian 2016
27. Patel 2019
28. Phillips 2016, Wu 2016
29. *Time* 2020, Wu 2016

CHAPTER SEVENTEEN: SHOULD WE EAT FAT?

1. DiNicolantonio 2016
2. Ludwig 2020
3. Leslie 2016
4. Dehghan 2017
5. Temple 2018
6. Steur 2021, Astrup 2020, Püschel 2019, Temple 2018, Dehghan 2017, Drouin-Chartier 2016, Mensink 2016, Morio 2016, Berger 2015, DiNicolantonio 2015, Forsythe 2010
7. Astrup 2020
8. Valsdottir 2019, Kosinski 2017, Morio 2016, Gower 2015
9. Löfvenborg 2021, Imamura 2016, Rohrmann 2013, Micha 2010
10. Löfvenborg 2021, Berry 2019, Temple 2018, Drouin-Chartier 2016, Imamura 2016, Morio 2016, Rohrmann 2013, Micha 2010

11. Temple 2018, Morio 2016
12. Wang 2021, Dehghan 2017
13. Ericson 2015
14. Alvarez-Bueno 2019, Mena-Sánchez 2019, Yu 2018, Gijsbers 2016, Kim 2016
15. Imamura 2016, Morio 2016, Mozaffarian 2016
16. Mozaffarian 2016
17. DiNicolantonio 2016
18. Mozaffarian 2016
19. Astrup 2020
20. Baynes 2018
21. Coletta 2010, Innis 2008, Oken 2008
22. Nakamura 2020, Carlsson 2019b, Jialal 2019, Baynes 2018, Bamberger 2017, Calder 2017, Chauhan 2017, Minihane 2016, Mozaffarian 2016, Wenxia 2016, Beydoun 2015, Chen C 2015, Jain 2015, Jeromson 2015, Logan 2015, Martínez-Fernández 2015, Marventano 2015, Wu 2014, Liu 2013, Parker 2012, Wang Q 2012, Kiecolt-Glaser 2011, Wall 2010, Banel 2009, Hartweg 2008, Ramel 2008, Spadaro 2008
23. Harvard Medical School 2019
24. Kirwan 2018, Daley 2010, Ponnampalam 2006
25. Hua 2020, Fan 2019, Baynes 2018, Calder 2017, Jeromson 2015, Logan 2015, Ramel 2008
26. Abbasnezhad 2020, Alarim 2020, Chen 2020, Choi 2020, Lichtash 2020, Ludwig 2020, Athinarayanan 2019, Bolla 2019, Hallberg 2019, Kuchkuntla 2019, Gershuni 2018, Lennerz 2018, Leow 2018, Sainsbury 2018, Wang LL 2018, Mancini 2016, Tay 2015, Tobias 2015, Yamada 2014, Bueno 2013, Krebs 2013, Hussain 2012
27. Forsythe 2010
28. Ota 2019, Taylor 2018
29. Ludwig 2020
30. Lennerz 2018
31. Ludwig 2020
32. Bolla 2019, Lennerz 2018, Leow 2018, Krebs 2016
33. Westman 2018
34. Püschel 2019
35. Sanllorente 2021

CHAPTER EIGHTEEN: PROS AND CONS OF SPECIFIC FOODS AND DIETS

1. Harjo 2021
2. Carlsson 2019b, Chauhan 2017, Del Gobbo 2016, Chen C 2015, Jain 2015, Marventano 2015, Mozaffarian 2006
3. US Environmental Protection Agency 2022, Scheer 2011
4. US Geological Survey 2022
5. Hyman 2018
6. Di Liberto 2020
7. Celiac Disease Foundation website
8. Bradford 2015
9. Prieto 2021

10. Goodwin 2019
11. Northwest Medicine Healthbeat website
12. Cohn 2014
13. Kaur 2018
14. Mishra 2019
15. Aneklaphakij 2021, Afshin 2014
16. Talib 2021, Tsao 2021, Salehi 2018, El-Sheikh 2017, Morstein 2017, Okla 2017, Mozaffarian 2016, Chen S 2015, Macedo 2015, Faghihzadeh 2014, Liu 2014, de la Lastra 2007
17. WHO 2018
18. Hyman 2018
19. *Time* 2020, Tousen 2020, Ramdath 2015
20. Hyman 2018
21. Carlsson 2019b, Löfvenborg 2016, Mozaffarian 2016, Malik 2010
22. Azad 2017, Laverty 2015, Yang 2010, Fowler 2008, Colditz 1990, Stellman 1986
23. NPR 2014
24. Talib 2021, Meng 2019, Kondo 2018, Mozaffarian 2016, Löfvenborg 2014
25. Talib 2021, Xu 2020, Kondo 2018, Li 2016, Mozaffarian 2016, Liu 2013, Yan 2013, Diepvens 2007, Nagao 2007
26. Bradford 2004
27. Mozaffarian 2016
28. Lipman 2014
29. Mao 2019, Rodríguez-García 2019, Mozaffarian 2016, Lee 2012
30. Gupta 2019, Gupta 2011
31. Fletcher 2020, Harvard Medical School 2018
32. Brady 2017
33. Schultz 2017, Mackinnon 2012
34. Hyman 2018
35. Hill-Briggs 2021, Kumar 2020, Groh 2019, Moffa 2019, Rodricks 2019, Hyman 2018, National Academies of Sciences 2018, Street 2018, Varshavsky 2018, Rosenfeld 2017, Evangelou 2016, Song 2016, Thompson 2015, Yang SN 2014, Bergman 2013, Thayer 2012, Neel 2011, Iavicoli 2009
36. Schug 2011
37. Varshavsky 2018, Evangelou 2016, Hartle 2016, Zota 2016, Haug 2011, Schecter 2010, Schecter 2004
38. Yang O 2015
39. Hill-Briggs 2021, Nguyen 2020, Evans 2002
40. Zota 2016, Zota 2014
41. Imamura 2016, Rohrmann 2013, Micha 2010
42. Löfvenborg 2021
43. Tromba 2021
44. Fée 2021, Greenberg 2021
45. Fée 2021
46. Greenberg 2021
47. Fée 2021

CHAPTER NINETEEN: THE LADA HONEYMOON DILEMMA

1. Stenström 2005
2. Harrar 2016, Turner 1997
3. Stenström 2005
4. Li 2020
5. Huang 2021, Rajkumar 2020, Leighton 2017, Huang 2016, Zampetti 2014, Zampetti 2012, Buzzetti 2007, Li 2003
6. Heath 2010

PART IV.

CHAPTER TWENTY: HUNGER

1. Gay 2018
2. Bungau 2020, Camacho 2017, Allison 2014
3. Kissileff 2012
4. Bungau 2020
5. Daghestani 2009
6. DiGruccio 2016
7. Vohl 2020, Barkan 2003
8. Tomiyama 2010
9. Klatzkin 2018, Epel 2001, Moyer 1994
10. Tara 2017
11. Kyriachenko 2019, Siddiqui 2009

CHAPTER TWENTY-ONE: CARBS AND OUR BRAIN, HEART, AND HERITAGE

1. Nabhan GP. *Coming Home to Eat: The Pleasures and Politics of Local Food* (WW Norton & Co, 2009)
2. Heath 2010
3. Egan 2017
4. From the websites of ANAD (National Association of Anorexia Nervosa and Associated Disorders) and Mirror Mirror
5. Gelman 2012
6. From the websites of ANAD (National Association of Anorexia Nervosa and Associated Disorders) and Mirror Mirror
7. Toni 2017
8. From the website of ANAD (National Association of Anorexia Nervosa and Associated Disorders)
9. Morales 2020, Wiss 2020, Cassin 2019, Jiménez-Murcia 2019, Wiss 2018, Loxton 2017, Volkow 2017, Criscitelli 2016, Schulte 2016, Volkow 2012
10. Bonder 2018
11. Nelder 2018, Yang 2018, Raevuori 2015
12. Grisel 2020
13. Lennerz 2018, Volkow 2017, Gearhardt 2012, Volkow 2012, Avena 2008, Avena 2006

14. Constant 2020, Wiss 2020
15. Wiss 2020, Burrows 2018, Leigh 2018, Schulte 2018
16. Constant 2020, de Vries 2016, Meule 2011
17. Nelder 2018, Pursey 2014, Meule 2011
18. Lennerz 2018
19. DiFeliceantonio 2018, Gordon 2018, Hoch 2015, Schulte 2015, Avena 2012, Avena 2011, Thornley 2008
20. Roth 2019
21. Constant 2020
22. Lennerz 2018, Figlewicz 2009, Anthony 2006
23. Kriz 2002

CHAPTER TWENTY-TWO: BUILDING A BETTER RELATIONSHIP WITH FOOD

1. Lean 2019, Lean 2018
2. Bolla 2019
3. Tara 2017
4. Heath 2010
5. Meule 2020
6. Bolte Taylor 2009
7. Roth 2019
8. Grisel 2020, Wiss 2020, Burrows 2018, Leigh 2018, Schulte 2018
9. Grisel 2020

CHAPTER TWENTY-THREE: COMPLETING THE JOURNEY

1. Brown 2021
2. *Time* 2020, Wu 2016

CHAPTER TWENTY-FOUR: FOOD FOR THOUGHT

1. Ewen 2015
2. *Time* 2020
3. Scheiner 2011
4. Bittman 2021
5. Wiss 2018
6. Bittman 2021, Moss 2021
7. Wiss 2018
8. Springmann 2022, Walls 2018, Franck 2013, Peterson 2009, Babcock 2001
9. *Food, Inc.* 2008
10. Prasad 2019
11. Pannett 2022
12. Sable-Smith 2018
13. Pannett 2022
14. Huetteman 2019
15. DiabetesMine 2021

16. T1International website, Dawkins 2020, Lancet Diabetes Endocrinology 2017, Perrin 2017, Hua 2016, Ramsey 2016, University of Michigan 2016, Greene 2015

17. Minaj 2019

18. Ewen 2015

19. Bettelheim 2022

20. Bakkila 2022, Pannett 2022

21. Conner 2019, T1International patient survey 2018

22. Luo 2020

23. Hill-Briggs 2021, Nhoung 2020, Conner 2019, Herkert 2019, Prasad 2019, Rosenthal 2019, Kang 2018, T1International patient survey 2018, Teare 2018, Patel 2016, Piette 2004

24. Randall 2011

25. Karlovitch 2019

26. Lindblom 2021, Bailey 2019, Daughtery 2019

27. See https://www.shaheen.senate.gov/imo/media/doc/Diabetes%20Groups %20INSULIN%20Act%20Letter.pdf

28. Beran 2018b

29. Chow 2018

30. Beran 2018b, Beran 2005

31. Ewen 2015

32. Rowland 2022

33. Hu 2021, den Braver 2018, Christine 2015, Sallis 2012, Morland 2009, Black 2008

34. Wilner 2020, Babar 2019, Stanley 2019, Beran 2018a, Quigley 2017, Beran 2016

35. Hill-Briggs 2021, Divers 2020, Burke 2019, Doucette 2017, Beckles 2016

36. US Bureau of Labor Statistics 2022

37. Cha 2022

38. Cha 2022

39. Cha 2022

40. Tolbert 2020

41. Tolbert 2020

42. Tolbert 2020

43. Hill-Briggs 2021

44. Caballero 2018

45. Patel 2016

46. Burke 2019

47. CDC 2020, Fortmann 2019, Yingling 2019, CDC 2017, López 2016

48. Saydah 2017

49. CDC 2020, Fortmann 2019, Yingling 2019, CDC 2017, Saydah 2017, López 2016, Link 2009

50. Blitstein 2021, Hill-Briggs 2021, Nguyen 2020, Arenas 2019, Gucciardi 2019, Orr 2019, Seliman 2018, Leung 2015, Seligman 2015, Silverman 2015, Gucciardi 2014, Evans 2002

51. Patel 2019

52. Minaj 2019
53. Shiva 2015
54. Hwang 2000
55. Nania 2019
56. Bittman 2021
57. Hill-Briggs 2021, Seligman 2018, Seligman 2015
58. Sallis 2012
59. Hill-Briggs 2021
60. McGhee 2021
61. Locklear 2022
62. Rowley 2017
63. Lappé 2020

CHAPTER TWENTY-FIVE: GO BIG AND GO HOME

1. Heath 2010
2. Scheiner 2011
3. Buzzetti 2020
4. FDA 2022, Carré 2021
5. Roep 2021, Brawerman 2020, Mallone 2020, Xu 2020, Zhong 2020, Atkinson 2019, Oram 2019, Thompson 2019, Balaji 2018, Cito 2018, Ovalle 2018, Cheng 2017
6. Brawerman 2020
7. Oram 2019
8. Jörns 2020

INDEX